i
o

Quick Reference to

Nursing Implications
of Diagnostic Tests

J. B. Lippincott Company Philadelphia/Toronto

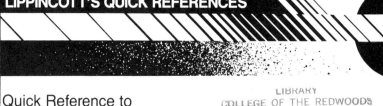

Quick Reference to

Nursing Implications of Diagnostic Tests

Patricia Gauntlett Beare, R.N., Ph.D.
Associate Professor
University of Texas School of Nursing at Galveston
University of Texas Medical Branch
Galveston, Texas

Virginia A. Rahr, R.N., M.S.N., Ed.D.
Associate Professor
University of Texas School of Nursing at Galveston
University of Texas Medical Branch
Galveston, Texas

Christina A. Ronshausen, R.N., M.S., N.S.
Assistant Professor
University of Texas School of Nursing at Galveston
University of Texas Medical Branch
and Staff Nurse
St. Mary's Hospital
Galveston, Texas

With 8 additional contributors

Sponsoring Editor: Diana Intenzo
Manuscript Editor: Don Reisman
Indexer: Deborah Ziwot
Art Director: Tracy Baldwin
Designer: William Boehm
Production Supervisor: N. Carol Kerr
Production Assistant: Susan A. Caldwell
Compositor: Hampton Graphics
Printer/Binder: R. R. Donnelley & Sons Company

6 5 4 3 2 1

Library of Congress Cataloging in Publication Data

Beare, Patricia G.
    Quick reference to nursing implications of diagnostic tests.
    (Lippincott quick references)
    Bibliography
    Includes index.
    1. Diagnosis.   2. Diagnosis, Laboratory.
3. Nursing.   I. Rahr, Virgina A.   II. Ronshausen,
Christina A.   III. Title.
RT48.B4   616.07'05   82-6565
ISBN 0-397-54366-2   AACR2

The authors and publisher have exerted every effort to ensure that drug selection and dosage set forth in this text are in accord with current recommendations and practice at the time of publication. However, in view of ongoing research, changes in government regulations, and the constant flow of information relating to drug therapy and drug reactions, the reader is urged to check the package insert for each drug for any change in indications and dosage and for added warnings and precautions. This is particularly important when the recommended agent is a new or infrequently employed drug.

To nursing students and practitioners, in the hope that they will be more knowledgeable and supportive in the care they provide for their patients and clients.

Contents

Contributors

Cathy C. Jones, R.N., M.S.N., CCRN, C.N.R.N.
Lecturer
San Jose State University
San Jose, California
Chapter 10: Tests Related to Neuromuscular Function

Janice B. Martin, B.S.N., M.N.
Instructor
University of Texas School of Nursing at Galveston
University of Texas Medical Branch
Galveston, Texas
Chapter 3: Tests Related to Renal Function

Barbara G. Mason, R.N., M.S.
Assistant Professor
University of Texas School of Nursing at Galveston
University of Texas Medical Branch
Galveston, Texas
Chapter 5: Tests Related to Digestive Function

Gayle Deets Miller, R.N., O.N.S.
Head Nurse, Orthopedics
The Greenville Hospital
Greenville, Pennsylvania
Chapter 11: Tests Related to Musculoskeletal Function

Connie L. Richardson, R.N., B.S., CCRN
Director of Staff Development/Patient Education
The Greenville Hospital
Greenville, Pennsylvania
Chapter 11: Tests Related to Musculoskeletal Function

Harriett L. Riggs, R.N., M.S.
Assistant Professor
University of Texas School of Nursing at Galveston
University of Texas Medical Branch
Galveston, Texas
Chapter 6: Tests Related to Metabolic Function

Mary Ellen Schweitzer, R.N., M.S.N.
West Nebraska General Hospital School of Nursing
Scottsbluff, Nebraska
Chapter 9: Tests Related to Immunology

Ruth Tucker, R.N., M.S.
Assistant Professor of Maternal-Child Health
University of Texas School of Nursing at Galveston
University of Texas Medical Branch
Galveston, Texas
Chapter 8: Tests Related to Reproductive Function

Preface

Quick Reference to Nursing Implications of Diagnostic Tests is designed to serve primarily as a basic reference for nursing students and practicing nurses. Nurse educators should also find this text a valuable aid for personal review and reference, as well as a teaching tool. Because nurses are expected to be knowledgeable about laboratory and diagnostic tests and to provide appropriate nursing care and patient teaching related to these tests, the need for a book of this nature has become increasingly important. It is the purpose of this book to assist the nursing student and the practicing nurse to meet these expectations and thereby improve patient care.

The book is organized according to the functions of the major systems of the body. Each chapter begins with an overview of the major pathophysiologic processes that affect the functioning of that particular system. The rationale for including this brief overview of pathophysiology is to provide a knowledge base for the laboratory and diagnostic tests that follow. For some readers this section will serve as a review.

The remainder of each chapter is then divided into Laboratory Tests and Diagnostic Tests. The section on Laboratory Tests is further subdivided into tests done on blood, urine, and feces, if pertinent. A consistent format is used for each laboratory test and includes a brief description of the test and its purpose, laboratory values (adult and pediatric), nursing implications, and the necessity for a signed consent form. The nursing implications section includes the procedure for collection and storage of the specimen, factors that may interfere with the test results, patient care, and patient education.

Each of the laboratory tests includes "normal values." The reader should be aware that these values may vary from one laboratory to another, depending upon the particular methods used, and that tests have more than one accepted normal value.

The section on diagnostic tests in each chapter also uses a consistent format and includes the following: a brief description of the test and its purpose, normal results of the test, nursing implications, and need for a signed consent. Nursing implications focus on patient care and education prior to, during, and after the procedure.

It is hoped that the nurses using this book will find greater confidence in their care of patients who are undergoing various laboratory and diagnostic tests. A further hope is that the patients and their families will receive better nursing care in relation to laboratory and diagnostic tests.

Patricia Gauntlett Beare
Virginia A. Rahr
Christina A. Ronshausen

Acknowledgments

We wish to acknowledge Joanna Huddleston, Sheila O'Connor, and Joan Drachenberg for their patience and invaluable help in typing, and in assisting us with other details in preparation of the manuscript.

List of Tests
by alphabetical order

1

Tests Related to Hematopoietic Function

Patricia Gauntlett Beare

2 TESTS RELATED TO HEMATOPOIETIC FUNCTION

OVERVIEW OF PHYSIOLOGY AND PATHOPHYSIOLOGY

The blood contains two major components. One component is a suspension of colloids, plasma, and electrolytes. The other component consists of the blood cells—erythrocytes or red blood cells (RBCs), leukocytes or white blood cells (WBCs), and platelets. Plasma constitutes 55% to 60% of the blood. Blood cells constitute about 40% to 45% of the total volume.

PLASMA ELECTROLYTES AND PROTEIN

The plasma components of major importance are the plasma electrolytes and plasma proteins. The positively charged electrolytes or cations are sodium, potassium, calcium, and magnesium. Negatively charged ions or anions are bicarbonate, chloride, organic acids, proteinates, phosphates, and sulfates.

Plasma proteins are of three basic types: albumins, fibrinogen, and globulins.

- *Albumins* are the major determinant of osmotic pressure of the blood, owing to their concentration and size. Lack of adequate albumin causes interstitial edema.

- *Fibrinogen* is a glycoprotein essential in the blood clotting process. Fibrinogen, or factor I, is converted to fibrin in the process of clot formation.

- The *globulin* components of the plasma proteins are designated as alpha one (α_1) alpha two (α_2), beta (β), and gamma (γ). The globulins are important for hemoglobin formation and for antibody response in immune reactions.

Albumin and fibrinogen are formed in the liver. About 50% of the globulins are formed in the liver, while the remainder are formed in the lymphoid tissues and other cells of the reticuloendothelial system. Blood proteins are important in acid–base balance, hormone actions, blood clotting, transport mechanisms, osmotic pressure, and blood viscosity. The plasma proteins act as a source for replacement of tissue proteins, especially during starvation or severe disease. Disease conditions such as burns or renal disease often cause rapid loss of plasma proteins.

RED BLOOD CELLS

The major function of red blood cells (RBCs) is to transport hemoglobin, which carries oxygen through the blood to the tissues. Red blood cells also contain carbonic anhydrase, which catalyzes the reaction between carbon dioxide and water. This allows the blood to react with carbon dioxide and transport it from the tissues to the lungs. The hemoglobin contained in the red blood cell is also important as an acid–base buffer.

Red Cell Formation

Red blood cells are produced after birth exclusively by the bone marrow. The stem cells in the bone marrow form hemocytoblasts which in turn form the basophil erythroblast that begins the synthesis of hemoglobin. The erythroblast then becomes a polychromatophil erythroblast. The nucleus of this cell shrinks, and greater quantities of hemoglobin are formed producing the cell known as a normoblast. Eventually, after the cells divide repeatedly, each cell becomes filled with hemoglobin and expels the nucleus of the erythroblast.

The final cell form, or the erythrocyte, contains no nucleus and passes into the blood capillaries through the process of diapedesis. Red blood cells are biconcave discs whose membranes are able to change shapes without rupturing as they pass through capillaries. Some of these erythrocytes, about 1%, continue to produce hemoglobin from small amounts of basophilic reticulum. These cells are known as reticulocytes.

Vitamin B$_{12}$

Certain vitamins, B$_{12}$ and folic acid, are needed for the formation of red blood cells. Vitamin B$_{12}$ in particular is required in the formation of DNA. Lack of this vitamin can cause failure of nuclear maturation and division. Its absence also inhibits the rate of red blood cell production and causes the cells to become larger than normal. These larger cells in the adult erythrocyte are called macrocytes. Macrocytes are irregular, large, and have oval-shaped membranes which cause them to have a shortened lifespan. The hemoglobin in these cells is normal; however, since the red blood cell is larger, the quantity of hemoglobin in these cells is considerably greater.

Failure to absorb B$_{12}$ from the gastrointestinal tract can also cause failure of the red blood cell to mature. The gastric mucosa may either fail to secrete normal gastric secretions, which contain intrinsic factor, or gastric mucosa may be removed or destroyed by disease or surgery. Intrinsic factor combines with B$_{12}$ and allows the vitamin to be absorbed.

Deficiencies of folic acid will also cause failure of the red blood cell to mature. Folic acid is required in the formation of DNA but is also required for RNA synthesis.

Hypoxia and Red Cell Production

Tissue oxygenation is the basic regulator of red blood cell production. Hypoxia (reduced amounts of oxygen at the tissue level) stimulates red blood cell production by stimulating increased amounts of erythropoietin. When the kidneys become hypoxic, they release an enzyme that acts on blood proteins to form the hormone erythropoietin. Erythropoietin acts on the bone marrow to increase the rate of red blood cell production.

- Any condition that causes hypoxia, such as hemorrhage, radiation therapy, high altitudes or heart or lung disease, will cause an increase in the rate of red blood cell formation.

HEMOGLOBIN

The primary function of hemoglobin is to combine with oxygen in the lungs and release the oxygen in the tissue capillaries. Hemoglobin is composed of two types of chemical units called polypeptide chains and heme groups.

Hemoglobin Structure

Each hemoglobin molecule contains two pairs of polypeptide chains, which generally are of four types: alpha (α), beta (β), gamma (γ), and delta (δ). Most adult hemoglobin consists of two alpha chains, two beta chains, and associated heme groups. Adult hemoglobin, or hemoglobin A, contains α_2, β_2 polypeptides. Fetal hemoglobin, or hemoglobin F, consists of two α chains and two γ chains and is designated α_2, γ_2.

- Genetic defects may affect hemoglobin synthesis and cause differences in the synthesis or structure of the chains.

In the disease of thalassemia there is a genetic impairment in hemoglobin A formation. Interference with either α or β formation causes increased amounts of fetal hemoglobin (α_2, γ_2), or A_2 hemoglobin (α_2, δ_2) or hemoglobin H (β_4).

Each molecule of hemoglobin contains four molecules of heme. One molecule of hemoglobin contains four iron atoms and can carry four molecules of oxygen. Oxygen binds loosely with the iron atom so that the combination is easily reversible, allowing oxygen to be released into interstitial tissue fluids.

- In patients with inadequate hemoglobin, such as in the patient with anemia, the blood cannot transport sufficient oxygen to meet the needs of the tissues.

Iron and Hemoglobin Formation

Formation of hemoglobin requires amino acids, iron, copper, pyridoxine, cobalt, and nickel. The total iron in the body is about four g, of which 65% is present in the hemoglobin.

Iron is absorbed from the small intestine in the ferrous form, where it immediately combines with the beta globulin, transferrin, and is transported in the blood plasma. When the body needs more iron, it absorbs more iron from the intestine; however, when the body is saturated with iron, iron is blocked from being absorbed and is excreted into the feces. Excess iron in the blood is deposited in all cells of the body, but especially in the liver in the form of ferritin. When the body's quantity of iron is more than the apoferritin storage pool can handle, some of it is stored in the tissue in an extremely insoluble form called hemosiderin.

DESTRUCTION OF RBCs

The red blood cell normally circulates in the blood for an average of 120 days. As the red blood cell becomes older, it becomes more fragile until it ruptures. Many red blood cells rupture in the spleen. When the cell ruptures, hemoglobin is released and subsequently phagocytized. The iron from the hemoglobin goes back to the bone marrow. The heme portion of the hemoglobin molecule is converted into bilirubin, which is released into the blood and later secreted by the liver into the bile.

POLYCYTHEMIA

Polycythemia is a hematologic disorder in which there are too many red blood cells in the circulation (erythrocytosis). Polycythemia is characterized by an increase in the red blood cell mass. This increased mass is associated with a high blood viscosity and sluggish flow of the circulation. This altered circulation results in decreased oxygen flow to the tissues. The body compensates for the high viscosity by an increase in blood volume. This compensation results in vasodilation and an increased oxygen flow to the tissues.

True polycythemia is defined as an increase in both hemoglobin concentration and red blood cell mass. It is a result of hypoxia (such as from high altitude), kidney disease, or an abnormality in regulation of erythropoiesis, such as proliferative diseases of the bone marrow (polycythemia vera). Increased blood viscosity requires increased cardiac work because the heart must work harder to circulate the extra blood.

ANEMIAS
Anemias may be defined as hematologic disorders when there are insufficient red blood cells in the circulation. The anemias are characterized by a reduced hemoglobin concentration in the red blood cell.

Types of Anemias

Based upon the red blood cell mass, anemias can be classed as relative or absolute. Relative anemias are caused by increases in the plasma volume such as in the anemias of pregnancy. Absolute anemias are caused by changes in the red blood cell mass. These absolute anemias can be further classified into anemias caused by decreased or abnormal production, or increased destruction or loss of red blood cells.

- Examples of anemias caused by decreased production or abnormal production of red blood cells are anemias resulting from decreased erythropoietin production, such as in renal disease, aplastic anemia, B_{12} or folic acid deficiency, iron deficiency, hemoglobinopathies, and thalassemia.

- Examples of anemias caused by increased destruction or loss of red blood cells are hereditary spherocytosis, G-6 PD deficiency, autoimmune hemolytic anemia, and blood loss anemia.

Compensatory Mechanisms

The body can compensate to alleviate the hypoxemia or reduced oxygen carrying capacity of the blood of anemia.

- The body shifts the oxygen dissociation curve to the right, which permits the tissues to extract increased amounts of oxygen from the red blood cells to meet the needs of the tissue.

- The body also redistributes blood from tissues with low oxygen requirements (such as in the skin or kidneys) to tissues with high oxygen requirements (such as the brain and heart). With severe anemia, the heart increases cardiac output in order to provide the tissues with oxygen.

- The slowest compensatory mechanism of the body is to increase the rate of red blood cell production. A compensatory increase in the number of red blood cells begins about 4 to 5 days after tissue hypoxia. This may be evidenced by increased erythropoietin in the serum and urine and large numbers of immature reticulocytes seen on the blood smear.

WHITE BLOOD CELLS (WBCs)

The primary function of the white blood cells is to provide a rapid and potent defense against foreign organisms. White blood cells are formed in the bone marrow and in the lymph tissues.

There are six types of white blood cells: neutrophils, eosinophils, basophils, monocytes, lymphocytes, and plasma cells. White blood cells are classified into two morphologic groups: agranulocytes and granulocytes. Neutrophils, eosinophils, and basophils are granulocytes because of their granular appearance. All granulocytes are produced in the bone marrow. Monocytes and lymphocytes are agranulocytes because their cytoplasm contains few granules.

The lifespan of the granulocytes in the blood is about 12 hours. Monocytes, which are agranulocytes, may live for weeks or months. Lymphocytes remain in the blood for only a few hours; however, they may have a lifespan as long as a few years. Since white blood cells that are present in the blood are transported from the bone marrow or lymphoid tissue to the site of body need, the lifespan and number of the white blood cells in the blood are limited.

White Blood Cell Disorders

- *Leukocytosis* is indicated by an increase in the number of white cells above normal.

  The terms eosinophilia, basophilia, monocytosis, lymphocytosis, and neutrophilia indicate increased numbers of the different white blood cell types.

- *Leukopenia* indicates a decrease in white blood cells below normal.

  The terms eosinopenia, basopenia, lymphocytopenia, monocytopenia, and neutropenia indicate decreased numbers of the different white blood cell types.

- *Leukemias* are conditions in which there is uncontrolled production of white blood cells originating from bone marrow or lymphoid tissue. Leukemias are usually characterized by greatly increased numbers of abnormal white blood cells in the circulating blood.

EOSINOPHILS

Eosinophils are the white blood cells important in antigen–antibody reactions in the tissues.

- The total number of eosinophils increases greatly during allergic reactions.

- Extremely large numbers of eosinophils in the blood also occur in parasitic infections.

BASOPHILS

Basophils have granules that contain heparin and histamine. Basophils, when liberating heparin into the blood, prevent blood coagulation and can speed the removal of fat particles from the blood.

- Basophils increase in number during the healing phase of inflammation and during prolonged chronic inflammation.
- Increases in basophils also occur in chronic myeloid leukemia and in polycythemia vera.

LYMPHOCYTES

The formation and the role of lymphocytes is described in the chapter on immunity.

MONOCYTES

Monocytes are phagocytic cells. Phagocytosis is the process of engulfing cells and debris. Initially, monocytes are released from the bone marrow as small immature cells. Within a few hours these immature cells begin to swell and develop large numbers of mitochondria and lysosomes. These mature forms of monocytes are called macrophages and can engulf and phagocytize many large bacteria and particles (such as pieces of necrotic tissue).

- Monocytes may increase in number during chronic infection, recovery from infection, and liver disease.

NEUTROPHILS

Neutrophils play numerous roles in the inflammatory process. Neutrophils, which enter the tissues to begin phagocytosis, are mature cells called "segs." Immature neutrophils, called "bands" or "stabs," are also seen in the peripheral blood.

- Most infections caused by pyrogenic bacteria are accompanied by an increase in neutrophils in the blood. This is owing to the bone marrow accelerating the release of cells from the bone marrow pool.
- This accelerated release of cells from the marrow storage pool is indicated by an increase in the ratio of band forms to segmented forms.

Occasionally in certain bacterial infections such as typhoid fever or severe pneumococcal infections, the bone marrow is unable to replenish the accelerated cell loss at the sites of tissue inflammation. When this occurs, there is a decrease in neutrophils called neutropenia.

Neutrophils are the first white blood cells to accumulate at the site of acute inflammation, sticking to damaged capillary walls and passing into tissue spaces. They then phagocytize bacteria and cellular debris.

PLATELETS

Platelets, which are also called thrombocytes, are cell fragments of a seventh type of white blood cell called a megakaryocyte. Megakaryocytes are also formed in the bone marrow. The chief function of platelets is the process of hemostasis.

Platelets in the blood survive for about 10 to 14 days. Approximately 15,000 to 30,000 platelets are formed each day for each cubic millimeter of blood. The control of platelet production is thought to be mediated through a hormone called thrombopoietin.

During the process of hemostasis, platelets will adhere to subendothelial surfaces (platelet adhesion), and accumulate (platelet aggregation) to form a platelet plug that walls off the ruptured blood vessel wall.

Platelets also release factors, such as serotonin, which cause blood vessel constriction and are responsible for clot retraction. These factors along with platelet factor III, which augment thrombin formation, result in the coating of the platelet plug with fibrin and the formation of a white thrombus. Final clot retraction is caused by thrombosthenin, a platelet protein.

- Decreases in platelet count, or thrombocytopenia, may occur during acute gram-negative or gram-positive bacterial infection or during viral infections.

- A decreased platelet count may be due to the tendency of platelets to stick together from the action of bacterial toxins on the platelet.

- Thrombocytopenia may also be inherited, congenital, or acquired.

- Drugs are the most common cause of defective platelet production.

Disseminated Intravascular Coagulation

Another coagulation defect that occurs as a complication of infections is disseminated intravascular coagulation (DIC).

In DIC, an infection sets off the normal clotting mechanism. The systemic infection causes damage to the walls of blood vessels and activates the coagulation sequence. Thrombin is generated, and there is activation of the fibrinolytic system against widespread clotting. Also, there is activation of both the intrinsic clotting system and the extrinsic system. Fibrin is deposited throughout the vascular system causing tissue necrosis and organ damage. Blood coagulation factors are depleted (II, V, VII, fibrinogen), and fibrin can no longer be formed.

Thrombocytosis

Thrombocytosis is the term used to describe increases in blood platelet levels above 500,000/mm³. Thrombocytosis may be secondary to some other dysfunction or trauma (such as after surgery or a splenectomy). Thrombocytosis, sometimes called thrombocythemia, which occurs as a primary disorder, often is accompanied by abnormal platelet function, causing a bleeding disorder.

Very high platelet counts usually cause thrombosis and increased bleeding tendencies. The thrombosis is probably caused by platelet aggregation and platelet factor III release. The cause of the bleeding tendency is unknown.

Qualitative abnormalities of platelet disorder may be hereditary or acquired. The acquired disorders of platelet dysfunction are associated with chronic renal failure or ingestion of aspirin.

BLOOD TESTS
BLEEDING TIME (Ivy's Technique)

The bleeding time is a screening test to distinguish disorders of primary hemostasis from disorders of coagulation defects. The bleeding time depends upon the quality and quantity of platelets and the ability of the blood vessel wall to constrict.

Laboratory Results

Normal Range

3 to 6 min

Nursing Implications

Procedure for Collection/Storage of Specimen

A sphygmomanometer cuff is placed around the patient's upper arm and the pressure is raised to 40 mm of mercury. Three small punctures are made along the outer (extensor) surface of the patient's forearm. Punctures are 5 mm deep and 1 mm wide. The three bleeding points are gently blotted with filter paper discs every 15 sec. The process is continued until bleeding ceases.

Possible Interfering Factors

1. Aspirin and other inhibitors of platelet function will prolong bleeding time.
2. When the puncture is not of uniform depth or width, the bleeding time will be affected.
3. Alcohol consumption may increase the bleeding time.
4. Dextran, mithramycin (Mithracin), and streptokinase will increase the bleeding time.

Patient Care

1. Explain the procedure and purpose of the test to the patient.
2. Instruct the patient to abstain from alcohol and aspirin for 1 wk prior to the test.

Patient Education

1. Instruct the patient with an increased bleeding time to avoid any interfering factors.
2. Instruct the patient to notify the physician prior to any surgery including dental surgery.
3. Instruct the patient not to take any over-the-counter medication without consulting the physician.
4. Instruct the patient to notify the physician prior to taking any prescribed drugs.
5. If the bleeding time is elevated, instruct the patient to avoid any trauma and explain how to apply pressure to control bleeding.

Signed Consent

Not required

BLOOD CROSSMATCHING

Blood crossmatching is a simple test to determine compatibility between donor and recipient blood. Actual blood types are unknown. Serum from the recipient is mixed with cells from the donor to determine if clumping (agglutination) occurs. This is called the major crossmatch. In a second test, the RBCs of the recipient are crossmatched against the serum of the donor. This is called the minor crossmatch. The major crossmatch is done to detect antibodies in the recipient's serum; the minor crossmatch is done to detect antibodies in the donor's serum.

Laboratory Results
Normal Results

Absence of clumping or hemolysis

Nursing Implications
Procedure for Collection/Storage of Specimen

A venous sample of 10 ml is obtained.

Possible Interfering Factors

None reported

Patient Care
See transfusion reaction (see below under Blood Typing)

Patient Education
See transfusion reaction (see below under Blood Typing)

Signed Consent
Not required

BLOOD TYPING

The main purpose of the blood typing test is to prevent the transfusion of incompatible blood. Blood has antigenic and immune properties. Because of this, antibodies in the plasma of one blood can react with antigens in the cells of another blood. These antigens are referred to as agglutinogens. Bloods are grouped and typed by major types of antigens, which are present or absent on the red blood cell membrane. When antigens (agglutinogens) from one blood react with antibodies (agglutinins) from another blood, clumping (agglutination) and hemolysis occur. This is the process that occurs in a transfusion reaction.

Some antigens are strong and regularly cause transfusion reactions. Two of these particular groups of strong antigens are the O–A–B system and the Rh–Hr system.

TYPE A AND TYPE B ANTIGENS

Type A and type B antigens occur in the cells of different persons. Since antigens are genetically determined, a person inherits the blood type. Because of this, a person may have no A or B antigens in his blood, have either A or B antigens, or have both A and B antigens.

- When only type A agglutinogen is present, the blood is group A.
- When only type B agglutinogen is present, the blood group is B.
- When both A and B agglutinogens are present the blood is group AB. Blood group AB is the universal recipient, and individuals can receive blood from all blood groups.
- When neither A or B agglutinogen is present, the blood group is group

O. Blood group O is called the universal donor, since it has no antigens and can donate to all blood groups.

When bloods are mismatched, so that anti-A or anti-B agglutinins are mixed with red blood cells containing either A or B agglutinogens, the red blood cells clump together.

- Prior to giving a transfusion, it is necessary to determine the blood groups of both the donor and recipient, so that a transfusion reaction will not occur.

Rh FACTORS AND Hr FACTORS

Blood is also typed according to the Rh system and Hr system according to the presence or absence of Rh antigen in the red blood cell membrane. Each of the Rh factors is also inherited. The Rh antigen, which is most likely to produce a reaction, is the D (Rh_o) antigen.

- Any time a person's blood reacts with anti-Rh_o serum, that person's blood is Rh positive.
- When blood does not react with anti-Rh_o serum, the blood is Rh negative.

Anti-Rh agglutinins are not produced until the person is exposed to Rh-positive cells. This may occur during pregnancy or after childbirth. The Rh-negative mother develops anti-Rh agglutinins when the fetus is Rh positive. Usually, the Rh-negative mother pregnant with the Rh-positive child does not develop sufficient anti-Rh agglutinins with her first baby to cause harm. However, the Rh-negative mother will develop a sensitivity to the Rh-positive factor as she receives antigens from fetal tissue after the baby is born. These anti-Rh antibodies will cause agglutination of the blood of the fetus in future pregnancies if the fetus is Rh positive. This disease state of the newborn is called *erythroblastosis fetalis.*

Hr factors are similar to Rh factors but are less likely to cause transfusion reactions. The three most important Hr factors are hr, hr′, and hr″.

Laboratory Results
Normal Values
ABO

Known serum	*Antibody present*	*Patient's serum*	*Major blood group*
Anti A	Anti B	none	O
none	Anti B	A	A
Anti A	none	B	B
none	none	AB	AB

Rh Factors

Percent of occurrence in whites and blacks
Whites: 85% Rh positive
15% Rh negative
Blacks: 90% Rh positive
10% Rh negative

Rh-negative agglutinogens (Wiener terms)	Reactions with Rh antisera		
	anti Rh_o	anti rh'	anti rh''
rh	−	−	−
rh'	−	+	−
rh''	−	−	+
rhy	−	+	+
Rh-positive agglutinogens			
Rh_o	+	−	−
Rh_1	+	+	−
Rh_2	+	−	+
RhZ	+	+	+

Nursing Implications
Procedure for Collection/Storage of Specimen

Obtain a venous blood sample of 10 ml. Determine Rh type by mixing antisera with a saline suspension of RBCs and plasma protein. To determine blood group, mix blood with saline; anti-agglutinin serum A and B are mixed separately with blood. Agglutination reactions are then observed.

Possible Interfering Factors

None reported

Patient Care
Blood Transfusions

1. Determine the patient's blood group prior to any transfusion.
2. Check the recipient's identified blood type with the type of blood to be administered with the aid of another qualified person to insure that the types match.
3. Obtain a baseline temperature reading, pulse, respiration, and blood pressure from the patient.
4. *If a transfusion reaction occurs,* observe for signs/symptoms of kidney shutdown. Acute kidney shutdown may occur within a few minutes, as toxic substances cause circulatory shock. Symptoms of transfusion reaction and procedures to follow are listed below:

   • The arterial blood pressure falls very low, urinary output decreases.

   • Rapid infusion of intravenous fluids, osmotic diuretics, and alkylating substances may be given as prescribed by the physician.

   • If a transfusion reaction is suspected, *stop* infusing the blood, keep the line open with saline solution, and notify the physician immediately.

5. *Observe for signs/symptoms of blood reaction.*

   • Fever is one of the most frequent transfusion reactions.

   • Flushing of the face, bleeding from operative wounds and other sites, constricting pain in the chest and lower back may occur.

   • Chills may also be present.

6. *Observe the patient for tetany.*
   - The usual anticoagulant for transfusion is citrate salt. Citrate combines with calcium.
   - If large quantities of blood containing citrate are infused rapidly, the patient may experience tetany.

7. *Patients with liver damage* are more likely to have citrate reactions.
   - Decrease the rate of transfusion with these patients.

8. Begin the blood transfusion with a saline solution and follow the blood transfusion with a saline solution.

9. Do not administer blood at the same time through the same intravenous line as antibiotics or other intravenous fluids or substances.

10. Start the IV with an 18-gauge needle to prevent breakdown of RBCs.

11. *Infectious diseases* such as hepatitis may be transmitted during blood transfusion. If the patient appears jaundiced, or if liver enzymes are elevated, observe for the presence of hepatitis.

12. *Observe for signs/symptoms of circulatory overload.* Circulatory overload can occur when the volume of blood is greater than what the heart can pump or when the blood transfusion is infused rapidly. Signs of this are those of pulmonary edema. The patients most likely to develop circulatory overload are infants, the aged, and those with cardiac injury or decreased cardiac reserve.

Patient Education

Rh typing

1. Inform the pregnant woman who has Rh-negative blood and is pregnant by a man who has Rh-positive blood that she should be Rh typed.

2. Rh antibodies can occur after antigenic initiation from the following:
   - pregnancy and abortions
   - blood transfusions
   - repeated IV injections of blood.
     Include this information in the history of patients with Rh-negative blood.

3. Explain to the Rh-negative mother the importance of frequent blood test monitoring during pregnancy. With subsequent Rh-positive pregnancies, antibodies in the mother's serum increase and may cause destruction of fetal RBCs.

4. If the newborn baby is suspected of having erythroblastosis, explain how the baby's blood will be tested as well as the procedure for an exchange transfusion if it becomes necessary.
   - The newborn erythroblastic baby is jaundiced at birth.
   - The hemoglobin level may fall for over a month after birth.
   - An exchange transfusion may be given, where the newborn infant's blood is replaced with Rh-negative blood.
   - Rh-negative blood (approximately 300 to 400 ml) is infused over a period of 1½ hr, while the infant's own Rh-positive blood is removed.

Signed Consent

Not required

BLOOD VOLUME AND RED CELL MASS

Blood volume and red cell mass studies are done on patients who undergo a rapidly changing fluid balance or who have experienced blood volume loss and replacement. These tests may also be done for the differential diagnosis of polycythemia. For direct measurement, either radiolabeled red cells (Cr^{51}) or ^{131}I albumin is used. When both the red cell mass and plasma volume are measured, the total blood volume is the simple sum of the red cell mass and plasma volume. Since measured volumes are expressed according to body weight (ml/kg), major errors may occur from lean body mass, obesity, or severe starvation. Increased plasma blood volume may occur with an increased secretion of anti-diuretic hormone.

Laboratory Results

Normal Values

Red cell mass

30 ± 3 ml/kg: the male adult

25 ml/kg: the female adult

Plasma volumes

98.0 ml/kg: premature infants

85.6 ml/kg: 1-yr-old

70.0 ml/kg: older child

40 ml/kg ± 4: adult male

40 ml/kg ± 4: adult female

Nursing Implications

Procedure for Collection/Storage of Specimen

1. Record the patient's height and weight.
2. Obtain a venous sample. The venous sample is mixed with the radio-isotope.
3. After 15 min, reinject the blood into the patient.
4. Obtain a venous sample in 15 min.

Possible Interfering Factors

Intravenous solutions being given at the time of the test may cause inaccurate results.

Patient Care

1. Observe the patient's hydration status. Note urine output and skin turgor.
2. Observe for signs and symptoms of hypovolemia or shock.

Patient Education

1. Explain the procedure to the patient.
2. If the blood volume and mass are decreased, prepare the patient for possible blood transfusion.

Signed Consent

Not required

BLOOD COAGULATION

Blood coagulation tests are used to measure the ability of the blood to clot. These tests are done to determine the cause of hemorrhagic disorders, to determine the effect of drugs such as anticoagulants on coagulation, and as screening tests to find individuals who are deficient in coagulation factors. Effective clotting is determined by the normality of both the extrinsic and intrinsic systems.

WHOLE BLOOD CLOTTING TIME (Lee and White Clotting Time, LWCT)

The whole blood clotting time (LWCT) can be used to detect severe deficiencies of clotting factors or to measure the effectiveness of heparin therapy. This test consists of placing a measured volume of blood into each of four glass tubes and recording the time that elapses before a solid clot appears.

Laboratory Results

Normal Range

3 to 6 min

Nursing Implications

Procedure for Collection/Storage of Specimen

1. Venous blood is collected in a plastic or siliconized syringe.
2. Any difficulty in obtaining the blood invalidates the test.
3. An 18- to 19- gauge needle should be used so that RBCs are not damaged.

Possible Interfering Factors

Standard apparatus and technique must be used. Test tubes rinsed in saline or test tubes that have been stoppered will affect the results. Plastic or silicone test tubes will lengthen results.

Patient Care

1. Record the results and note any consistent trend in normal values.
2. The test is done at the patient's bedside. Since it is a timed test, time the test immediately after the blood comes into contact with the glass test tube.
3. If the patient is on heparin therapy be aware of the following:
   - The antidote is protamine sulfate—1 mg neutralizes 100 u of heparin.
   - The LWCT is maintained at 2 to 3 times the normal limit or between 20 to 30 min.
   - Heparin acts by keeping thrombin from forming and acts quickly to block blood clotting reactions.
   - Intracranial hemorrhage, ocular surgery, intestinal obstruction, gas-

trointestinal ulceration, threatened abortion are contraindications
for heparin therapy.

Patient Education

Inform the patient to report any discolored urine, black stools, or excessive
menstrual bleeding.

Signed Consent

Not required

COAGULATION FACTORS

Coagulation factors are identified by roman numerals. Adequate concentration of all coagulation factors are necessary to maintain adequate hemostasis. Deficiencies of all factors except III, IV, XII are associated with hemorrhagic disorders.

Factor I deficiency (a deficiency in fibrinogen) may be congenital or acquired.

Congenital	Fibrin	Acquired	Cause
Afibrinogenemia	No measured fibrin	Impaired fibrinogen production	Disorders of liver, terminal cancer, chronic tuberculosis
Hypofibrinogenemia	levels lower than 100 mg/dl	Fibrinogen destruction	Complications of surgery, abnormal obstetric cases
Dysfibrinogenemia	Fibrin present is functionally abnormal	Excess utilization of fibrinogen	Widespread blood clotting

Factor II deficiencies are deficiencies of prothrombin and are usually acquired. Prothrombin is dependent upon vitamin K for its synthesis. Factor II deficiencies are almost always seen with deficiencies of factors VII, IX, and X.

Factor III, or thromboplastin, deficiency is not normally seen in plasma. Deficiency of plasma thromboplastin is due to the absence of or deficiency of one or more of the coagulation factors. Tissue thromboplastin is contained in the cells of connective tissues and in the lungs, brain, and placenta. Thromboplastin is released by the tissues immediately upon injury.

Factor IV is calcium and normally is present in the blood. Plasma calcium deficiencies seldom cause bleeding tendencies.

Factor V is the factor known as proaccelerin. Factor V is essential for converting prothrombin in stage II of the clotting process, for plasma thromboplastin generation in stage I of the clotting process, and as a cofactor with factor VII to activate extrinsic tissue thromboplastin. Decreased factor V is seen in the following conditions:

Congenital—parahemophilia

Acquired—liver disease, fibrinolysis, surgery, circulating V inhibitors, and acute leukemia

Factor VII is known as proconvertin and is essential for activating factor X in the presence of thromboplastin. Factor VII also helps convert prothrombin to thrombin during stage II and is the first factor to be depressed following coumarin therapy. Decreased levels occur in the following conditions:

Congenital—rare

Acquired—liver disease, vitamin K deficiency, hemorrhagic disease of the newborn, prolonged administration of antibiotics

Factor VIII is known as the antihemophilic factor and is required for the generation of intrinsic plasma thromboplastin in stage I. Decreased levels are seen in hemophiliacs. The amount of factor VIII present generally parallels the severity of the bleeding symptoms in hemophilia.

Decreased factor VIII occurs in the following:

Congenital—hemophilia A, Von Willebrand disease

Acquired—DIC, fibrinolysis, factor VIII inhibitors

Increased factor VIII may occur in the following:

adrenalin therapy

hyperthyroidism

muscular exercise

oral contraceptives

pregnancy

sudden cessation of coumadin therapy

Factor IX is known as the plasma thromboplastin component. It is also known as hemophilic B or Christmas factor. This factor influences the amount of thromboplastin available to convert prothrombin to thrombin. Decreased factor IX is seen in the following conditions:

Congenital—hemophilia B

Acquired—liver disease, nephrotic syndrome, vitamin K deficiencies, dicoumarol therapy

Factor X is known as the Stuart–Prower factor and is essential for the conversion of prothrombin to thrombin. Decreased factor X occurs in these conditions:

Congenital—rarely

Acquired—hemorrhagic disease of the newborn, liver disease, vitamin K deficiency, and in coumarin therapy

Factor XI or plasma thromboplastin antecedent (PTA) is known as hemophilic factor C. Factor XI continues the cascade effect in the coagulation sequence. Decreased plasma XI occurs in these conditions:

Congenital—autosomal dominant trait

Acquired—intestinal malabsorption of vitamin K, liver disease, newborn infants with circulating factor XI inhibitors

Factor XII is known as the Hageman factor, and it initiates the entire coagulation sequence. Factor XII is essential for the generation of intrinsic plasma thromboplastin. It is unique in that there are no significant clinical abnormalities including no bleeding tendencies associated with factor XII.

Factor XIII, known as the fibrin stabilizing factor (FSF), is an enzyme that is necessary to stabilize the cross-linkage of fibrin strands to form a firm clot. A deficiency of factor XIII results in a weak clot that can cause delayed or poor wound healing, abnormal scar formation, and prolonged bleeding. Decreased levels are seen in these conditions:

Congenital—rare

Acquired—lead poisoning, myeloma, pernicious anemia, liver disease, circulating inhibitors, and agammaglobulinemia

Blood Coagulation Factors

Plasma Coagulation Factors and Their Synonyms

Factor I	fibrinogen
Factor II	prothrombin
Factor III	tissue thromboplastin
Factor IV	calcium
Factor V	proaccelerin
Factor VII	proconvertin
Factor VIII	antihemophilic globulin (AHB)
Factor IX	plasma thromboplastin component (Christmas factor)
Factor X	Stuart–Prower factor
Factor XI	plasma thromboplastin antecedent
Factor XII	Hageman factor
Factor XIII	fibrin stabilizing factor

Normal Values	*Range (Mg/100 ML)*
I	150–350
II	70–130
V	7–130
VII	7–150
VIII	50–200
IX	70–130
X	70–130
XI	70–130
XII	30–225

Laboratory Results

The normal or abnormal factors are determined by the use of other tests.

Factor I normal   Fibrinogen titer
1:728 to 1:256

Factor II deficiencies	Prolonged prothrombin time, coagulation time, partial thromboplastin time
Factor III normal	Thromboplastin generation test
Factor IV normal	Normal plasma calcium levels
Factor V deficiencies	Abnormal prothrombin, partial thromboplastin, and prothrombin consumption test
	Factor V assay 50% to 200%
Factor VII deficiencies	Prolonged prothrombin time test
Factors VIII and IX normal	50% to 200% assay
Factor X deficiencies	Abnormal coagulation time, prothrombin time, partial thromboplastin time, prothrombin consumption time
Factor XI deficiencies	Prolonged clotting times, partial thromboplastin time, prothrombin consumption time and thromboplastin generation times
Factor XII	Prolonged prothrombin consumption time, partial thromboplastin time, coagulation time, thromboplastin generation time
Factor XIII abnormal	Formation of a weak clot

Nursing Implications

Procedure for Collection/Storage of Specimen

1. See specific coagulation test for collection of specimen.
2. Perform an atraumatic venipuncture.
3. Withdraw 5 ml of blood into a plastic or siliconized glass syringe.
4. Remove the tourniquet.
5. Collect the entire specimen in a second syringe or vacuum tube.
6. Transfer blood into the appropriate containers.
7. Send all the tubes to the laboratory promptly. Some specimens may need to be refrigerated or quick frozen by the laboratory.

Patient Care

1. In patients with suspected bleeding tendencies, apply firm pressure to the specimen collection site to avoid blood seepage or hematoma formation.
2. Withhold aspirin or aspirin-containing drugs for 1 wk prior to the test.
3. Obtain a clinical history from the patient and family to identify any personal or family episodes of bleeding.
4. Describe bleeding episodes in terms of type, degree, and duration of bleeding.
5. Obtain a list of all medications the patient is taking.
6. Obtain a history of the patient's pattern of alcohol use.

7. Obtain a dietary history from the patient. Ascertain whether dietary deficiencies in protein or vitamin K occur.
8. Obtain a surgical history. Note whether any recent surgeries have occurred, particularly gastrointestinal surgeries in which part of the stomach may have been removed.

Patient Education

1. Relate the patient education to the specific disease or problem identified.
2. In diseases in which hemorrhage is possible, instruct the patient on the following:
   - how to observe for bleeding
   - to wear an ID bracelet
   - to avoid injury, especially contact sports
   - which drugs will affect bleeding
   - to notify the physician of his factor defect prior to dental extraction or any other surgical procedure
   - not to take aspirin or over-the-counter drugs without permission of the physician

Signed Consent

Not required

CLOT RETRACTION

The clot retraction test is a test that measures the ability of clotted blood to contract. A normal blood clot normally undergoes contraction when serum is expressed from the clot and thrombosthenin is released. The degree of clot retraction is also due to the number of platelets present. Poor clot retraction will occur when platelets are decreased below normal $(100,000/\mu l)$ or when there is an abnormality in the platelets themselves. Clot retraction is decreased as fibrinogen and erythrocyte concentrations increase. Hypofibrinogenemic conditions or excessive fibrinolysis within the clot will cause a small, firm, completely retracted clot with unclotted red cells. Clot retraction tests are useful in diagnosing platelet deficiency and decreased/increased fibrinolytic activity.

Laboratory Results

A normal clot will retract from 3 sides of a test tube in 1 to 2 hr. The clot will be inspected at 1, 2, 4, and 24 hr for the presence of a retracted clot.

Nursing Implications

Procedure for Collection/Storage of Specimen

A specimen of 5 ml of whole blood is placed in a glass test tube.

Possible Interfering Factors

1. Shaking or jarring the test tube will lead to a shortened clot retraction time.
2. Red cell mass will affect clot retraction. In blood containing a large

mass of red cells, clot retraction is limited owing to the large volume. The degree of clot retraction is decreased in anemia.

3. Increased plasma fibrinogen levels will cause poor clot retraction.
4. The clot used for clot retraction may be examined for lysis. Normally the clot will not undergo lysis before 72 hr. The time at which lysis does occur is reported as the clot lysis time.

Patient Care

Patient care is related to the specific disease entity.

Patient Education

1. There is no specific patient education related to the test.
2. If an abnormal test result is found, teach the patient about protection from injury. Bleeding tendencies may be increased.

Signed Consent

Not required

COMPLETE BLOOD COUNT (CBC)

The complete blood count is a laboratory test that consists of the following:

- White blood cell count (WBC or Leukocytes)
- Differential white cell count (Diff)
- Red blood count (RBC)
- Hemoglobin (Hgb)
- Hematocrit (Hct)
- Red blood cell indices
  - Mean corpuscular hemoglobin (MCH)
  - Mean corpuscular hemoglobin concentration (MCHC)
  - Mean corpuscular volume (MCV)

WHITE BLOOD CELL COUNT (WBC or Leukocytes)

The leukocyte count is the total number of circulating white blood cells. The leukocyte count serves as a guide to the severity of the disease process and must be related to the clinical condition of the patient. The leukocyte count is normally higher in the newborn infant than in the adult.

Factors that increase leukocyte count include emotional stress, strenuous exercise with a rise proportional to the intensity, after administration of steroids to a patient with severe infection, and in disease states.

Leukopenia (decrease in leukocytes) occurs during and after bone marrow depression, viral infections, and hypersplenism.

The white blood cells or circulating leukocytes are counted as part of the complete blood count. Many diseases are accompanied by an increase or decrease in a specific type of white blood cell. The leukocyte count serves as a guide to the severity of the disease.

Leukocytosis, or an increase in white blood cells above 10,000 per cu mm, occurs in measles, pertussis, sepsis, acute infections, malignant disease, tissue necrosis, and trauma or tissue injury.

Leukopenia, or a decrease in white blood cells below 4,000 per cu mm, may occur in viral infections, radiation therapy, bone marrow depression, agranulocytosis, and aplastic anemia.

Laboratory Results
Normal Values

Age	Normal Leukocyte Count (cells per cu mm) Average	Leukocyte count SI. unit Average
At birth	18,100	18.1
12 hr	22,800	22.8
24 hr	18,900	18.9
1 wk	12,200	12.2
2 wk	11,400	11.4
4 wk	10,800	10.8
2 mo	11,000	11.0
4 mo	11,500	11.5
6 mo	11,900	11.9
8 mo	12,200	12.2
10 mo	12,000	12.0
12 mo	11,400	11.4
2 yr	10,600	10.6
4 yr	9,100	9.1
6 yr	8,500	8.5
8 yr	8,300	8.3
10 yr	8,100	8.1
12 yr	8,000	8.0
14 yr	7,900	7.9
16 yr	7,800	7.8
18 yr	7,700	7.7
20 yr	7,500	7.5
21 yr	7,400	7.1

Nursing Implications
Procedure for Collection/Storage of Specimen

A venous blood sample of 7 ml is obtained.

Possible Interfering Factors

1. Strenuous exercise may cause a transient rise in WBC.
2. Emotional stress and epinephrine may cause a temporary rise in WBC.
3. Stress may increase count.
4. Drug therapy (bone marrow depressants) may decrease count.
5. Anesthetic agents may increase count.

6. Time of day (early morning, low level; late afternoon high peak) may vary count.
7. Convulsions may increase count.
8. Paroxsymal tachycardia may increase count.

Patient Care

1. Observe and record any sign of infection.
2. Protect the patient with leukopenia from infection, since the body is unprotected from infectious agents.
3. Observe and record any factor that may increase or decrease WBC counts.
4. Since ACTH masks the symptoms of infection in a patient, infection can spread rapidly. Leukocytosis may or may not be present. Observe the patient who is on steroid therapy for increases in temperature, respiratory moistness, or any other signs of infection.

Patient Education

1. Patient instruction centers around teaching related to the specific disease entity.
2. Teach the patient with leukopenia good handwashing techniques and other measures to protect self from infection.

Signed Consent

Not required

DIFFERENTIAL WHITE BLOOD CELL COUNT (Diff)

The leukocyte count of circulating white blood cells is differentiated according to five types of cells. These types of white blood cells are neutrophils, eosinophils, basophils, lymphocytes, and monocytes. The differential white cell count is performed in order to determine the relative number of each type of white cell present in the blood.

- Increases in neutrophils (segs) occur in bacterial infections, metabolic or drug intoxication, and in appendicitis.
- Neutropenia occurs in massive bacterial invasions.
- Eosinophilia occurs in allergies, parasitic infections, and in scarlet fever.
- Eosinopenia occurs in stress and in response to ACTH.
- Lymphocytosis occurs in viral infections, whooping cough, and infectious mononucleosis.
- Lymphopenia occurs in thymic hypoplasia.
- Monocytosis occurs in tuberculosis, monocytic leukemia, subacute bacterial endocarditis, collagen diseases, and ulcerative colitis.

Laboratory Results

Normal Results
See Table 1-1.

Segmented Neutrophils		Band Neutrophils		Eosinophils		Basophils		Lymphocytes		Monocytes	
Age	Percent	Age	Percent	Age	Percent	Age	Percent	Age	Percent	Age	Percent
Birth	47 ± 10	Birth	14.1 ± 4	Birth	2.2	Birth	0.6	Birth	31 ± 5	Birth	5.8
12 hr	56	12 hr	15.2	12 hr	2.0	12 hr	0.4	12 hr	24	12 hr	5.3
24 hr	47	24 hr	14.2	24 hr	2.4	24 hr	0.5	24 hr	31	24 hr	5.8
1 wk	34	1 wk	11.8	1 wk	4.1	1 wk	0.4	1 wk	41	1 wk	9.1
2 wk	29	2 wk	10.5	2 wk	3.1	2 wk	0.4	2 wk	48	2 wk	8.8
4 wk	25 ± 10	4 wk	9.5 ± 3	4 wk	2.8	4 wk	0.5	4 wk	56 ± 15	4 wk	6.5
2 mo	25	2 mo	8.4	2 mo	2.7	2 mo	0.5	2 mo	57	2 mo	5.9
4 mo	24	4 mo	8.9	4 mo	2.6	4 mo	0.4	4 mo	59	4 mo	5.2
6 mo	23	6 mo	8.8	6 mo	2.5	6 mo	0.4	6 mo	61	6 mo	4.8
8 mo	22	8 mo	8.3	8 mo	2.5	8 mo	0.4	8 mo	62	8 mo	4.7
10 mo	22	10 mo	8.3	10 mo	2.5	10 mo	0.4	10 mo	63	10 mo	4.6
12 mo	23	12 mo	8.1	12 mo	2.6	12 mo	0.4	12 mo	61	12 mo	4.8
2 yr	25	2 yr	8.0	2 yr	2.6	2 yr	0.5	2 yr	59	2 yr	5.0
4 yr	34 ± 10	4 yr	8.0 ± 3	4 yr	2.8	4 yr	0.6	4 yr	50 ± 15	4 yr	5.0
6 yr	43	6 yr	8.0	6 yr	2.7	6 yr	0.6	6 yr	42	6 yr	4.7
8 yr	45	8 yr	8.0	8 yr	2.4	8 yr	0.6	8 yr	39	8 yr	4.2
10 yr	46 ± 15	10 yr	8.0 ± 3	10 yr	2.4	10 yr	0.5	10 yr	38 ± 10	10 yr	4.3
12 yr	47	12 yr	8.0	12 yr	2.5	12 yr	0.5	12 yr	38	12 yr	4.4
14 yr	48	14 yr	8.0	14 yr	2.5	14 yr	0.5	14 yr	37	14 yr	4.7
16 yr	49 ± 15	16 yr	8.0 ± 3	16 yr	2.6	16 yr	0.5	16 yr	35 ± 10	16 yr	5.1
18 yr	49	18 yr	8.0	18 yr	2.6	18 yr	0.5	18 yr	35	18 yr	5.2
20 yr	51	20 yr	8.0	20 yr	2.7	20 yr	0.5	20 yr	33	20 yr	5.0
21 yr	51 ± 15	21 yr	8.0 ± 3	21 yr	2.7	21 yr	0.5	21 yr	34 ± 10	21 yr	4.0

Nursing Implications
Procedure for Collection/Storage of the Specimen

Obtain a venous blood sample. A stained blood smear is obtained from the sample and is examined.

Possible Interfering Factors
None reported

Patient Care

Observe for and record any signs and symptoms of conditions that may increase or decrease the patient's white cell counts.

Patient Education

Patient education is related to the disease process identified.

Signed Consent

Not required

RED BLOOD CELL MORPHOLOGY

Red cells are examined by means of a blood smear to detect abnormal cells. Red cell morphology can evaluate erythropoietin stimulation, cell maturation abnormalities, and specific disease entities. There are unique abnormalities of cell shape in various disorders.

Laboratory Results
Normal Results

Normal size, shape (biconcave discs), and hemoglobin concentration

Abnormal Results

Macrocytosis—increases in cell size without a change in the concentration of hemoglobin in the cell (seen in maturation abnormalities)

Microcytosis—decrease in cell size (seen in anemias)

Elliptocytes—oval deformity of cells (seen in hereditary ovalocytosis)

Spherocytes—microcytic/hyperchromic round cells (seen in hereditary spherocytosis)

Spiculated cells—cells with dart-like or needle-like cells (seen in liver disease, lipid disease, renal disease. Indicates RBC membrane damage)

Target cells—cells with an increase in membrane to cell content (seen in the hemoglobinopathies C and S)

Sickle cells—sickle-shaped deformed cells (seen in sickle cell anemia)

Nucleated red cells—late normoblasts (indicates disorganization of RBC delivery or absence of splenic function

Red cells with Howel Jolly bodies—cells contain nuclear fragments (seen in patients with a poorly functioning or absent spleen)

Basophilic stippling—the reticulocytes basophilia is punctate, not diffused (seen in increased erythropoietin stimulation. Heavy stippling may indicate lead poisoning)

Sidenocytes—presence of small, irregular granules in the red cell (may be seen in malaria and other diseases)

Porkilocytes—large, irregular fragmented RBCs (seen in severe maturation defects)

Nursing Implications
Procedure for Collection/Storage of Specimen

1. Collect a drop of blood from a finger stick.
2. Place the blood on a clean slide. Use a second slide to draw the drop the length of the slide.
   or
3. Place a drop of blood between two coverslips and rapidly pull them apart.
4. Slides and coverslips are then stained and mounted by the laboratory.

Possible Interfering Factors

None reported

Patient Care
Observe for and record any signs and symptoms of conditions that may alter the size and shape of the RBCs.

Patient Education
1. Instruct the patient about the test and its purpose.
2. If altered cell size or shape is found, instruct the patient in the treatment of the disorder identified.

Signed Consent
Not required

HEMATOCRIT (HcT)
The hematocrit measures the volume percent of blood that is composed of red cells. Changes in blood volume affect the hematocrit. Immediately following an acute hemorrhage, the HcT may be normal; in the recovery phase, it is decreased.

Dehydration states will increase the HcT. Since it has a diurnal variation, the HcT can be as much as 10% lower in the evening than in the morning.

Laboratory Results

Normal hematocrit values—micro hematocrit method

Age	Average (%)	Age	Average (%)
Children		*Men*	
Birth	56.6	14	44
End 1st wk	52.7	18	47
2nd wk	49.6	18–50	47
3rd wk	46.6	50–60	45
4th wk	44.6	60–70	43
2 mo	38.9	70–80	40
4 mo	36.5	*Women*	
6 mo	36.2	14–50	42
8 mo	35.8	50–80	40
10 mo	35.5	*Pregnant women*	
1st yr	35.2	4 mo	42
2nd yr	35.5	5 mo	40
4th yr	37.1	6 mo	37
6th yr	37.9	7 mo	37
8th yr	38.9	8 mo	39
12th yr	39.6	9 mo	40

Nursing Implications

Procedure for Collection/Storage of Specimen

Venous blood sample may be obtained by venipuncture or by a capillary blood stick from a finger or ear.

Possible Interfering Factors
1. Failure to fill the test tube entirely with the blood specimen.
2. Prolonged stasis owing to vasoconstriction by the tourniquet.
3. Severe burns, polycythemia, and hemoconcentration may elevate the HcT.

Patient Care
1. Assess the hydration status of the patient because dehydration may elevate results.
2. Assess the patient for anemia if a decreased HcT occurs.

Patient Education

Relate patient education to the problem diagnosed.

Signed Consent

Not required

HEMOGLOBIN (Hgb)

This test measures the amount of hemoglobin in the blood. A normal hemoglobin is essential to transport oxygen from the lungs to the body tissues. Increased blood hemoglobin occurs with decreased cardiac output, increased red blood cell volume, dehydration, and impaired pulmonary gas exchange. Decreased blood hemoglobin occurs with decreased red blood cell volume, blood loss, decreased red blood cell oxygenation, and malnutrition. Severe hemolysis from any cause elevates the plasma hemoglobin concentration. The laboratory diagnosis of polycythemia is based on hemoglobin concentration. Hemoglobin determinations are important in the evaluation of anemia.

Laboratory Results
Mean Normal Values*

Age	Hemoglobin (g/100 ml)
Birth	17.0
1 to 3 mo	14.0
3 mo to 5 yr	12.0
6 to 10 yr	12.0
11 to 15 yr	13.0
Adult male	15.0
Menstruating female	13.5
Pregnancy (last trimester)	12.0

*The physiologic normal for the individual is increased by altitude or by any condition in which the arterial O_2 saturation is decreased.

Nursing Implications
Procedure for Collection/Storage of Specimen

Obtain a venous blood sample of two ml or a capillary blood sample from a finger puncture.

Possible Interfering Factors

1. Blood specimens drawn from a hand or arm receiving an intravenous infusion.
2. Hemoglobin values may be falsely increased by venous stasis owing to prolonged vasoconstriction from the tourniquet.

Patient Care

1. With decreased hemoglobin concentrations, assess the patient for signs of anemia.
2. Assess the hydration status of the patient.

Patient Education

Relate patient education to the problem diagnosed.

Signed Consent

Not required

RED BLOOD CELL COUNT (RBC)

Red blood cell count determines the total number of erythrocytes in a cubic millimeter of blood. Increased erythrocyte counts occur with decreased cardiac output, impaired pulmonary gas exchange, excessive red blood cell production, and as a steroid therapy side effect. Decreased erythrocyte counts occur in vitamin deficiencies (B_6 and $B_{1,2}$), iron deficiency, chronic infections, chronic renal diseases, and bone marrow depression. Physiologic and environmental variations that may affect erythrocyte counts are posture, exercise or excitement, dehydration, age, sex, and altitude.

Laboratory Results

Mean Normal Values for the Red Blood Cell Compartment*

Subjects	Hgb (gm/dl)	RBC (millions/ cu/mm+)	HcT (%)	MCV (μ^3)	MCH ($\mu\mu$g)	MCHC (%)
Adult men	15.1	5.1	47	90	30	34
Adult women	13.5	4.5	42	88	30	33
Boys						
Birth	20.0	5.6	59	105	36	33
1 mo	17.0	5.2	50	101	36	32
3 mo	15.0	4.5	45	100	33	33
6 mo	14.0	4.6	46	100	30	30
9 mo	13.0	4.6	45	97	28	28
1 yr	12.1	4.2	41	95	27	29
2 yr	12.3	4.2	40	88	28	30
4 yr	12.6	4.2	37	89	28	28
8 yr	13.4	4.6	41	87	29	29
14 yr	14.0	4.7	41	88	29	30
Girls						
Birth	19.5	5.6	58	103	34	34
1 mo	17.0	5.2	49	102	36	32
3 mo	14.8	4.4	44	104	33	33
6 mo	13.8	4.2	44	100	30	32
9 mo	12.8	4.2	43	98	28	30
1 yr	12.2	4.2	43	95	27	30
2 yr	12.2	4.2	43	94	27	30
4 yr	12.7	4.4	43	88	28	28
8 yr	13.0	4.5	40	89	29	28
14 yr	13.2	4.5	40	87	29	29

*Values represent the mean and 95%.

Nursing Implications

Procedure for Collection/Storage of Specimen

A venous blood sample is obtained. Capillary blood may also be used.

Possible Interfering Factors

Administration of an intravenous infusion in the same arm being used to obtain the specimen

Patient Care

1. Decreased levels of RBCs commonly characterize anemia. Assess the patient for other signs of anemia by obtaining a complete dietary history, physical assessment, and assessment of other signs and symptoms of anemia.
2. Assess the patient for the presence of any physiologic factor that may affect laboratory values.
3. Increases in RBC, not owing to altitude or strong emotions, may be indicative of polycythemia. Assess the patient for signs and symptoms of polycythemia.
4. Assess the patient for a history of chronic illnesses or infections that may cause a decrease in RBCs.
5. Since acute blood loss owing to hemorrhage may cause decreased RBCs, assess the patient for recent bleeding or trauma.

Patient Education

Teach the patient according to the problem or disease identified.

Signed Consent

Not required

RED BLOOD CELL INDICES

- Mean Corpuscular Hemoglobin (MCH)
- Mean Corpuscular Hemoglobin Concentration (MCHC)
- Mean Corpuscular Volume (MCV)

Mean corpuscular hemoglobin (MCH) is a test that measures the average weight of the hemoglobin contained in a red blood cell. The MCH is higher in newborns and infants and is found to be higher in uncomplicated macrocytic anemias; it is decreased in iron deficiency anemias and in newly treated pernicious anemia.

Mean corpuscular hemoglobin concentration (MCHC) represents the mean concentration of hemoglobin in each red blood cell. Cells that are hypochromic have a low hemoglobin concentration. Normal cells are normochromic.

Mean corpuscular volume (MCV) represents the mean volume of red blood cells. The MCV is usually higher than normal in the newborn and infant. Diameters of a large number of red blood cells are determined and plotted as to frequency. A distribution curve is obtained. Macrocytosis or microcytosis will shift the curve to one side or the other. Results below 80 μ (2 standard deviations) indicate microcytosis (small RBCs), while results 100 μ or above

(2 standard deviations) indicate macrocytosis (large RBCs). Normal cells are normocytic.

Laboratory Results

	MCV	MCHC (%)	Disease or condition
Normocytic, normochromic	76–100	30–38	Acute blood loss, aplastic anemias, acquired hemolytic anemias
Microcytic, hypochromic	60–76	20–30	Iron deficiency anemia, sideroblastic anemia
Microcytic, normochromic	60–76	30–38	Drugs, infection, kidney disease, liver disease, radiation
Macrocytic, normochromic	100–160	30–38	Anticonvulsant drugs, folic acid deficiency, pernicious anemia, hypothyroidism, metabolic drugs

Nursing Implications

Procedure for Collection/Storage of Specimen

Obtain a venous blood sample.

Possible Interfering Factors

None reported

Patient Care

Observe for and record any of the factors that may increase or decrease test results.

Patient Education

1. Explain the procedure to the patient.
2. Relate patient education to the disease entity diagnosed.

Signed Consent

Not required

EOSINOPHIL COUNT

Although the relative number of eosinophils in the blood may be determined by the differential white count, a direct method for counting eosinophils is done in this test. A low eosinophil count is found in Cushing's disease, shock, and following the administration of ACTH. Increased amounts occur in allergic reactions, certain leukemias, and parasitic infections.

Laboratory Results

Normal Range

150 to 300 eosinophils per cu mm

Nursing Implications
Procedure for Collection/Storage of Specimen

1. Collect 1 ml of whole blood by a capillary stick of the heel, toe, or finger.
2. Eosinophil counts may be ordered in conjunction with the thorn ACTH test. A fasting eosinophil count is done. The patient is given an injection of ACTH. A second eosinophil count is performed 4 hr after the injection.

Possible Interfering Factors

None reported

Patient Care

1. Observe and record any sign of infection or allergic reaction.
2. Obtain a patient history of allergies, infections, or other medical disorders.

Patient Education
Teach the patient according to the disease entity identified.

Signed Consent
Not required

COMPLEMENT

The complement test is used to demonstrate the occurrence of a blood group antigen–antibody interaction. The complement system is involved in the humoral part of the inflammatory response and interacts with portions of the clotting sequence and fibrinolytic system. The complement system consists of at least nine globulins that exert their effect by enzymatic activity. Components are designated C1–C9. Complex proteins are activated in sequence in the complement system. In the classical complement pathway, appropriate antibodies, when altered by combination with the antigen, bind complement. Eventually all nine complement components of the complement system are subsequently bound, culminating in the hemolysis of the red blood cell. Complement-binding antibodies may be IgM, three of the subclasses of IgG, but not IgA or IgE.

Laboratory Results
Normal Values

No hemolysis of blood

Abnormal Values

Hemolysis or complement components that are bound to the red cell. C_4 and C_3 are the principal complement components detected.

Nursing Implications
Possible Interfering Factors

1. Serum must be fresh or stored at -90 C° to 55 C° for no longer than 3 mo; 2 wk at $+4$ C°; less than 36 hr when stored at room temperature.
2. Heparin therapy may interfere with results of the test.

Patient Care and Education

Patient care and instruction is related to the diagnosis and management of the disease entity. Abnormal complement has been found in systemic lupus, glomerulonephritis, paroxsymal hemoglobinuria, dermatologic disorders, sickle cell anemia, and bacteremia.

Signed Consent

Not required

HEINZ BODY TEST

Heinz bodies are single or multiple, round or oval, serrated granules in the red blood cell. Heinz bodies are precipitated hemoglobin and are present in hemolytic disorders. Certain drugs that cause oxidative reactions cause precipitation of hemoglobin in glucose-6-phosphate dehydrogenase (G-6-PD) deficiency. Unstable hemoglobins such as hemoglobin H or Zurnick often cause increased numbers of Heinz bodies.

Laboratory Results

Normal Values

Occasional Heinz bodies (owing to normal aging of the RBC)

Nursing Implications

Procedure for Collection/Storage of Specimen

1. Whole blood is collected using heparin or some other additive as an anticoagulant.
2. The whole blood is mixed with a crystal violet stain. The red cells are examined for Heinz bodies.

Possible Interfering Factors
Drug Therapy

- antimalarials
- sulfonamides
- analgesics
- antipyretics
- phenacetin

- nitrofurans
- vitamin K
- chloromycetin
- thiazide diuretics

Patient Care

1. Obtain a history of the patient's ancestry. The American Black has a 20% incidence of G-6 PD, with the incidence of C-6 PD highest in the tropical and semitropical regions.
2. Obtain a drug history for patients who might have taken those drugs listed under Interfering Factors.
3. Observe the patient's fluid and electrolyte balance. Fluids may have to be increased to promote elimination of wastes caused by RBC breakdown.

Patient Education

Relate patient education to the specific disease process identified.

Signed Consent
Not required

HEMOGLOBIN ELECTROPHORESIS

There are numerous types of hemoglobin based upon the structure of the globin chains. The hemoglobin electrophoresis test is used to detect the types of hemoglobin present in the red blood cell. The electrophoresis may also classify the hemoglobin structure as normal or abnormal. Abnormal hemoglobins may be found in the hemoglobinopathies such as in sickle cell disease.

Laboratory Results
Normal Values

Hgb A_1	95% to 98%	total adult Hgb
Hgb A_2	2% to 3%	total adult Hgb
Hgb F	2%	first 2 yr life
	0.8%	after 3 yr through adulthood

Abnormal Variants

Hgb S, Hgb C, Hgb H, Hgb D, and Hgb E

Nursing Implications
Procedure for Collection/Storage of Specimen
1. Obtain a venous blood sample of 10 ml. Capillary blood may also be used.
2. Send the specimen to the laboratory immediately, since some of the abnormal hemoglobins are unstable.

Possible Interfering Factors
1. A blood specimen that is not fresh.
2. Transfusions using blood containing abnormal Hgb.

Patient Care
1. Increased levels of fetal hemoglobin (Hgb F) indicate abnormality after 6 mo of age—usually thalassemia. Obtain a family history and check ancestry for Mediterranean descent.
2. The presence of an increased *hemoglobin S* indicates sickle cell anemia. Sickle cell anemia is genetically transmitted by a recessive gene, so obtain a family history. Further testing may need to be done by means of a sickle cell test. Persons with sickle cell trait will have Hgb S, 20% to 40%; Hgb A, 60% to 80%; Hgb F, small amount. Sickle cell anemia will have the homozygous pattern of Hgb S 80% to 100%. Sickle cell disease causes a more rapid sickling of cells than cells having only the trait.
3. Hemoglobin H disease may be characterized by abnormal levels of Hgb H. Observe the patient and give care related to anemia.
4. Hemoglobin C can occur in the homozygous state to produce a mild anemia. In the heterozygous state (A/C), the disease is asymptomatic. If the patient has hemoglobin C disease, observe for signs and symptoms of anemia.
5. Check if the patient has received a transfusion in the last 3 to 4 mo.

Patient Education

Relate patient instruction to the problem or disease diagnosed.

Signed Consent

Not required

OSMOTIC FRAGILITY

Osmotic fragility tests indicate the ability of the red blood cell to withstand the influx of water into the cell. The main factor affecting this red blood cell ability is the shape of the cell. Increased osmotic fragility is found in hemolytic anemias and hereditary spherocytosis. Decreased osmotic fragility is found in postsplenectomy patients, in sickle cell anemia, iron-deficiency anemia, thalassemia, and polycythemia vera. The technique for testing osmotic fragility involves placing red blood cells in sodium chloride solutions of specific concentrations. The amount of hemolysis of the red blood cells is then compared against a blood sample used as a control.

Laboratory Results

Osmotic fragility curves shifted to the left indicate less fragile cells; to the right, indicate more fragile cells (Fig. 1-1).

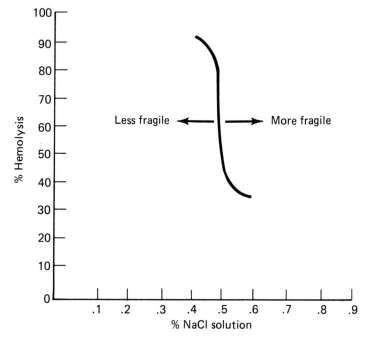

FIG.1-1. *Osmotic fragility curves.*

Nursing Implications
Procedure for Collection/Storage of Specimen
1. Collect 15 to 20 ml of heparinized venous blood.
2. Collect a blood sample from a normal control group at the same time.

Possible Interfering Factors
None reported

Patient Care
There is no specific patient care required related to the test.

Patient Education
1. Instruct the patient about the purpose of the test.
2. If there is increased RBC fragility, instruct the patient in the treatment of the disorder identified.

Signed Consent
Not required

PLATELET COUNT
Following damage to a blood vessel, platelets migrate to the injured area. The young platelets attach to the collagen fibers in the epithelial lining. ADP is released, and more platelets aggregate at the site. The platelets swell and serotonin and electrolytes appear. The swelling mass of platelets plugs the damaged wall; the serotonin causes vasoconstriction. The membranes of the aggregated platelets have platelet factor III activity upon which the coagulation proteins become activated. Coagulation occurs. Thrombin enhances further aggregation. The platelet aggregates undergo consolidation and contraction by the action of thrombin on the contractile protein, thrombosthenin. Platelet fibrinogen is converted to fibrin, which strengthens the platelet.

Platelets will be increased during hemorrhage, hemolysis, and steroid administration postsplenectomy. A sustained elevation may be seen in myeloproliferative syndromes such as polycythemia. Thrombocytopenia, a low platelet level, is seen in diseases in which there is a decrease or absence of megakaryocytes—the platelet precursors in bone marrow. Decreased platelets are also seen in patients with normal megakaryocytes in the bone marrow as in aplastic anemia, leukemia, drug toxicity, or pernicious anemia. The low platelet count may be due to increased destruction such as idiopathic thrombocytopenia purpura.

Drugs that decrease platelet count are quinidine, chlorthiazides, sulfa, and antihistamines. Viruses may cause thrombocytopenia in the acute phase or during convalescence.

Laboratory Results
Normal Range
150,000 to 250,000 per cu mm

Nursing Implications

Procedure for Collection/Storage of Specimen

1. Warm the patient's ear or finger.
2. With a sterile lancet make a small incision. Wipe away the first drop of blood. Capillary blood is drawn into a pipette from the second drop.

Possible Interfering Factors

None reported

Patient Care

1. Protect patients with decreased platelet count from injury. Easy bruising may occur.
2. The count in patients with thrombocythemia or sustained rises in platelets may be in millions per cubic millimeter. Thrombosis and hemorrhage may be present at the same time. Observe the patient for signs of thrombosis or hemorrhage.
3. Patients with decreased platelets may develop bleeding during infections or stress.
4. Observe for signs of bleeding from body orifices.

Patient Education

Educate the patient as to the importance of protecting self from injury.

Signed Consent

Not required

PARTIAL THROMBOPLASTIN TIME (PTT)

The PTT tests for abnormalities involving the coagulation proteins of the intrinsic pathway. The test cannot measure abnormalities of factor III, factor VII, or platelets; however, the PTT is prolonged in deficiencies of factors VIII, IX, X, XI, and XII. The test is done by adding plasma to calcium chloride and partial thromboplastin. The PTT is used for routine screening of coagulation disorders. (For details related to this test, see page 60.)

PORPHOBILINOGENS AND PORPHYRINS

The porphyrin synthesis begins in the mitochondria of the cell with the formation of delta-aminolevulinic acid (ALA). It continues in the cytoplasm with the combination of two molecules of ALA to form porphobilinogen (PBG). Normally little porphyrin is formed. Porphyrins are formed when excess porphyrinogen production occurs as in the porphyrias. Porphyrins are excreted in the bile or urine. Tests are done on both urine and blood specimens. Lead poisoning may or may not cause porphyrins to be present in the urine. Benzene toxicity, cirrhosis, hepatitis, and Hodgkin's disease may cause increased levels of porphyrins.

Laboratory Results

Normal

Urine delta-aminolevulinic acid—less than 4.9 mg/liter for persons under age 15

Signed Consent
Not required

PROTHROMBIN TIME (PT, Pro–Time)

The prothrombin time is done by adding plasma to a tube containing thromboplastin and calcium. Deficiencies of factors VIII, IX, XI, and XII are not detected by the prothrombin time. The prothrombin time is prolonged in deficiencies of factors I, II, V, VII, and X or in the presence of an antithrombin such as heparin. It is a useful screening procedure for deficiencies of factors II, V, VII, and X and is used to monitor anticoagulant therapy in patients receiving this drug therapy. Coumarin drugs inhibit factors II, VII, IX, and X. (For details related to this test, see page 58.)

SCHILLING TEST

The Schilling test is done to determine malabsorption of B_{12} owing to a lack of intrinsic factor or other abnormalities. The test may also be done after the patient has been given oral porcine intrinsic factor. If excretion of the intrinsic factor is then normal, it is concluded that the patient has intrinsic factor deficiency. If not, the malabsorption is due to intestinal abnormalities.

Laboratory Results
Normal Results

The patient will excrete a large proportion of the radioactive B_{12} in the urine.

Abnormal Results

The patient will excrete little radioactive material (0% to 3%) in the urine.

Nursing Implications
Procedure for Collection/Storage of Specimen

1. Keep the patient NPO after midnight.
2. Have the patient discard the first voided urine specimen of the morning.
3. Have the patient drink 24 ml of radioactive B_{12} in water. Note the time the B_{12} was administered.
4. Begin collection of the 24-hr urine specimen.
5. Give a flushing dose of vitamin B_{12}, 1 mg IM 2 hr after beginning the 24-hr urine specimen.
6. Allow the patient to have food and water after the B_{12} injection is given.
7. Collect a second 24-hr urine specimen.
8. Measure the urine volume.
9. If the excretion of the radioactivity is low (<7%) the Schilling test is repeated after seven days. The procedure is the same except that 60 mg of hog intrinsic factor is given orally with the radioactive B_{12}.

Possible Interfering Factors

The following factors or conditions may cause an abnormally low excretion of radioactive vitamin B_{12}:

- decreased renal function with impaired glomerular filtration
- elderly patients
- incomplete collection of the urine specimen

Patient Care

1. Observe the patient's urinary output. Renal insufficiency may occur after administration of the radioactive B_{12}.
2. Do not administer any laxatives to the patient during the test.

Patient Education

1. Explain the procedure to the patient. Instruct the patient to collect *all* of the urine.
2. If the patient's probable diagnosis of pernicious anemia is confirmed, teach the patient and family how to administer B_{12} injections.

Signed Consent

Required

SERUM IRON

This test measures serum transport of iron. All sera contain iron that is derived from the physiologic breakdown of red cells; however, transport or plasma iron is bound to plasma iron-binding β-globulin transferrin. In this test, the iron is split away from the transferrin in such a way that hemoglobin iron is not liberated from the red cells. Serum iron will be decreased in iron deficiency and infection. Increases of serum iron will be seen in viral hepatitis, untreated drug-induced bone marrow failure, idiopathic hemochromatosis, hereditary iron-loading anemia, pernicious anemia, and hemolytic anemia.

Laboratory Results

Normal Range

> 100 to   150 μg/100 ml–adults
>
> 1100 to 2700 μg/liter at birth
>
> 300 to   700 μg/liter 4–10 mo
>
> 530 to 1190 μg/liter 3–10 yr

Nursing Implications

Procedure for Collection/Storage of Specimen

1. Ten ml of blood is collected in iron-free glassware by syringe or vacutainer method.
2. Serum must be refrigerated if not tested immediately.
3. Serum must be collected in the morning. Later samples show a significant physiologic decrease in iron concentration.

Possible Interfering Factors

- use of iron-containing collection material
- iron dextran (Imferon)
- ingestion of ferrous sulfate

Patient Care

1. Ask the patient for the date of her last menstrual period. Serum iron is lower during menstruation than during the intermenstrual stage.
2. Be aware that subnormal levels of the plasma iron may occur in the later part of pregnancy.
3. Assess the patient's dietary history; a diet low in iron-rich foods can decrease serum iron.
4. Assess the patient for history of recent infection, which can decrease serum iron.

Patient Education

See Total iron binding capacity (p. 44).

Signed Consent

Not required

THROMBIN TIME

The thrombin time tests the third stage of coagulation, or the conversion of fibrinogen to fibrin. The test is useful when evaluating defects or alterations in fibrinogen structure such as with dysfibrinogenemia. Thrombin time is used to detect and monitor heparin therapy. Thrombin times may be measured in emergency situations to detect life-threatening fibrinogen deficiencies. Thrombin times may be increased in afibrinogenemia, hemolytic diseases of the newborn, DIC, certain obstetric complications, and with poor nutrition.

Laboratory Results

Normal Values

15 to 20 sec (normals vary widely)

Nursing Implications

Procedure for Collection/Storage of the Specimen

1. Collect 10 ml of fresh whole blood.
2. If the test is used to monitor heparin therapy, the blood is drawn 1 hr before administration of the anticoagulant.
3. Deliver the specimen to the laboratory promptly.

Possible Interfering Factors

1. The thrombin time may be prolonged *normally* in the newborn and in multiple myeloma.
2. Heparin anticoagulant therapy causes an increased thrombin time.

Patient Care

Observe the patient for bleeding and protect the patient from injury.

Patient Education

Relate patient teaching to the disease or problem identified.

Signed Consent

Not required

TOTAL IRON BINDING CAPACITY (TIBC)

The amount of transferrin protein in the blood is measured as the total iron-binding capacity. The test measures the total amount of iron that can be bound to the sum of apotransferrin and transferrin present in the blood. Circulating transferrin is normally about one-third saturated. The TIBC is helpful in separating iron-deficient patients without iron stores from those patients who develop internal iron blockage owing to inflammation.

TIBC will be higher than normal with absolute iron deficiency. Marrow damage, ineffective erythropoiesis, or iron overload in the organs and tissues causes a full saturation of the TIBC and an elevated TIBC. An increase in the TIBC may occur also in the later part of pregnancy. Decreases in TIBC are seen in cancer, hepatic disease, chronic infection, and hemolytic anemias. Lower levels may also occur in nephrosis, uremia, and starvation.

Laboratory Results
Normal Range

3 to 10 yr	3860–5220 µg/liter
Adult	300–400 µg/100 ml

Serum Iron and Serum Iron-Binding Capacity in Various Pathologic States

Disease	Serum Iron (µg/dl)	Total Iron-Binding Capacity (µg/dl)
Normal	65–185	300–350
Iron-deficiency anemia (dietary and blood loss)	Low (7–60)	Increased (450–500)
Anemia of chronic infection	Low (14–36)	Decreased (150–200)
Pernicious anemia		
Relapse	High (150–350)	Normal
Treated	Low (40–100)	Normal
Hemolytic anemia		
Congenital syphilis	Mod. increased	Mod. Increased
Sickle cell anemia	Mod. increased	Mod. Increased
Thalassemia	Increased	Decreased
Pyridoxine-responsive anemia	Increased	Normal
Refractory sideroblastic anemia	Normal or increased	Normal or mod. increased
Hereditary sex-linked anemia	Increased	Normal or mod. decreased
Hypochromic anemia responsive to crude liver extract	Increased	Normal
Transferrin deficiency	Very low	Very low
Anemia of azotemia	Low	Mod. reduced

(Continued)

Serum Iron and Serum Iron-Binding Capacity in Various Pathologic States (*Continued*)

Disease	Serum Iron (μg/dl)	Total Iron-Binding Capacity (μg/dl)
Hemochromatosis (primary)	Normal	Mod. reduced
Idiopathic pulmonary hemosiderosis	Low	Normal
Nephrotic syndrome	Low	Low

Nursing Implications

Procedure for Collection/Storage of Specimen

Obtain a venous blood sample of 10 ml.

Possible Interfering Factors

- altered protein or hormonal balance
- estrogen therapy
- hydroxyurea
- ACTH

Patient Care

Observe the patient for signs or symptoms of disorders usually diagnosed by this test, such as infection and hemolytic anemias.

Patient Education

1. Explain the test and its purpose to the patient.
2. Teach the patient according to the disease or disorder diagnosed.

Signed Consent

Not required

PROCEDURES

BLOOD CULTURES

Preprocedure

Label the laboratory slip with the time, antibiotic therapy, and rectal temperature of the patient.

During Procedure

1. Cleanse the tops of the culture medium tubes, the venipuncture site, and the probing finger with the same solution. Use a 70% alcohol wipe, allow to dry, apply tincture of iodine, and allow to dry.
2. Obtain at least 5 ml of blood. Aerobic, anaerobic, and fungal cultures require a separate sample and different culture media.
3. Change the needle each time a culture medium is inoculated. The culture is inoculated with one part blood to 10 parts culture medium.

Postprocedure

Send the specimen to the laboratory immediately.

BLOOD SAMPLING (Syringe Technique)

Nursing Implications

Preprocedure

1. Select a large syringe with an 18- to 20-gauge needle for the adult, 19- to 23-gauge for a child.
2. Prepare the site. See Vacutainer technique (p. 46).

During Procedure

1. Enter the vein with the needle. When the vein is entered, *gently* pull back on the plunger to obtain the sample.
2. Place a small dry dressing on the site.

Postprocedure

1. Remove the needle from the syringe after the sample is obtained.
2. Quickly transfer the sample into vacuum tubes. Do not force blood through the needle. This causes hemolysis of the cells in the sample.

BLOOD SAMPLING (Vacutainer Technique)

Nursing Implications

Preprocedure

1. Explain the procedure to the patient.
2. Assist the patient to lie down or sit in a comfortable position.
3. Wash your hands.
4. Locate a large peripheral vein, preferably in the antecubital fossa. Forearms and back of hands may be used. These sites are more sensitive to pain, and the veins collapse more easily.
5. The femoral vein may be used in emergencies. The femoral vein lies medial to the femoral artery. Locate the femoral artery and make the puncture at a 90° angle, 1 to 2 cm medial to the pulsation.

During Procedure

1. Distend the vein by means of a tourniquet or blood pressure cuff.
2. Palpate the vein. Check pulses distal to the site for circulatory impairment.
3. Lightly slap the site or allow the arm to become dependent. Warm towels may be used also.
4. Assemble the vacuum device.
5. Clean the site with an alcohol swab or iodine swab using a circular motion. Permit these agents to dry.
6. Re-palpate the vein above the needle entry point to avoid contamination of the insertion site.
7. Instruct the patient to open and close his fist.
8. Stabilize the vein with your thumb and draw the skin taut.
9. Insert the needle of the vacuum tube into the vein with the bevel of the needle up.
10. With the vein still stabilized, remove the tourniquet and allow the container to fill.

11. The tube should fill completely, since additives used for the test that are in the tube must be in the correct proportion to the blood collected.
12. Remove the needle, apply pressure with a dry dressing. Maintain pressure for 2 to 4 min to prevent a hematoma.

Postprocedure

Gently mix the blood in the tube by inverting the tube 8 to 10 times. Do *not* shake the tube.

DRAWING BLOOD FOR BLOOD GAS MEASUREMENT (ABGs)

Nursing Implications

Preprocedure

1. Choose the radial, brachial, or femoral artery.
2. If the radial artery is used, check for a positive Allen's test as follows:
   a. Palpate both the radial and the ulnar arteries.
   b. Firmly occlude both arteries. Raise the arm.
   c. Release the ulnar artery and assess for return of color to the hand.
   d. If the color does not return to the hand, it indicates that the ulnar artery is not capable of perfusing the hand. *Do not* do a radial artery puncture.
3. Collect equipment
   - container of crushed ice
   - 5-ml glass syringe
   - two 22-inch needles, alcohol swabs
   - 0.5 ml of sodium heparin
4. Explain the procedure to the patient.
5. Explain to the patient that this procedure may cause a sharp pain in the hand.
6. Note the concentration of oxygen the patient is receiving and record on lab requisition.
7. Obtain a baseline rectal temperature. Elevations in temperature will affect oxygen saturation results.

During Procedure

1. Draw 0.5 ml heparin into a glass syringe.
2. Flush the syringe with heparin.
3. Position the arm on a firm surface, palpate the artery.
4. Cleanse the site with alcohol swabs.
5. Immobilize the artery between two fingers.
6. Holding the syringe like a pencil and at a 40° to 90° angle, penetrate both the skin and artery.
7. Note the color of the blood. The sample should be bright red.
8. Obtain 3 to 5 ml of blood and withdraw the needle.
9. Apply pressure for 5 min to the site.

Postprocedure
1. Immediately expel *all* of the air bubbles from the specimen.
2. Place the syringe with the specimen in the crushed ice.
3. Send to the laboratory immediately.

BONE MARROW ASPIRATION

The bone marrow aspiration or biopsy is a test used to determine if the bone marrow is manufacturing normal red cells, white cells, and platelets.

Normal Values

The bone marrow is rust red with visible amounts of fatty substances and grey-white marrow fragments.

Formed cell elements	Normal mean percent
Reticulum cell	up to 2%
Proerythroblast	up to 5%
Early normoblast	up to 20%
Late normoblast	up to 15%
Myeloblast	up to 3%
Myelocyte	10 to 20%
Stab forms	8 to 35%
Polymorphonuclear leukocyte	10 to 20%
Eosinophil myelocyte	up to 4%
Mature eosinophil	up to 4%
Mature basophil	up to 1%
Lymphocyte	up to 25%
Plasma cell	up to 5%
Monocyte	up to 1%
Megakaryocyte	up to 1%

Abnormal Results

Most disorders of erythropoiesis are characterized by an increase in red cell precursors. Greater than 25% lymphocytes in the marrow is abnormal. Greater than 15% monocytes is abnormal.

Nursing Implications

Preprocedure
1. Explain the procedure to the patient. The bone marrow aspiration is performed by inserting a bone marrow needle into the sternum, iliac crest, or tibia for the purpose of removing marrow from the bone for laboratory examination. The stylus is removed once the needle is in the bone marrow. A syringe is attached to the needle, 1 to 2 ml of the bone marrow is withdrawn.
2. Position the patient on the back or side according to the site selected.
3. Shave the skin around the site.

4. Cleanse the skin around the site with an antiseptic such as Betadine.
5. Place sterile towels around the site.

During Procedure

1. The site is anesthesized with procaine by the physician.
2. Explain to the patient that the initial sensation will be one of pressure as the bone marrow is entered. Some pain will occur when the needle enters the bone, and marrow is withdrawn in the syringe.
3. Ask the patient to lie as still as possible during the procedure.

Postprocedure

1. Carefully label the slides and send to the laboratory.
2. Apply pressure over the aspiration site to control bleeding.
3. Place an adhesive bandage over the site.
4. Observe the patient for marked bleeding at the puncture site or for continued pain, which may indicate a fracture.
5. Observe the patient for 2 to 3 dy following the procedure for redness or tenderness at the site. This may indicate infection.

Signed Consent

Required

BIBLIOGRAPHY

Beck W: Hematology. Cambridge, MIT Press, 1977

Brown B: Hematology Principles and Procedures. Philadelphia, Lea & Febiger, 1980

Byrne J: Hematologic studies: part I—a review of the CBC: the quantitative tests. Nursing 76, No. 6, 10:11–12, 1976

Byrne J: Hematologic studies: part II—a review of the CBC: the differential white cell count. Nursing 76, No. 6, 11:15–17, 1976

Byrne J: Hematologic studies: part III—a review of the CBC: stained red cell examination. Nursing 76, No. 6, 12:15, 1976

Byrne J, et al: Laboratory Tests: Implications for Nurses and Allied Health Professionals. Menlo Park, California, Addison-Wesley, 1981

England JM: Prospects for automated differential leucocyte counting in the routine laboratory. Clin Lab Hemat No. 1, 4:263–73, 1979

Fischbach F: A Manual of Laboratory Diagnostic Tests. Philadelphia, JB Lippincott, 1980

Freedman ML, Marcus DL: Anemia and the elderly: is it physiology or pathology? Am J Med Sci No. 280, 2:81–85, 1980

Guyton A: Textbook of Medical Physiology, 5th ed. Philadelphia, WB Saunders, 1976

Leavell B, Thorup O: Fundamentals of Clinical Hematology. Philadelphia, WB Saunders, 1976

Morens DM: WBC and differential: value in predicting bacterial diseases in children. Am J Dis Child No. 133, 1:25–27, 1979

Prober CG, Stevenson DK, Neu J, Johnson JD: The white cell ratio in the very low birth weight infant. Clin Ped No. 18, 8:481–86, 1979

Weinstein JS, Foster JD, Stinson LE: The platelet estimate: is it being ignored? Postgrad Med No. 68, 2:63–64, 1980

Ziesler FD, Rich SA, Fasco MJ, Russell C, Kelly JH: Reappraisal of thromboplastin. Ann Clin Lab Sci No. 8, 11:202–11, 1981

2

Tests Related to Cardiovascular Function

Patricia Gauntlett Beare

Virginia A. Rahr

Christina A. Ronshausen

OVERVIEW OF PHYSIOLOGY AND PATHOPHYSIOLOGY

The purpose of the cardiovascular system is to transport oxygen and nutrients to the cells of the body and to remove carbon dioxide and other wastes from those cells. Clinical signs and symptoms of dysfunction of the cardiovascular system depend on the metabolic needs of the tissue cells and the ability of the system to function adequately to meet those needs.

Factors that can produce dysfunction include the following:

- decreased cardiac output
- high or low blood volumes
- altered blood viscosity
- increased or decreased peripheral resistance
- irregularity of heart rate or rhythm
- abnormal electrolyte balance
- influence of the sympathetic or parasympathetic nervous systems
- inflammatory or infectious processes

CARDIAC OUTPUT

Cardiac output is the volume of blood ejected by the left ventricle; it is determined by the formula of the heart rate multiplied by the stroke volume. Cardiac output varies according to the requirements of the tissues for oxygen and the amount of blood that must be pumped to that area.

- Major causes of decreased cardiac output are (1) impairment of the pumping function of the heart, and (2) decreased blood volume in the system.
- Impairment of the pumping function of the heart can be altered by (1) inadequate oxygenation of the myocardial tissue, (2) altered blood volume/blood flow in the system, (3) altered distensibility of the heart muscle, (4) altered neural regulation, (5) altered contractibility of the heart muscle, and (6) alteration in blood components.

ATHEROSCLEROSIS AND ISCHEMIC HEART DISEASE

The primary cause of impairment of the pumping function of the heart is ischemic heart disease, which is usually secondary to atherosclerosis of the coronary arteries. Atherosclerosis occurs in individuals with a genetic predisposition or in those who eat a diet high in cholesterol and other fats.

The ingested cholesterol and fats are deposited in the intima of the arteries, creating atherosclerotic plaques. In time, these plaques are replaced with fibrous tissue and may even become calcified. The results of these pathologic changes are a decrease in lumen size and loss of elasticity of the arteries. In the presence of decreased lumen size and loss of elasticity of the coronary arteries, less blood, and consequently less oxygen, is delivered to the heart muscle. This is true particularly when the workload of the heart is increased.

Collateral Circulation

Collateral circulation of the small branches of the coronary arteries develops to compensate for the decreased coronary blood flow. The development of collateral circulation may, for a period of time, keep up with decreased blood flow from the atherosclerosed coronary arteries. The extent of damage to the heart muscle may be determined in part by the presence and extent of the collateral circulation.

Coronary Occlusion

Blood flow to the heart muscle may be obstructed partially or totally by occlusion of the vessel lumen by an atherosclerotic plaque, spasm of the vessel musculature, or by thrombus development on the thickened and roughened edges of the internal layer of the artery. Occlusion of a coronary artery may cause ischemia, infarction, or pump failure. The degree of tissue injury to the heart muscle depends upon which artery is occluded and the location of the occlusion within the artery.

Angina

If the flow of blood to the heart muscle is acutely diminished or not sufficient to meet myocardial need for oxygen, a state of ischemia exists. With ischemia the heart muscle is injured but not permanently damaged, and pain is produced. This clinical state is known as angina pectoris. When the demand for oxygen is reduced, as with rest, or the flow of blood is increased, as with the use of nitrates, the assault to the ischemic area is relieved.

Myocardial Infarction

When the occlusion to blood flow occurs for a longer period (over 30 minutes), some tissue cells sustain permanent damage and cannot maintain cardiac function. The cells, which are permanently damaged, die resulting in necrosis. This state of cell death is called a myocardial infarction. The necrotic tissue is surrounded by an area of ischemia.

The final size of the infarction will depend on (1) the duration of anoxia, (2) the size of the vessel involved, and (3) the presence of collateral circulation. If the ischemic area begins to receive adequate oxygen and nutrition, the cells will heal without residual effect.

Cardiac Enzymes

As the cells die, the necrotic tissue releases enzymes from within the cells into the bloodstream. The cardiac enzymes include the following:

- creatine phosphokinase (CPK)
- lactic dehydrogenase (LDH)
- serum glutamic-oxaloacetic transaminase (SGOT)

The levels of these enzymes in the blood are an indicator of the degree of damage to the myocardium.

Cardiac Output

The pumping function of the heart, and thus the cardiac output, is influenced by the location and the extent of the myocardial infarction.

The left ventricle is the most common site of a myocardial infarction because the left coronary artery, which supplies its blood, is most often occluded. Because some of the muscle fibers within the left ventricle are not functioning, while others are unable to contract with much force, the pumping ability is decreased.

The pumping ability is further compromised by the phenomenon of "systolic stretch." During the systole, when all the muscle fibers should be contracting, the damaged fibers do not contract, but instead bulge outward. Consequently the force of contraction is not as strong. Some blood remains within the ventricle, and cardiac output is further decreased.

The cardiac output may also be affected if the infarcted area involves part of the normal electrical pathway of the heart. Damaged cells are unable to conduct electrical impulses. This results in alterations in heart rate and rhythm and variances in ventricular output.

PUMP FAILURE

If the pumping function of the ventricles is impaired in such a way that the cardiac output is less than the volume of blood received, pump failure is said to exist. Pump failure is a secondary process of heart disease affecting the left or right side of the heart. In addition to atherosclerosis, valvular disease, pulmonary or systemic hypertension, renal failure, and hepatic disease may also be precursers to pump failure.

Cardiac output may or may not be altered in pump failure depending on the compensatory mechanisms of the body. If cardiac output is not decreased, a state of compensated pump failure exists. In the event of decreased cardiac output, or in the event of vessel demand for increased blood supply, immediate as well as long-term compensation occurs.

• The immediate and long-term compensatory mechanisms for pump failure are increased heart rate and force of contraction, ventricular dilatation, and hypertrophy of the ventricles.

Increased Heart Rate

The heart rate normally will increase in response to demands from the tissues for more oxygen. Tissue demand for oxygen will be increased due to exercise, an increased metabolic rate, or when blood cells themselves are unable to carry sufficient oxygen. The heart rate may also increase in conditions such as anemia, thyroid disease, or pregnancy. The heart cannot maintain its increased rate indefinitely and eventually begins to fail.

Myocardial infarction may also cause the heart to fail, with a subsequent decrease in cardiac output. Within a few seconds after the fall in cardiac output, sympathetic stimulation occurs. This stimulation increases the heart rate and force of contraction and constricts peripheral vessels. Peripheral venous constriction increases return of venous blood to the heart. At the same time, the parasympathetic nervous system is inhibited, which allows the heart rate to increase. The increased force and rate of contraction, along with the larger venous return, increases cardiac output.

Ventricular Dilatation

The left ventricle dilates in response to chronic volume overload. Ventricular dilatation prevents a backlog of fluid from entering into a relatively noncompliant pulmonary vascular bed. The ventricle stretches to accommodate the increased blood volume. This increase in stretch causes an increased force of contraction. Over-stretch occurs when the muscle fibers are stretched by the increased blood volume beyond their capacity. This acts adversely on the heart causing a decreased strength or force of contraction.

Ventricular Hypertrophy

Stimulation for increased heart rate and increased force of contraction over a period of time will cause muscles of the involved ventricle to hypertrophy. The blood vessels within the ventricle proliferate as the muscle hypertrophies, but not to the same extent. When the hypertrophied heart responds to an increased workload, there are still insufficient numbers of blood vessels to supply adequate amounts of oxygen and nutrients. The ventricle cannot continue to pump effectively without oxygen. If the workload continues, ischemia, infarction, or further pump failure can occur.

AFFECTED KIDNEY FUNCTION

A decreased cardiac output decreases blood supply to the kidneys. This decreases the glomerular filtration rate, which in turn increases the blood volume by retaining fluid and decreasing the excretion of urine. The decreased cardiac output also increases aldosterone secretion, which results in an increased reabsorption of sodium and water. The secretion of the antidiuretic hormone is also increased as a result of the reabsorbed sodium increasing the osmotic concentration of the cellular fluid. The effect of this compensatory mechanism is to increase fluid retention, and by doing so, increase the venous return to the heart. This increased blood volume can cause the heart to fail. Decreased blood supply to the kidneys stimulates the release of the hormone erythropoietin which in turn stimulates the body to produce more red blood cells.

HYPERTENSION

Hypertension places an increased workload on the heart and can lead to pump failure. The increased workload on the heart causes the left ventricle to hypertrophy and possibly to dilate. Since blood supply by the coronary arteries does not keep up with the increasing heart mass, the hypertrophied heart can become anoxic, especially under stress. Hypertension is the clinical state in which the arterial pressure (either systolic or diastolic, or both) is elevated.

As hypertension becomes more advanced, a negative cycle evolves in which blood flow to the kidneys decreases. The excretory function of the kidney is altered so that sodium and water are retained. This additional extracellular volume causes the blood pressure to rise and further increases the workload on the heart. Thus the chance of development of pump failure is increased.

ARRHYTHMIAS

Alterations in the rate and rhythm of the heart can influence the functioning of the heart. Irregularities in rate and rhythm originate from disturbances in impulse formation or impulse conduction. The irregularities may be temporary or permanent and can vary in severity. The site of impulse formation is determined by the rapidity with which the cardiac cells reach impulse threshold during the phase of depolarization. The sinoatrial (SA) node's rate of impulse formation is the fastest of the cardiac cells and is considered the pacemaker of the heart. The SA node also provides stimulation for contraction of both the atria and the ventricles.

The site and rate of impulse formation can be influenced by (1) electrolyte imbalance, (2) tissue damage, and (3) neural innervation.

- With increased levels of sodium in the body in the presence of pump failure, the rate of impulse formation is decreased, further compounding the pump failure.

- The rate can also be decreased in the presence of elevated levels of potassium, which may occur with supplemental potassium therapy.

In the event of cell damage at the SA node, a new pacemaker will evolve. Depending on the irritability of the heart from tissue injury or an electrolyte imbalance, one or more new sites of impulse formation may arise. Other sites of impulse formation decrease the effectiveness of the pumping function of the heart.

Conduction of the impulses through the heart can be impaired as a result of tissue damage and electrolyte imbalance. If the infarcted area involves the electrical pathway, the damaged cells will be unable to conduct the impulses. Either the impulse must take another pathway, or, if the impulse is blocked completely, another impulse must be initiated beyond the blockage to complete the circuit. The impulse can also be blocked, especially at the atrioventricular (AV) node, by the presence of an elevated potassium level.

The rate of impulse formation is directly influenced by the sympathetic and parasympathetic nervous systems, primarily the sympathetic system. Stimulation of the sympathetic system will cause the heart rate to increase. Stimulation of the parasympathetic system will cause the heart rate to decrease.

The electrocardiogram (ECG) is the principal means of identifying irregularities in heart beat. Because of the complexity of this subject, ECGs will not be covered in this book. The reader is referred to the numerous sources available on this subject.

BLOOD VISCOSITY

The viscosity of the blood can decrease the pumping function of the heart and the cardiac output. In response to tissue hypoxia, such as in pump failure and secondary polycythemia, the body increases the number of red blood cells (RBC) available to carry oxygen. The increased number of red blood cells increases the viscosity of the blood, thus making it harder for the heart to pump the blood. If there is a chronic increase in the blood viscosity, pump failure might result.

INFECTIOUS CONDITIONS

Cardiac output can be altered by inflammatory and infectious processes of the heart. Such processes involving the heart valves may cause decreased cardiac output. This is owing to difficulty in pumping blood through narrowed, stenosed valves, or owing to blood regurgitation into the atria by ineffective closure of the valves. Inflammation involving the valves of the heart may cause incompetency or stenosis of the mitral, aortic, or tricuspid valves. This often occurs as a result of rheumatic fever. In addition, inflammatory or infectious processes can involve the muscle layers on the heart. This occurs in endocarditis and pericarditis and can interfere with the pumping function of the heart.

BLOOD TESTS
ANTICOAGULANTS

There are several cardiovascular conditions in which it is desirable to prolong the clotting time of the blood. Some of the more common indications for using anticoagulants are to decrease the possibility of (1) formation of thrombi, (2) extension of a thrombus or thrombi, and (3) emboli formation. Some of the most common conditions under which thrombi tend to form are in patients with the following:

- severe atherosclerosis, especially coronary artery disease
- inflammatory processes, such as thrombophlebitis
- stasis of blood, such as in atrial fibrillation, shock, or immobility
- coagulopathies, such as thrombocytosis or disseminated intravascular coagulation (DIC)

Extension of thrombi is a possible complication in patients with any of the above conditions. Prevention of this complication is sought by the use of anticoagulant therapy.

Another complication of the formation of thrombi is emboli formation. Fragments of thrombi may become dislodged and are carried in the bloodstream. They may lodge in vital organs such as the lungs, causing pulmonary embolism; the brain, causing a stroke; or the heart, causing a myocardial infarction.

The purpose of anticoagulant therapy is to prolong the clotting time of the blood. Increased blood clotting time reduces the incidences of thrombi formation, extension of thrombi, and emboli formation.

The most frequently administered anticoagulants are heparin and the coumarin derivatives which include bishydroxycoumarin (Dicumarol) and warfarin sodium (Coumadin). The laboratory tests used to monitor patients on anticoagulant therapy are (1) prothrombin time (pro-time, PT), (2) partial thromboplastin time (PTT), and (3) activated partial thromboplastin time (aPTT). The oldest, but least accurate, coagulation test is the Lee–White clotting time. It may be used on occasion to monitor patients on heparin therapy. Many factors reduce its accuracy and hence its usefulness.

Other tests related to blood coagulation are used primarily in patients who have dysfunctions in blood coagulation. These tests, such as bleeding times (Duke and Ivy), capillary coagulation time, and fibrinogen are discussed in the chapter on the hematopoietic system.

PROTHROMBIN TIME (PT, Pro–Time)

Prothrombin, also known as clotting factor II, is a glycoprotein produced in the liver. It requires fat-soluble vitamin K for synthesis.

Prothrombin time measures the time required for clotting to occur after thromboplastin and calcium are added to decalcified plasma. The most common use of PT is to judge the effect of coumarin derivatives, especially Coumadin.

Prothrombin time is prolonged in the following conditions: anticoagulant therapy, severe liver disease, dietary deficiency of vitamin K, premature infants or newborn infants deficient in vitamin K, in malabsorption of fats (vitamin K is fat-soluble), and in rare cases, such as idiopathic familial hypoprothrombinemia or hypofibrinogenemia (acquired or inherited).

Laboratory Results

Normal Range

12 to 14 sec (this value is known as the "control")

Therapeutic Range

2 to 2½ times the normal or control

Nursing Implications

Procedure for Collection/Storage of Specimen

1. The PT should be performed within 4 hr after collection of the blood specimen.
2. Excessive room temperature or refrigeration of the specimen should be avoided.

Possible Interfering Factors

1. Many drugs enhance or antagonize the effect of Coumadin and thus increase or decrease the PT. Some drugs taken alone or in combination with Coumadin may alter the PT (Table 2-1).
2. Foods may decrease PT, especially diets high in vitamin K and high in fats.

Patient Care

1. Observe the patients with a prolonged prothrombin time for any unusual bleeding. Bleeding gums, prolonged bleeding from minor cuts, petechiae, and bruising from minor traumas are all important observations to make. The possibility of covert or nonobvious bleeding sources, such as gastrointestinal or other bleeding, should also be considered. The antidote to reverse the anticoagulant effect of Coumadin is vitamin K.
2. Before giving an anticoagulant, the nurse should check the most recent PT report and recognize values that are normal, therapeutic, or abnormal.
3. Notify the physician of abnormally high pro-times, because hemorrhage is a danger.

TABLE 2-1. **Most Common Drugs Affecting PT**

May Increase PT	May Decrease PT
Acetaminophen	Antacids
Allopurinol	Antihistamines
Alcohol	Ascorbic acid
Aspirin (in large doses)	Barbiturates
Chloramphenicol	Colchicine
Corticosteroids	Griseofulvin
Disulfiram (Antabuse)	Oral contraceptives
Erythromycin	Tetracycline
Glucagon	Vitamin K
Guanethidine	
Indomethacin	
Mercaptopurine	
Methyldopa	
Monoamine oxidase (MAO) inhibitors	
Neomycin	
Propylthiouracil	
Quinidine	
Streptomycin	
Sulfonamides	
Sulfonurea	
Thyroid preparations	

Patient Education

1. Instruct the patient about what the test measures and why it is necessary. When the therapeutic dose is being determined, daily PTs are usually ordered. After a maintenance dose is achieved, PTs are monitored less frequently, such as once a week.
2. Teach the patient to observe for unusual or abnormal bleeding tendencies. They should notify a designated health professional if they note any unusual bleeding.
3. Caution the patient not to take other prescriptions or over-the-counter drugs unless the physician ordering the anticoagulant has taken this into consideration.
4. Minor surgeries or dental procedures, such as teeth extractions, may be followed by prolonged bleeding. Instruct the patient to avoid these procedures, if possible, while the PT is elevated.
5. Alcohol consumption may increase the effect of Coumadin. Teach the patient to avoid alcohol or to use it with extreme moderation.
6. Help the patient to assess activities of daily living to identify potential injuries that might cause prolonged bleeding. Some examples of minor

alterations in activities of daily living are to use a soft toothbrush to avoid bleeding gums or to use an electric razor to avoid nicking of skin.

7. Instruct the patient in modification of daily diet. The patient's present diet is usually maintained, but diets high in foods containing vitamin K may need to be modified, since vitamin K decreases the pro-time. Excessive fats, which enhance the absorption of vitamin K, should also be avoided.

8. Have the patient wear a Medic-Alert bracelet stating which of the anticoagulants is being taken.

Signed Consent

Not required

PARTIAL THROMBOPLASTIN TIME (PTT)

Thromboplastin is clotting factor III, although the numerical designation is not commonly used. It is present in both the blood and in tissue. Thromboplastin is required for the normal clotting of blood.

Partial thromboplastin time measures the time required for clotting to occur after a "partial thromboplastin reagent" is added to blood plasma.

The PTT is prolonged in anticoagulant therapy using heparin and by defects in clotting factor I (fibrinogen), factor II (prothrombin), and factors V, VII, IX, X, XI, and XII. The PTT is the best single screening test for disorders of coagulation.

Laboratory Results

Normal Range

50 to 90 sec (this is called "control")

Therapeutic Range

2½ to 3 times the control

Nursing Implications

Procedure for Collection/Storage of Specimen

The blood specimen should be collected at the same time each day, preferably one-half hour after administration of heparin.

Possible Interfering Factors

Drugs that may antagonize the anticoagulant effects of heparin, thus decreasing the PTT, are

- antihistamines
- digitalis preparations
- tetracycline

Drugs that may decrease the adhesiveness of platelets, thus prolonging the clotting time are

- aspirin
- persantine
- Robitussin

Patient Care

1. Observe the patients on heparin or with an abnormally prolonged PTT for any unusual bleeding, such as bruising from minor trauma, nosebleeds, or bleeding gums.
2. Internal bleeding should also be considered a possibility, especially in patients with a history of peptic ulcer disease. The nurse should be alert to early signs and symptoms of shock as well as to blood in the urine and tarry stools.
3. Monitor PTT reports and recognize therapeutic and abnormal findings. In the presence of an abnormally prolonged clotting time, anticoagulants should be withheld pending notification of the physician.
4. Hold heparin or discontinue prior to surgery. The heparin may be given up to 4 hr prior to surgery. Evaluate the PTT or aPTT before surgery.

Patient Education

1. When the PTT is prolonged, as with heparin therapy, the patient should be taught to observe for and report any unusual or abnormal bleeding.
2. Heparin is usually administered to hospitalized persons, but occasionally a patient may be discharged while still receiving heparin. In that event, careful teaching regarding administration of heparin is required.

Signed Consent

Not required

ACTIVATED PARTIAL THROMBOPLASTIN TIME (aPTT)

The aPTT is a modification of the PTT, which allows for greater reliability of results. The aPTT is also less time consuming to perform. The modification is the addition of particulate matter or a chemical reagent to the thromboplastin reagent. This addition rapidly activates the contact factors.

The aPTT is indicated for the same conditions as the PTT. It is commonly used to monitor heparin dosage. The aPTT reflects fairly sensitively changes in the heparin level.

Laboratory Results
Normal Range

The aPTT is usually standardized so that the normal (control) is between 35 to 45 sec.

Therapeutic Range

2 times the control

Nursing Implications
Procedure for Collection/Storage of Specimen

The blood specimen should be collected at the same time each day, preferably ½ hr after administration of heparin.

Possible Interfering Factors

Drugs that may antagonize the anticoagulant effects of heparin, thus decreasing the aPTT are

- antihistamines
- digitalis preparations
- tetracycline

Drugs that may decrease the adhesiveness of platelets, thus prolonging the clotting time are

- aspirin
- persantine
- Robitussin

Patient Care

1. Patients on heparin or with an abnormally prolonged aPTT should be observed for any unusual bleeding, such as bruising from minor trauma, nosebleeds, or bleeding gums.
2. Internal bleeding should also be considered a possibility, especially in patients with a history of peptic ulcer disease. The nurse should be alert to early signs and symptoms of shock as well as to blood in the urine and tarry stools.
3. aPTT reports should be monitored and therapeutic and abnormal findings recognized. In the presence of an abnormally prolonged clotting time, anticoagulants should be withheld pending notification of the physician.
4. Patients scheduled for surgery should have either the heparin held or discontinued prior to surgery or the aPTT or PTT should be carefully evaluated before surgery.

Patient Education

1. When the aPTT is prolonged, as with heparin therapy, the patient should be taught to observe for and report any unusual or abnormal bleeding.
2. Heparin is usually administered to hospitalized persons, but occasionally a patient may be discharged while still receiving heparin. In that event, careful teaching regarding administration of heparin is required.

Signed Consent

Not required

CARDIAC ENZYMES

Enzymes are proteins that modify or promote biochemical processes within cells of the body. Enzymes are found within all body tissues and are contained within the cells. Normally, the blood contains small amounts of the enzymes. Damage or necrosis or the cell membrane causes an increased release of certain enzymes into the blood. Five main enzymes are abnormally high with necrosis of cardiac tissue—creatine phosphokinase (CPK), serum glutamic-oxaloacetic transaminase (SGOT), serum glutamic-pyruvic transaminase (SGPT), lactic dehydrogenase (LDH), and alpha-hydroxybutyrate dehydrogenase (α-HBD). Total enzyme elevations may occur with cardioversion, defibrillation, hypotension, and trauma owing to falls or to multiple injections. Certain drugs such as morphine sulfate, anticoagulants, anabolic steroids, streptomycin, penicillin, cephalothin sodium (Keflin), and methyldopa (Aldomet) may cause transient elevation of some of these enzymes.

ALPHA-HYDROXYBUTERIC DEHYDROGENASE (α-HBD)

The enzyme alpha hydroxybuteric dehydrogenase (α-HBD) is elevated after a myocardial infarction. An increase in α-HBD is always accompanied by an increase in the lactic dehydrogenase (LDH) levels. The α-HBD remains elevated for a long period of time, even after the other enzymes have returned to normal. α-HBD may be especially valuable in determining if a patient has had a "silent" myocardial infarction or an infarction without associated chest pain. This is possible owing to the long duration of elevation of α-HBD. Heart failure and nephrosis may cause an increase in α-HBD, whereas angina pectoris will not. The HBD/LDH ratio may be increased in myocardial infarction, progressive muscular dystrophy, and megaloblastic disease. The ratio of HDB/LDH is depressed in liver disease.

Laboratory Results
Normal Range

140 to 350 u

Range with Myocardial Infarction

Rises	10 to 12 hr
Peak level	48 to 72 hr
Returns to normal	12 to 13 dy

Nursing Implications
Procedure for Collection/Storage of Specimen

Collect a venous blood sample.

Possible Interfering Factors

None reported

Patient Care
Instruct the patient with an elevated α-HBD accompanied by an increased LDH to avoid any activity that may increase the workload on the heart until a diagnosis is made.

Patient Education
None

Signed Consent
Not required

CREATINE PHOSPHOKINASE (CPK)

Creatine phosphokinase is a muscle enzyme released upon damage or injury to muscle tissue. There are three sources of CPK in human serum: muscle, heart, and brain. Damage to any of the three sources elevates total CPK. CPK is a two-peptide chain that identifies its origin of muscle tissue. Heart, brain, and muscle CPK can be separated from each other by electrophoresis. These peptide chains are called isoenzymes. CPK isoenzymes can be used to differentiate heart muscle damage from brain or skeletal muscle activity or damage: CPK isoenzyme I (BB) is of brain tissue origin; CPK isoenzyme II (MB) is of heart tissue origin; CPK isoenzyme III (MM) is of skeletal muscle origin.

The CPK is the first of the cardiac enzymes to elevate after a myocardial infarction. Since it returns to normal rapidly after the initial infarction, new elevations of the enzymes may indicate extension of the infarction, especially if chest pain continues. CPK isoenzymes can also be used to detect and follow therapy in patients suffering from muscle degenerative diseases. They have been used also to determine reactions from anesthesia.

Total CPK serum enzyme elevations may occur with the following:

- muscle disease, muscle damage, or trauma
- lung disease (slight elevation)
- acute brain damage
- dissecting aneurysm
- head injury
- cerebral infarction
- hypothyroidism
- unusual athletic activity or muscle overactivity
- myocarditis
- repeated intramuscular injections
- anticoagulants
- morphine sulfate
- acute alcoholism
- newborn children with tricuspid insufficiency
- black people
- last trimester of pregnancy
- infantile muscular atrophy. Congenital muscular dystrophy, only CPK II (MB) will be elevated by age 2 to 8 mo
- operative procedures

Total CPK serum enzyme may be falsely decreased during the following:

- first two trimesters of pregnancy
- hypothyroidism

Laboratory Results*

Normal Range

Adult	<75 u/liter
Children	<100 u/liter

Range with Myocardial Infarction

Initial elevation	2 to 5 hr
Peak period elevation	16 to 24 hr
Total period elevation	24 to 72 hr
Return to normal	2 to 3 dy

Nursing Implications

Procedure for Collection/Storage of Specimen

1. Perform the laboratory test on fresh blood serum.
2. Do not refrigerate or store specimen.
3. Isoenzymes in persons suspected of having a myocardial infarction should be run immediately upon admission and every 6 hr for 24 to 30 hr.

Possible Interfering Factors

- athletic activity
- intramuscular injections
- morphine
- anticoagulants
- alcohol

Patient Care

1. Assess for recent trauma, history of convulsions, or history of chest pain.
2. In presence of increased CPK, observe for possible signs/symptoms indicating tissue damage (*e.g.,* chest pain).
3. In children with no history of trauma or convulsions, assess for family history of degenerative muscle disease.

Patient Education

If elevation of total enzymes exists, avoid any activity that may increase workload of heart until diagnosis is made.

Signed Consent

Not required

---

*Varies according to specific laboratory test, race, sex.

LACTIC DEHYDROGENASE (LDH)

Lactic dehydrogenase (LDH) consists of five different components called isoenzymes. All five are normally present in human plasma. The first two isoenzymes (LDH_1, LDH_2) are found in cardiac muscle, renal cortex, cerebrum, and erythrocytes. The third isoenzyme (LDH_3) is found in lymphatics, spleen, leukocytes, pancreas, platelets, and lung tissue. The fourth and fifth isoenzymes (LDH_4, LDH_5) are found in the liver, skeletal muscle, and skin (Table 2-2).

Laboratory Results

Normal Range

150 to 325 u/liter

Range with a Myocardial Infarction

Onset	12 to 24 hr
Peak	48 to 72 hr
Diagnostic level	2 to 4 times normal
Return to normal	7 to 1 dy

TABLE 2-2. **Serum Enzyme Elevations with Various Disease Processes**

	LDH_1	LDH_2	LDH_3	LDH_4	LDH_5	Total LDH
Myocardial infarction	X					
Myocardial infarction with congestive heart failure	X				X	
Hepatitis					X	
Liver damage					X	X
Hemolytic anemia						X
Pernicious anemia						X
Leukemia						X
Pulmonary embolus	X	X	X			X
Pulmonary infarction	X	X	X			X
Muscular dystrophy	X	X				
Abdominal pain						X
Neoplastic disease						X
Granulocytic leukemia						X
Patients with artificial heart valves						X
Patients with cardiopulmonary bypass						X

Nursing Implications
Procedure for Storage/Collection of Specimen

1. Fresh whole blood is collected by venipuncture.
2. Avoid hemolysis of blood when collecting sample, since isoenzymes are found in erythrocytes.
3. Specimen should not stand for over 1 hr.
4. Specimen should not be analyzed after 24 hr.

Possible Interfering Factors

Factors which may increase serum LDH are the following:

- hemolysis of red blood cells
- standing of specimen over 1 hr
- anabolic steroids
- anesthetic agents
- aspirin
- ethanol
- fluorides
- codeine, demerol, morphine
- hemodialysis
- muscle exercise
- pregnancy
- starvation
- acute alcohol intoxication

Factors that may decrease serum LDH are the following:

- storage after 24 hr
- ascorbic acid

Patient Care

1. Note that laboratory levels > 2000 u indicate a poor prognosis.
2. Observe the LDH_1/LDH_2 ratio. Flipped LDH_1/LDH_2, or the ratio of LDH_1 to LDH_2 which is greater than one, may occur in myocardial infarction between 12 to 24 hr and remains elevated for 48 hr after infarction.

Patient Education

1. Instruct the patient to avoid any activities that may increase workload of heart until diagnosis is made.
2. Instruct the patient to eat a normal diet and avoid alcohol and strenuous activity prior to having blood sample drawn.
3. Instruct the patient to avoid aspirin prior to having blood sample drawn.

Signed Consent

Not required

SERUM GLUTAMIC-OXALOACETIC TRANSAMINASE (SGOT)

Serum glutamic-oxaloacetic transaminase is an enzyme found in red blood cells, heart, liver, skeletal muscle, kidney, brain, pancreas, and lung tissue. An elevated enzyme level is a manifestation of tissue necrosis.

Increased levels of SGOT occur in the following:

- degenerative diseases of the central nervous system
- convulsive disorders
- following head injury
- cerebral infarction
- liver disease/injury
- musculoskeletal diseases
- trauma
- intramuscular injections
- cardioversion

Falsely decreased levels of enzymes occur during the following:

- ketoacidosis
- beriberi
- uremia
- hemodialysis

A rise in SGOT 6 to 8 hr after chest pain may indicate extension of the infarction.

Laboratory Results

Normal Range

12 to 40 u

Diagnostic Level

200 u

Range With a Myocardial Infarction

Initial elevation	4 to 6 hr
Peaks	24 to 48 hr
Return to normal	3 to 6 dy

Nursing Implications

Procedure for Collection/Storage of Specimen

1. Collect fresh whole blood by venipuncture.
2. Do not refrigerate or store specimen.
3. Storage of blood may falsely increase or decrease laboratory results.

Possible Interfering Factors

Drug therapy

- narcotics
- anticoagulants
- oxacillin sodium (Prostaphlin)
- ampicillin (Polycillin)
- opiates
- erythromycin
- secobarbital sodium (Seconal)
- diuretics
- digoxin
- lidocaine
- morphine
- diazepam (Valium)

Patient Care

1. Observe the patient for signs of extension of the infarction. Take additional rhythm strips. A rise in SGOT 6 to 8 hr after chest pain may indicate extension of the infarction.
2. Observe for an elevation in SGOT with liver damage as a result of congestive heart failure or shock.
3. Observe the level of serum enzymes. Enzyme levels higher than 5 times normal or elevated over a prolonged period of time may suggest a poorer prognosis for the patient with myocardial infarction.

Patient Education

1. Avoid any activities that increase workload on the heart until diagnosis is made.
2. Instruct the patient to avoid the use of salicylates if the patient has liver damage.

Signed Consent

Not required

OTHER BLOOD SERUM TESTS
ANTISTREPTOLYSIN O TITER (ASO)

Antistreptolysin O titer (ASO) is a blood serum test that indicates a recent hemolytic streptococcus infection and validates clinical findings of rheumatic fever.

Laboratory Results

Normal titer	250 u
Increased titer	2 to 4 dy after infection
Peak rise	4 to 6 wk after infection
Diagnostic level of titer	400 to 500 u

Nursing Implications

Procedure for Collection/Storage of Specimen

Fresh whole blood is collected by venipuncture.

Possible Interfering Factors

None reported

Patient Care

Observe the patient for signs and symptoms of rheumatic fever. Assess the heart for any abnormal sounds, such as murmurs.

Patient Education

Relate patient education to the diagnosis made.

Signed Consent

Not required

BLOOD CULTURES

Blood for cultures may be obtained from the patient and sent to the lab for culture. Aerobic and anaerobic growth may be observed for the presence of *Streptococcus viridans, enterococcus, staphylococcus,* or other gram-negative or gram-positive bacteria.

Laboratory Results

Normal Results

No bacteria present in culture

Positive Results

Presence of bacteria in culture

Nursing Implications

Procedure for Collection/Storage of Specimen (See hematology chapter)

1. Temperature of the culture must remain at a constant 101°F or higher.
2. Blood cultures must be sent immediately to the laboratory after collection. (For further details related to this test, see p. 45)

Possible Interfering Factors

None reported

Patient Care

1. Be aware that a negative culture may occur if patient has been placed on an antibiotic therapy.
2. Transient bacteremia may occur following dental procedures or tonsillectomies, giving a false indication of bacterial endocarditis.
3. Blood cultures will be negative when *Rickettsia burnetii* are the organisms causing bacterial endocarditis.
4. Blood cultures must be taken over a period of several days.
5. The period of observation for bacterial growth may be several days to three weeks.

6. Two or more positive cultures for the organism are considered diagnostic.

Patient Education

Instruct the patient to notify the nurse if symptoms of infection, such as chills, fever, or pain occur.

Signed Consent

Not required

DIGITALIS BLOOD LEVEL

Digitalis is given when there is a need to strengthen the force of myocardial contraction, to decrease the heart rate, or to allow greater relaxation of the ventricles for better filling. Pump failure, or congestive heart failure, is the most common indication for the use of digitalis.

Digitalis blood level measures the amount of digitalis currently in the bloodstream. Digitalis has a cumulative effect and is eliminated slowly from the body. Measurement of blood levels may be used to evaluate drug therapy of drug toxicity.

Laboratory Results

Drug	Therapeutic level	Potentially toxic level
Digitoxin	14–30 ng/ml	Over 30 ng/ml
Digoxin	1–2 ng/ml	Over 3 ng/ml

Nursing Implications
Procedure for Collection/Storage of Specimen
1. Whole blood is collected.
2. Wait 6 hr after the drug is administered, or draw blood before the drug is given.

Patient Care
1. Notify physician of toxic or less than therapeutic blood levels.
2. Observe for signs and symptoms of digitalis toxicity. These include loss of appetite, nausea, vomiting, diarrhea, bradycardia, arrhythmias, blurred vision, flickering lights, yellow borders around dark objects, mental confusion, headache, or fatigue.
3. If a potentially toxic blood level is noted, withhold any further dosages of digitalis and notify the physician. In the presence of decreased urinary output, blood samples should be tested more frequently.

Patient Education

Assess the patient's knowledge about digitalis treatment, such as beneficial effects and possible toxic effects, and give individualized instruction about drug regimen.

Signed Consent

Not required

ERYTHROCYTE SEDIMENTATION RATE (ESR, SED Rate)

The erythrocyte sedimentation rate is the speed at which red blood cells settle in uncoagulated blood. It is a nonspecific indicator of the presence of inflammation somewhere in the body. It is used to determine the progress of previously diagnosed diseases, or to assist in diagnosing a disorder in which symptoms may be vague, or to confirm a diagnosis. ESR is elevated in numerous diseases where inflammation or tissue injury occurs. Extremely high ESR levels are found with malignancy, collagen diseases (rheumatoid arthritis, systemic lupus erythematosus), and renal disease. In cardiovascular diseases, ESR is increased in myocardial infarctions (but not in angina pectoris), in active rheumatic fever, and post-commissurotomy syndrome. The ESR will be decreased with sickle cell anemia, polycythemia, hypoproteinemia, and congestive heart failure owing to decreased serum fibrinogen.

Laboratory Results

Normal ranges vary widely according to the method used. Consult your laboratory for normal ranges.

Nursing Implications

Procedure for Collection/Storage of Specimen

Laboratory test is performed on fresh blood serum.

Possible Interfering Factors

None reported

Patient Care

1. In situations where the patient is demonstrating vague symptomology, observe for signs and symptoms of inflammatory processes, such as fever or pain.
2. In myocardial infarction, the ESR usually is increased within 2 or 3 dy after infarction. Peak rate is 4 to 5 dy and duration 2 to 6 mo. The degree of ESR elevation does not correlate with severity or prognosis.

Patient Education

None

Signed Consent

Not required

BLOOD LIPIDS

The blood lipids circulate in blood plasma bound to proteins. These complexes of proteins and lipids are called lipoproteins. Lipoproteins include cholesterol, triglycerides, phospholipids, and fatty acids. Electrophoresis is the method used to separate the lipoproteins. This separation of lipoproteins and distinction between glycerides of dietary and endogenous origin has been very helpful in detecting hyperlipidemia of genetic origin.

The two lipoproteins of clinical significance in the management of atherosclerosis are cholesterol and triglycerides. Two types of hyperlipidemia are important in cardiac disease: type 2, in which the cholesterol is elevated and the triglycerides are normal or mildly elevated; and type 4, in which the cholesterol is normal and the triglycerides are elevated.

CHOLESTEROL

Cholesterol is a lipoprotein widely distributed in various tissues. Large amounts of cholesterol are found in many foods, such as egg yolks and various oils and fats, especially those of animal origin. Cholesterol can be synthesized by the liver and is a normal constituent of bile. It is important also in metabolism, serving as a precursor of various steroid hormones. The association of abnormally increased blood lipids and atherosclerosis is well established. Cholesterol is markedly increased in hypercholesterolemia of unknown origin. It is also usually increased in the following:

- biliary obstruction
- hypothyroidism
- pancreatic disease
- pregnancy
- nephrosis
- diabetes mellitus

  Cholesterol is usually decreased in the following:

- hyperthyroidism
- malnutrition, starvation, malabsorption syndrome
- chronic anemia
- cortisone therapy
- severe liver disease from chemicals, hepatitis, drugs

Laboratory Results
Normal Range

150 to 250 mg/dl. The normal cholesterol level varies among populations and age groups. Some authorities suggest that 200 mg/dl should be considered the upper desirable level.

Age-related acceptable cholesterol levels are the following:

0–19 yr	120–130
20–29 yr	120–240
30–39 yr	140–270
40–49 yr	150–310
50–59 yr	160–330

Nursing Implications
Procedure for Collection/Storage of Specimen

1. The patient must be fasting, preferably for 12 to 14 hr, before the blood specimen is drawn.
2. The patient should have been eating a normal diet for 2 wk before the test.

3. The patient should have several measurements of cholesterol before a definite diagnosis of hyperlipidemia is made, since there can be marked day-to-day fluctuations in the same patient.

Possible Interfering Factors

Drugs that may cause increased serum cholesterol are the following:

- phenytoin sodium (Dilantin)
- corticosteroids
- oral contraceptives
- androgens
- thiazides
- sulfonamides
- promazine and chlorpromazine
- bromides
- iodides
- vitamins A and C

Drugs that may cause decreased serum cholesterol are the following:

- allopurinol
- tetracyclines
- erythromycin
- isoniazid
- MAO inhibitors
- androgens*
- kanamycin
- neomycin
- estrogens
- cholrestyromine
- thiouracil
- nitrates and nitrites

Patient Care

Nursing care is usually related to the patient's need for instruction regarding diet, drugs, weight control, and exercise to decrease blood lipids.

Patient Education

1. The patient should be taught the importance of eating a normal diet for 2 wk prior to the test and fasting 12 to 14 hr before having the test done.
2. Teach the patient how to modify daily diets. Patients with high choles-

---

*May increase or decrease cholesterol levels

terol levels are likely to be placed on low cholesterol diets and require dietary instruction.

3. Teach the patient about other therapeutic measures to decrease cholesterol levels. Drug therapy to decrease cholesterol levels, along with exercise and weight control, are often indicated for patients with elevated cholesterol levels.

4. Inform the families with a history of hereditary hyperlipidemia or familial hypercholesterolemia to have their children tested at an early age.

Signed Consent

Not required

TRIGLYCERIDES

Triglycerides are a combination of glycerol and the three fatty acids. Most animal and vegetable fats are triglycerides. Many triglycerides are synthesized by the intestinal mucosa, which absorbs dietary fatty acids. Triglycerides, along with cholesterol, are important in the development of atherosclerosis. Triglycerides are increased in the following:

- familial hyperlipidemia
- liver diseases
- nephrotic syndrome
- hypothyroidism
- diabetes mellitus (higher values are seen with hyperglycemia and poorer control of diabetes; the levels are reduced by insulin therapy and better control)
- alcoholism
- gout
- pancreatitis
- acute myocardial infarction

    Triglycerides are decreased in the following:
- congenital α-beta-lipoproteinemia
- malnutrition

Laboratory Results

Concentrations of triglycerides above these levels are considered abnormal:

20–25 yr	120 mg/dl
26–29 yr	140 mg/dl
30–39 yr	150 mg/dl
40–49 yr	160 mg/dl
50+ yr	190 mg/dl

Nursing Implications
Procedure for Collection/Storage of Specimen

1. Valid triglyceride determinations require a 12- to 14-hr fast before the specimen is drawn.
2. Dietary fat intake promptly and directly affects the triglyceride level; therefore, a fasting baseline is necessary.
3. The patient should be relaxed and seated at least 10 min before the test is done.
4. The patient should, if possible, avoid thyroid medication, steroidal contraceptives, or lipid-lowering drugs for 3 wk and should not have gained or lost weight in the preceding month.
5. It is inappropriate to perform lipid studies while a patient is hospitalized for a heart attack, because myocardial infarction causes an increase in very low-density lipoproteins and a fall in low-density lipoproteins.

Patient Care
Nursing care is usually related to the patient's need for instruction regarding diet, drugs, weight control, and exercise to decrease blood lipids.

Patient Education

1. Before the test is done, the patient should have been instructed in the need to fast for 12 to 14 hr before the test and to avoid physical and psychological stress.
2. Drugs that increase or decrease blood triglycerides should not be taken prior to the test.

Signed Consent
Not required

DIAGNOSTIC TESTS
ANGIOGRAPHY (Arteriography)

Angiography or arteriography is an x-ray procedure used to visualize the vascular structure of various areas of the body. Vascular abnormalities such as calcified atherosclerotic plaques, strictures, occlusions, masses, or vascular deformities such as aneurysms can be demonstrated by angiography.

A radiopaque substance such as Hypaque or Renografin is injected into an artery. During the last few seconds of dye injection and immediately afterward, a rapid succession of serial radiographs are taken. In some cases a cutdown on the artery is done to inject the dye. A catheter may need to be threaded into the artery and guided to the area that is to be visualized. In addition to the coronary arteries (see Cardiac catheterization procedure), the most common angiograms are of the renal system, the peripheral vascular system of the legs, and the carotid and cerebral vessels.

Normal Results
Normal vascular structure

Nursing Implications

Preprocedure

1. Explain the procedure to the patient and family in simple terms. Include in your explanation that the procedure will be somewhat uncomfortable and that at the time of injection of the dye a very hot, flushing sensation will be felt for approximately 30 to 60 sec.
2. Ask the patient if he is allergic to iodine, as the radiopaque substance contains iodine. Notify the physician of any suspected allergy to iodine.
3. Obtain baseline vital signs and assess the peripheral vascular system for comparison postprocedure.
4. Explain to the patient that foods and fluids may be restricted for several hours prior to the test, depending on the type of angiography to be done.
5. Administer a sedative, analgesic, or tranquilizer as prescribed by the physician.

During Procedure

1. The patient is taken to a special procedure room or to the x-ray department.
2. After injection of the radiopaque substance, observe the patient carefully for any sign of allergic reaction, such as dyspnea, nausea, vomiting, tachycardia, and diaphoresis. Antihistamine drugs, oxygen, and epinephrine should be on hand.
3. Explain the activities being performed by the physician and by the radiologic technicians.

Postprocedure

1. Assess the injection site for bleeding. There will be a pressure dressing over the injection site, and an ice pack may be used.
2. Assess the involved limb. Check the pulse distal to the injection site, such as the pedal pulse when the femerol artery is injected, every hour for 4 to 8 hr after the procedure. Report any signs of vascular occlusion immediately.
3. Take vital signs every 30 min or every hour for several hours.
4. Explain any special orders left by the physician. When the femerol artery is injected the affected limb must be kept straight for a number of hours. Bedrest may be ordered for 12 to 24 hr, depending on the type of angiography.
5. Institute safety measures until the preprocedure sedation has worn off.
6. Assess the patient for a possible late hypersensitivity reaction to the radiopaque substance.
7. Encourage the patient to drink fluids in order to hasten the excretion of the dye from the kidneys.

Signed Consent

Required

CARDIAC CATHETERIZATION

Cardiac catheterization is a procedure in which catheters are introduced into the chambers of the heart. During the procedure blood samples are taken, cardiac output is assessed, pressures within the great vessels and chambers are measured to assess valvular competency and myocardial function. Special catheters may be used to record intracardiac electrocardiograms and phonocardiograms. Cardiac catheterization may be indicated for preoperative evaluation of valvular dysfunction, congenital heart disease, myocardial infarctions, chest pain, and pulmonary hypertension or ischemic heart disease. Cardiac catheterization may also be done postoperatively to assess the effectiveness of cardiac surgery.

Normal Results

- Normal anatomic structure and function of heart and coronary arteries
- Normal pressures within heart chambers and normal cardiac output
- Normal percentage of oxygen saturation and content of blood

Nursing Implications

Preprocedure
1. Explain the basic cardiac anatomy and the procedure.
2. Place the patient on no food after midnight (may have fluids).
3. Shave both inguinal areas.
4. Have the patient empty bladder prior to procedure.
5. Give a preoperative sedative if prescribed by the physician.
6. Answer any questions the patient or family might ask.

During Procedure
1. Inform the patient that he will have an intravenous line and will lie flat on a hard table.
2. Prep the catheter insertion site with a surgical scrub using a local anesthetic only. The catheterization is a sterile procedure.
3. X-ray films will be taken during procedure. The patient may watch the film on an overhead screen.
4. Explain to the patient that he may be asked to cough and take deep breaths during the procedure.
5. Explain to the patient that he may feel "hot" as the dye is injected.
6. The procedure takes 1 to 4 hr.

Postprocedure
1. Check blood pressure and pulse every 15 min. Notify the physician if there is a 10 mg Hg decrease or rise in blood pressure.
2. Check the peripheral pulses distal to insertion site. Observe for numbness, tingling, and color of the extremity.
3. Check the dressing for bleeding. If bleeding occurs, apply pressure and notify the physician.
4. Assess the level of consciousness of the patient.

5. Maintain the patient on bedrest for 24 hr. The patient may turn from side to side. The leg on the same side as the catheterization should be kept straight or extended. Encourage the patient to wiggle toes and dorsiflex feet every hour.

Signed Consent
Required

EXERCISE TESTING (Stress Test)
Exercise testing is a procedure in which the patient's cardiovascular response to progressive stressful exercise is measured; it measures a person's capacity to exercise. During exercise the cardiac output increases to meet the increasing demands of the body's tissues for oxygen. The ability of the heart to increase the cardiac output to meet increased oxygen demands determines a person's maximal exercise capacity. Factors that may influence this exercise capacity include age, sex, physical conditioning, and integrity of the cardiovascular system.

Exercise testing may be done as part of the annual physical examination to determine impairment of heart function owing to cardiac disease and to determine a patient's response to medical or surgical treatment of cardiac dysfunction.

Three common types of exercise tests are the step test, the bicycle ergometer, and the treadmill (Table 2-3).

Normal Results
Performance values are 10% above or below a normal comparable person's exercise results. There should be no significant ECG abnormalities, arrhythmias, or symptoms.

Nursing Implications
Preprocedure

1. Explain the procedure to the patient. Explain to the patient that he will be tested in stages as he walks at progressive speeds and elevations in an effort to increase the heart rate.
2. Answer any questions the patient or family may have.
3. Encourage the patient to get adequate rest before the test.
4. Encourage the patient to eat a light meal at least 2 hr before the test.
5. Instruct the patient to avoid consumption of alcohol, coffee, or tea before the test.
6. Inform the patient to wear loose-fitting clothes which are not nylon. (nylon interferes with ECG monitoring). A woman should wear a blouse which buttons in front, and a bra.
7. Instruct the patient to wear comfortable, rubber-soled, well-fitting shoes (no slippers or clogs).
8. Withhold medications prior to the test as prescribed by the physician.
9. Assess the patient for chest pain or anginal attacks. Notify the physician prior to the test if the patient is experiencing chest pain.

TABLE 2-3. **Advantages and Disadvantages of the Step Test, the Bicycle Ergometer, and the Treadmill**

Test	Advantages	Disadvantages
Step test	Simple to use Least expensive to purchase	Excessive body movement alters ECG tracings The patient needs to keep a steady pace during the test Maximum exercise capacity hard to achieve Test may be long in duration
Bicycle ergometer	Moderately expensive to purchase Easy to obtain physiologic readings	Equipment needs to be calibrated frequently Patient must pedal at a constant speed Leg muscles may fatigue easily Patient must be encouraged to keep pedaling
Treadmill	Easy for patient to keep the same speed Readings are easier to obtain Results are more easily reproduced	Most expensive to purchase Patient may lose balance Patient can develop increased endurance with repeated testing More effort is required of the overweight patient

During Procedure

1. Tell the patient that a blood pressure reading and an ECG will be done before the test is begun. During an exercise test, blood pressure readings, and the ECG are monitored to evaluate a person's response to the exercise.
2. Assist the patient if necessary to assume the correct position to begin the test.
3. Place the recording electrodes on the patient's chest.
4. The workload of the heart will increase gradually during the test. Instruct the patient to indicate to the staff when any of the following occur:
   - chest pain
   - pain in the legs
   - shortness of breath
5. Inform the patient that the test will end if the following occurs:
   - the patient develops any symptoms

- when the patient has performed the required exercise with no adverse effects
- any severe changes in the blood pressure or ECG occur

6. Have emergency equipment available.

Postprocedure

1. Have the patient rest lying down for approximately 5 min. Advise the patient to avoid taking a warm or hot shower for at least 2 hr, since vasodilation and orthostatic venous pooling may occur.
2. Monitor the patient's vital signs for at least 30 min postprocedure.

Signed Consent

Required

BIBLIOGRAPHY

Arbert S, Fielder S, Landau T, Rubin I: Recognizing digitalis toxicity. Am J Nurs 77, No. 12:1935–1937, 1943–1945, 1977

Aspinau MJ: A simplified guide to managing patients with hyponatremia. Nursing 78, No. 8, 12:32–35, 1978

Chamberlain SL: Low-dose heparin therapy. Am J Nurs 80, No. 6:1115–1117, 1980

Cohen S: New concepts in understanding congestive heart failure. Am J Nurs 81, No. 1:Pt1:119–142, 1981; No. 2:Pt 2:357–380, 1981

Dracup KA: Unraveling the mysteries of cardiomyopathy. Nursing 79, No. 9, 5:84–87, 1979

Felver L: Understanding the electrolyte maze. Am J Nurs 80, No. 9:1591–1595, 1980

Finesilver C: Reducing stress for cardiac catheterization patients. Am J Nurs 80, No. 8:1805–1807, 1980

Fischbach F: A Manual of Laboratory Tests. Philadelphia, JB Lippincott, 1980

Guyton AC: Textbook of Medical Physiology, 5th ed. Philadelphia, WB Saunders, 1976

Houser D: What to do first when a patient complains of chest pain. Nursing 76, No. 11:54–56, 1976

Kee J: Clinical implications of laboratory studies in critical care. Crit Care Quart No. 2, 3:1–17, 1979

Kumpuris AG, Raizner AE, Luchi RJ: The role of serum digitalis levels in clinical practice. Heart and Lung No. 8, 4:711–715, 1979

Lanuza DM, Jennrich JA: The amount of blood withdrawn for diagnostic tests in critically-ill patients. Heart and Lung No. 5, 6:933–938, 1976

Mancini RE, Cavanaugh AL: Drug interactions and digitalis toxicity. Am J Nurs 80, No. 12:2169–2170, 1980

Moore K: How patient education can reduce the hazards of anticoagulation. Nursing 77, No. 9:24–29, 1977

Phipps W, Long B, Woods NB: Medical-Surgical Nursing: Concepts and Clinical Practice. St Louis, CV Mosby, 1970

Sivarajan E S, Halpenny CJ: Exercise testing. Am J Nurs 79, No. 12:2162–2170, 1979

Sodeman W Jr, Sodeman W: Pathologic Physiology: Mechanisms of Disease. Philadelphia, WB Saunders, 1974

Spooner B, Gross BW, Hasko BA: Diverse implications of laboratory values in congestive heart failure. Crit Care Quart No. 2, 3:37–45, 1979

Tanner G: Heart failure in the MI patient. Am J Nurs 77, No. 2:230–234, 1977

Tiongson JG: Cardiac Isoenzymes: clinical implications and limitations. Crit Care Quart No. 2, 3:47–51, 1979

Zeluff GW, Suki WN, Jackson D: Hypercalcemia: Etiology, manifestations, and management. Heart and Lung No. 9, 1:146–151, 1980

3

Tests Related to Renal Function

Janice B. Martin

OVERVIEW OF PHYSIOLOGY AND PATHOPHYSIOLOGY

The major responsibility of the renal system is to maintain a stable, internal environment for the body. To maintain this stability, the kidneys produce urine which is transported, stored, and discharged by way of the ureters, bladder, and urethra. With renal dysfunction, the ability of the kidneys to perform regulatory functions is impaired. Inadequate regulation of metabolic waste excretion, acid–base balance, electrolyte levels, and extracellular fluid volumes occur with dysfunction of the renal system.

Factors that can produce renal dysfunction include the following:

- increased permeability of the glomeruli
- decreased glomerular filtration rate
- reduced numbers of nephrons
- impairment of the tubular transport mechanisms
- acute, generalized injury of the renal tubules
- obstruction of urine outflow

NEPHRON STRUCTURE

Nephrons are the structural and functional units of the kidneys. Individual nephrons are composed of a glomerulus and a renal tubule. Each glomerulus consists of a tuft of capillaries that filter water, electrolytes, and waste products from the blood. Surrounding the glomerulus is Bowman's capsule, which leads into the renal tubule. The tubule is composed of the proximal tubule, loop of Henle, distal tubule, and collecting duct. These structures function to reabsorb many of the filtered substances.

Nephrons regulate the composition and volume of the extracellular fluid through the processes of filtration, tubular reabsorption, and tubular secretion.

RENAL FILTRATION

Urine formation begins in the glomeruli, which filters fluid from the blood. Approximately one fourth of the cardiac output, or 1200 ml of blood, flows through the renal arteries to the kidneys each minute. About 120 ml of fluid is filtered each minute from the total renal blood flow. This fluid is called the glomerular filtrate and consists predominantly of water, hydrogen ions, bicarbonate ions, waste products from metabolic activity, and electrolytes.

- *Urea, creatinine,* and *uric acid* are the end products of protein metabolism filtered by the glomeruli.
- *Electrolytes* passing into the filtrate include sodium, chloride, potassium, calcium, phosphorus, and magnesium.
- The glomerular filtrate may contain *glucose* if the serum level of glucose exceeds a certain level, the renal threshold.
- Since *proteins* and *blood cells* are too large to filter through the glomeruli, these substances do not appear in the filtrate.

GLOMERULAR FILTRATION RATE (GFR)

The amount of glomerular filtrate formed during a given time period is the glomerular filtration rate. The renal clearance is the volume of plasma from which the amount of a substance is cleared from the blood by the kidneys per unit of time. Glomerular filtration is basically a passive process and is influenced by the concentration of plasma proteins and the blood pressure.

The plasma protein concentration directly affects the colloid osmotic pressure (COP). COP is the pressure exerted by the protein concentration of the blood.

- Plasma protein concentration, or COP, has an inverse relationship with the GFR.
- A rise in the plasma protein concentration decreases the amount of filtrate. A low plasma protein concentration increases the amount of filtrate.

Blood Pressure Mechanisms and GFR

Extracellular fluid volume has a direct relationship with the GFR.

- Increases in extracellular fluid volume, which cause a rise in blood pressure, increases the rate of filtration.
- Decreases in extracellular fluid volume, which cause a decrease in blood pressure, decreases the filtration rate.

The enzyme *renin* influences the relationship between the GFR and blood pressure. When the GFR is lowered, the distal tubules respond by increasing the blood pressure by secreting renin. *Renin* stimulates the formation of angiotensin and the secretion of aldosterone. *Angiotensin* is a powerful vasoconstrictor, which increases the blood pressure by decreasing the renal blood flow further reducing the GFR. *Aldosterone,* a hormone produced by the adrenal cortex, stimulates the renal tubules to return filtered *sodium* to the extracellular fluid. Along with the sodium, water is returned to the extracellular fluid.

- Thus, the renin-angiotensin-aldosterone system is a mechanism for the kidneys to maintain the extracellular fluid volume.

Age and GFR

Age influences the GFR. At birth, the infant's kidneys are functionally immature. Renal blood flow and the GFR are low. The GFR and renal blood flow gradually decline after age 45. By age 85, the GFR and renal blood flow values are about two-thirds of their values at age 45.

GLOMERULAR FILTRATION IMPAIRMENT

The major causes of renal dysfunction resulting from glomerular filtration impairment are:
- increased permeability of the glomeruli
- decreased glomerular filtration rate
- reduced numbers of nephrons

Increased Glomerular Permeability

Increased permeability of the glomeruli allows small plasma proteins and some blood cells to pass into the filtrate. The predominant plasma protein entering the filtrate is *albumin,* since it is the smallest in size of the major plasma proteins. Loss of albumin results in a reduced plasma protein concentration and decreased colloid osmotic pressure. A decrease in colloid osmotic pressure of the blood allows leakage of fluid from the blood into the interstitial tissues. As a consequence, the blood pressure is lowered and the renin-angiotensin-aldosterone system is stimulated. However, this compensative mechanism cannot effectively restore the blood volume, since the retained water also accumulates in the interstitial tissues because of the decreased plasma protein concentration.

A decreased cardiac output and lowered blood volumes result in a decreased blood supply to the kidneys and a decreased GFR. With decreased blood perfusion, the renin-angiotensin-aldosterone system begins to conserve *sodium* and *water,* thus limiting the body's ability to excrete sodium and water. This retention of water can cause congestive heart failure from the fluid overload. *Oliguria* (urine production of less than 30 ml per hour) results from the decreased glomerular filtration and the kidney's conservation of sodium and water.

Reduced Glomerular Filtration

As glomerular filtration is reduced, the filtering of *urea, creatinine,* and *uric acid* is decreased. Prolonged reduction of the GFR results in *azotemia.* Azotemia is defined as high blood levels of the waste products of protein metabolism. Excretion of *potassium* and *hydrogen ions* is dependent upon the presence of sodium in the glomerular filtrate. Since a reduced GFR results in a limited amount of sodium in the filtrate, potassium and hydrogen ions are retained.

- Thus, a decreased blood supply to the kidneys can cause *hyperkalemia* and *metabolic acidosis.*

TUBULAR REABSORPTION

During filtration many essential substances pass indiscriminately from the glomeruli into the renal tubules. The process of tubular reabsorption returns these substances to the extracellular fluid. Tubular reabsorption may be either passive or active. Passive reabsorption requires no energy use. Active reabsorption requires the use of energy.

PASSIVE REABSORPTION

Tubular reabsorption of *water* and *urea* is accomplished by passive reabsorption. Ninety-nine percent of the water in the glomerular filtrate is normally reabsorbed.

Water reabsorption is influenced by the antidiuretic hormone (ADH). *ADH* is produced in response to baroreceptor cell stimulation of the anterior hypothalamus.

- The presence of ADH results in greater permeability of the distal tubules and collecting ducts to water; thus reabsorption increases.
- Absence of ADH causes increased loss of water in the urine.

Urea is absorbed in minimal amounts, since urea molecules are too large to pass easily through the renal tubules.

Creatinine in the glomerular filtrate is not reabsorbed by the renal tubules; thus the amount of creatinine filtered is equal to the amount of creatinine in the urine.

ACTIVE REABSORPTION

The transport mechanisms for active reabsorption have established maximum amounts of substances that can be reabsorbed each minute. Active reabsorption provides for the return of *glucose, potassium, proteins, sodium, chloride, calcium, magnesium, bicarbonate, phosphates,* and *uric acid* to the extracellular fluid. If the filtrate levels of these substances exceed the maximum amounts for the transport mechanisms, the excess is excreted in the urine.

In addition to ADH, *aldosterone* and *parathyroid hormone* influence tubular reabsorption. Aldosterone causes an increased reabsorption of *sodium* and *water.* The parathyroid hormone, which is produced by the parathyroid gland, influences the transport of *calcium* and *phosphorus.* Parathyroid hormone production is stimulated by a lowered extracellular calcium concentration. This hormone functions to increase extracellular calcium by enhancing calcium reabsorption and reducing phosphorus reabsorption in the renal tubules.

TUBULAR SECRETION

The final process used by the kidneys in urine production is secretion. Tubular secretion transports substances from the extracellular fluid into the renal tubules. Secretion differs from filtration in that substances are transported directly into the tubules and are not filtered through the glomeruli. Filtration removes substances that need to be conserved or eliminated from the blood. Secretion removes only substances that are to be eliminated from the blood.

POTASSIUM, HYDROGEN, AND AMMONIA SECRETION

Potassium, hydrogen, and ammonia are substances secreted by the renal tubules.

Potassium secretion is controlled by the extracellular potassium concentration and by the hormone aldosterone. An increased extracellular potassium concentration enhances potassium secretion into the renal tubules and increases potassium excretion. A lowered extracellular potassium concentration decreases aldosterone production and inhibits tubular potassium secretion. When aldosterone increases sodium reabsorption, tubular secretion of potassium is simultaneously enhanced.

Hydrogen ions and *ammonia secretion* is dependent upon the extracellular *p*H.

- In acidosis the extracellular *p*H is lowered and the secretion of hydrogen ions and ammonia is increased.

- In alkalosis the extracellular pH is increased and tubular secretion of hydrogen ions and ammonia is decreased. Urine composition is adjusted to maintain a stable, internal environment.

TUBULAR DYSFUNCTION

Major causes of renal tubular dysfunction include reduced numbers of nephrons, impairment of the tubular transport mechanisms, and acute generalized injury of the renal tubules.

NEPHRON DESTRUCTION

The major disease processes affecting the kidneys totally destroy some nephrons but leave other nephrons intact. The intact nephrons enlarge and carry increased amounts of electrolytes and waste products.

Water and Sodium Excretion

When nephron destruction is not extensive, the intact nephrons excrete large amounts of water to dilute their increased loads of electrolytes and waste products. The body's water and sodium stores can easily be depleted unless water intake is increased.

With severe reduction in the number of nephrons, the opposite problem occurs with sodium and water. When this occurs, the amount of filtrate formed is decreased and water and sodium excretion is limited. Urine production may be less than 30 ml per hour (oliguria) or production of urine may cease (anuria).

Serum Creatinine and Urea

When nephron destruction is extensive, the remaining intact nephrons cannot compensate. The intact nephrons are unable to clear the same amounts of substances from the blood as did all the nephrons. The waste products from *protein* metabolism accumulate in the blood, and serum levels of *creatinine* and *urea* rise.

Potassium and Hydrogen Ion Secretion

With extensive nephron destruction, the renal tubules also become ineffective in the secretion of potassium and hydrogen ions. *High serum levels of potassium occur. Metabolic acidosis* results as hydrogen ion excretion is reduced. As a consequence, plasma stores of bicarbonate combine with the retained hydrogen ions to form carbonic acid. This results in a decrease in plasma bicarbonate levels. The respiratory system attempts to restore the acid–base balance by eliminating the carbon dioxide formed during the disassociation of the carbonic acid.

IMPAIRED TUBULAR TRANSPORT

Impairment of the tubular transport mechanisms can result from inherited tubular disorders or from acquired renal diseases. This type of renal dysfunction affects the kidneys' ability to regulate substances that are reabsorbed or secreted. Water, bicarbonate, hydrogen, glucose, sodium, and amino acids are among these substances.

Water Reabsorption

Diabetes insipidus is a disease characterized by an inability of the kidney to reabsorb water. In this disorder, the distal tubules and collecting ducts are not responsive to ADH. The kidneys are unable to concentrate urine. Polyuria can cause severe dehydration.

Bicarbonate and Hydrogen

Metabolic acidosis occurs with dysfunction of bicarbonate or hydrogen transport mechanisms. A defect in the proximal tubular transport mechanism for bicarbonate reabsorption causes increased urinary loss of this ion. A defect in the distal tubular transport mechanism for hydrogen impairs the ability of the kidney to secrete hydrogen. With this distal tubular defect, the kidneys are able to reabsorb bicarbonate. The metabolic acidosis is not as severe as with the proximal tubular defect.

Glucose

Damage of the proximal tubular transport mechanism for glucose reabsorption results in excretion of excessive amounts of glucose. This inherited disorder is associated with a lowered renal threshold for glucose and not abnormal blood glucose levels.

Sodium

Loss of sodium in the urine is increased with dysfunction of the sodium reabsorption mechanism of the distal tubules. This disorder is predominantly associated with chronic pyelonephritis. With this dysfunction, the kidneys are unable to conserve sodium and serum sodium levels are lowered.

Amino Acids (Cystine)

Dysfunction of the tubular transport mechanisms for amino acid reabsorption leads to excretion of amino acids. The most frequent amino acid excreted is *cystine*. Damage from cystine excretion results from the tendency of cystine to form stones, which obstruct the urinary tract.

TUBULAR DAMAGE

Inadequate blood supply, kidney infections, poisons, transfusion reactions, and crush injuries are among the causes of acute, generalized damage of renal tubules.

- This type of tubular damage leads to *acute renal failure* with an abrupt decrease in the GFR and extensive impairment of tubular reabsorption and secretion.

URINE EXCRETION

After urine formation, the ureters, bladder, and urethra transport urine out of the body. Peristalsis in the ureters and a valve between the ureters and bladder ensures a unidirectional flow of urine to the bladder. The bladder increases in size to allow storage of urine. The immature nervous system of infants responds to a rise in bladder pressure. Voiding is spontaneous. When the nervous system matures the infant gains voluntary control of bladder emptying. Nerve signals indicate the need to void when bladder volume and pressure are increased.

Urine exits the body through the urethra. As a protection against infection, the urethra produces a bacteriostatic substance that limits the entrance of bacteria to the urinary system.

URINARY TRACT OBSTRUCTION

Renal dysfunction can result from an obstruction in the urinary tract. Increased pressure occurs in the urinary tract from the nephrons to the obstruction site. The accompanying stasis of urine predisposes the individual to the development of stones and infection. As a consequence of increased pressure in the nephrons, renal structures dilate and renal blood flow is decreased. The decreased renal blood and infection can result in progressive nephron destruction.

BLOOD TESTS
ALDOSTERONE

Aldosterone, a hormone produced by the adrenal cortex, causes conservation of sodium and excretion of potassium by the kidneys. With a decreased glomerular filtration rate (GFR), aldosterone production is increased. An increased GFR reduces production of aldosterone. Elevated aldosterone levels result from increased renin production, which occurs with decreased renal blood flow.

Laboratory Results
Normal Range

Adult   5 to 15 mg/100 ml

Nursing Implications
Procedure for Collection/Storage of Specimen

1. The patient must be supine for at least 2 hr prior to collection of the specimen.
2. Prior to collection of the specimen, intake of sodium and potassium must be within normal ranges.

Possible Interfering Factors

Increase test results

- low sodium diet
- dehydration
- exercise
- upright posture
- diuretics

Decrease test results

- increased sodium intake
- increased potassium intake

Influence test results

- pregnancy
- oral contraceptives

Patient Care

1. Maintain normal intake of sodium and potassium prior to collection of the specimen.
2. Keep the patient on bedrest for 2 hr prior to collection.
3. Assess blood pressure for elevations as increased aldosterone levels result in sodium and water retention.

Patient Education

1. Inform the patient about dietary and activity controls for the test.
2. If the patient has hypertension related to elevated aldosterone levels, provide instruction about salt-restricted diet and antihypertensive drugs.

Signed Consent

Not required

ELECTROLYTES

The kidneys are the primary regulators of electrolytes in the serum. The major electrolytes include calcium, chloride, magnesium, phosphate, potassium, and sodium.

CALCIUM (Ca)

Within the blood, calcium predominantly exists in a protein-bound form and in an ionized form. Ionized forms possess electrical charges. Ionized calcium performs a major role in the regulation of cell membrane permeability, blood clotting, heart contraction, muscular activity, and nerve impulse transmission.

The parathyroid hormone influences the concentration of serum calcium. Lowered serum calcium levels stimulate secretion of the parathyroid hormone. This hormone acts to increase serum calcium levels by releasing bone calcium into the extracellular fluid. Decreased serum calcium levels cause an increased tubular reabsorption of calcium and a decreased tubular reabsorption of phosphorus. Calcitonin, a hormone produced by the thyroid gland, causes an increase in the renal excretion of calcium.

Although decreased calcium levels frequently are associated with renal dysfunction, increased calcium levels may occur also in renal disease. Hypercalcemia, or an increased serum calcium, results when chronic renal failure and associated secondary hyperparathyroidism cause parathyroid adenomas. Other causes of hypercalcemia include bone-damaging diseases and primary hyperparathyroidism.

Hypocalcemia, a low serum calcium level, is associated with decreased renal clearance of phosphorus and the inability of the kidney to activate vitamin D. Hypocalcemia also occurs with vitamin D deficiency and decreased secretion of the parathyroid hormone.

Laboratory Results
Normal Ranges

Total serum calcium

Adult	9.0 to 11.0 mg/100 ml
Child	9.0 to 12.0 mg/100 ml
Neonate	7.4 to 12.0 mg/100 ml

Ionized serum calcium

Adult	4.5 to 5.5 mg/100 ml
Child	4.5 to 5.4 mg/100 ml

Nursing Implications
Procedure for Collection/Storage of Specimen

1. Fresh whole blood is collected by venipuncture.
2. Prolonged venous stasis increases calcium levels. After the venipuncture needle is inserted, remove the tourniquet.
3. Have the patient fast overnight, since food intake affects serum calcium levels.

Possible Interfering Factors

- heparin
- insulin
- prolonged ambulatory activity
- magnesium salts

Patient Care

1. Have the patient maintain supine position for 30 min prior to obtaining the specimen.
2. Increase fluid intake when blood levels of calcium are increased. This assists in decreasing tubular reabsorption of calcium and preventing formation of calcium stones.
3. Inform physicians immediately of an acute onset of symptoms indicating hypocalcemia. The major symptom of hypocalcemia is tetany. Calcium gluconate should be available.

Patient Education

1. Instruct patients with a history of renal calcium stones to avoid milk and milk products. If such intake is not contraindicated, these patients should increase fluid intake.
2. Since milk has high levels of sodium and phosphorus, milk may need to be limited in the diets of patients with renal dysfunction. Assess the patient for calcium imbalance. Renal patients having low calcium levels may require calcium supplements and vitamin D. Instruct the patient to take calcium after meals for better utilization.
3. Administer aluminum hydroxide gel (a phosphate-binding medication for regulation of calcium and phosphorus levels in patients with renal diseases) as prescribed.

Signed Consent
Not required

CHLORIDE (CI)
Chloride is reabsorbed by the kidneys. Chloride ions influence maintenance of normal electrolyte balance, water distribution, and colloid osmotic pressure.

Metabolic acidosis, caused by dysfunction of the proximal tubular transport mechanism for bicarbonate, can produce a high concentration of chloride (hyperchloremia). In this disorder, bicarbonate ions are excreted and chloride ions are returned to the extracellular fluid. Factors that reduce renal blood flow can also cause hyperchloremia by decreasing the amounts of chloride excreted.

A decreased chloride level (hypochloremia) is associated with metabolic acidosis in which bicarbonate is reabsorbed by the kidneys and chloride is excreted. Other causes of hypochloremia include prolonged vomiting and uncontrolled diabetes.

Laboratory Results
Normal Range

Adult	98–106 mEq/L
Child	98–105 mEq/L

Nursing Implications
Procedure for Collection/Storage of Specimen

Venous blood is collected for specimen.

Possible Interfering Factors

Increase test results

• medications containing bromides

Patient Care
Monitor abnormal chloride levels in conjunction with serum indicators of acid–base balance.

Patient Education
None

Signed Consent
Not required

MAGNESIUM (Mg)
Large portions of the body's magnesium stores are located in the bones and within cells. Magnesium has a vital role in activating many enzymes and in regulating muscular activity. Renal excretion of magnesium may be enhanced by the hormone aldosterone.

A high level of magnesium (hypermagnesemia) is most commonly associated with renal failure. Renal failure impairs the excretion of magnesium. Hypomagnesemia, a low serum magnesium, can result from increased renal excretion of magnesium and can occur in conjunction with diabetic keto-acidosis and hyperthyroidism. Other causes of hypomagnesemia include gastrointestinal malabsorption, alcoholism, and diuretic usage.

Laboratory Results
Normal Range

Adult	1.5 to 2.1 mEq/L
Child	1.7 to 2.2 mEq/L

Nursing Implications
Procedure for Collection/Storage of Specimen

Venous blood is collected for specimen.

Possible Interfering Factors

None reported

Patient Care

Do not give patients with renal dysfunction magnesium-containing laxatives (milk of magnesia) or antacids (magnesium hydroxide). However, dietary restriction of magnesium usually is not required in renal dysfunction.

Patient Education

Instruct the patient with renal failure to avoid magnesium-containing medicines. Over-the-counter laxatives and antacids commonly contain magnesium.

Signed Consent
Not required

PHOSPHORUS (P)

Phosphorus in the body exists in two forms: organic phosphate and inorganic phosphate. Laboratory tests measure inorganic phosphate, which is primarily located in the extracellular fluid. Additional phosphate stores are found within bones and cells. Phosphate is important in the formation of bones, metabolism of fat and carbohydrates, and maintenance of acid–base balance.

An increased serum phosphorus level occurs (hyperphosphatemia) in renal dysfunction because of the kidneys' inability to excrete phosphate. Another disorder leading to increased phosphate levels is hypoparathyroidism. Depression of phosphate levels (hypophosphatemia) is associated with hyperparathyroidism and vitamin D deficiency. In rare cases, hypophosphatemia results from dysfunction of the renal tubular transport mechanisms for phosphate reabsorption.

Laboratory Results

Normal Range

Adult	3.0 to 4.5 mg/dl or 1.8 to 2.6 mEq/L
Child	4.0 to 7.0 mg/dl or 2.4 to 4.1 mEq/L
Neonate	4.0 to 10.0 mg/dl or 2.4 to 5.9 mEq/L

Nursing Implications

Procedure for Collection/Storage of Specimen

1. Venous blood is collected.
2. Avoid hemolysis by using a vacuum container to obtain the specimen.
3. Do not refrigerate or store the specimen.
4. Specimen should be obtained after the patient has fasted overnight.

Possible Interfering Factors

Increase test results

- diphenylhydantoin
- heparin
- pituitrin
- vitamin D
- epinephrine
- insulin

Patient Care

1. Restrict dietary phosphorus in patients with renal dysfunction as prescribed.
2. In hyperphosphatemia, aluminum hydroxide is administered to increase phosphorus excretion in the feces.
3. If drug therapy includes aluminum hydroxide monitor the number and type of stools.

Patient Education

1. Teach the patient about dietary and drug regimens.
2. Do not substitute antacids containing magnesium for aluminum hydroxide.
3. Renal patients should not take milk of magnesia for constipation.

Signed Consent

Not required

POTASSIUM (K)

Potassium is the dominant intracellular electrolyte. Extracellular potassium levels are much smaller than intracellular levels. Potassium plays a major role in nerve stimulus conduction, smooth muscle activity, and skeletal muscle activity. Abnormally high or low levels of potassium result in dangerous cardiac arrhythmias and death.

Factors influencing the excretion of potassium by the kidneys are aldosterone secretion, potassium content of the plasma and cells, and the pH of body fluids. An increase in aldosterone results in an increased potassium excretion as the kidneys exchange potassium for sodium. The potassium levels in body fluids are directly associated with the amount of potassium filtered and secreted by the kidneys. An increase in the potassium level results in an increased excretion of potassium. A decrease in potassium level results in a decreased excretion of potassium. In acidosis, potassium ions are retained as the kidneys excrete excess hydrogen ions.

Hyperkalemia, or excess potassium levels, can result from decreased urinary excretion in renal failure or tubular transport dysfunction. Other causes of hyperkalemia include decreased aldosterone production in adrenal cortical dysfunction or increased release of intracellular potassium in acidosis, surgery, crushing injuries, and massive hemolysis.

Decreased concentration of potassium *(hypokalemia)* results from increased urinary losses occurring during the diuretic phase of acute renal failure, impairment of the hydrogen tubular transport mechanism, use of diuretics containing thiazides, and increased aldosterone levels. Other causes of hypokalemia include gastrointestinal loss with diarrhea, vomiting, or nasogastric suction, and decreased intake of potassium.

Laboratory Results

Normal Range

Adult	3.5 to 5.0 mEq/L
Child	3.5 to 5.0 mEq/L

Nursing Implications

Procedure for Collection/Storage of Specimen

1. Avoid hemolysis during collection by using vacuum containers.
2. Do not store or refrigerate specimen.

Possible Interfering Factors

Increase test results

- tobacco smoke
- potassium-sparing diuretics
- blood transfusion
- fever
- intravascular hemolysis

Decrease test results

- Potassium-excreting diuretics

Patient Care

1. Assess the patient for medications that affect potassium levels, such as diuretics containing thiazides, ACTH, cortisone, acetazolamide, and para-aminosalicylic acid.

2. Assess for symptoms of hyperkalemia and hypokalemia.
3. Immediately notify physician of abnormal potassium levels.
4. Restrict potassium intake in hyperkalemia.
5. Potassium penicillin should not be used if potassium intake is restricted.
6. Administration of calcium in the treatment for hyperkalemia counteracts the effects of potassium on the heart. Sodium bicarbonate and glucose–insulin infusions may be administered to shift extracellular potassium into the cells. Sodium polystyrene sulfonate (Kayexalate) may be administered to increase potassium loss by way of the gastrointestinal tract.
7. In administering intravenous potassium to treat hypokalemia, dilute the potassium in intravenous solution. Intravenous potassium should not be administered faster than 20 mEq per hour. Prior to the administration of K^+, renal output should be assessed.
8. Assess heart rate prior to administering digitalis, as abnormal potassium levels can cause digitalis toxicity.
9. Assess for symptoms of hyperkalemia if a patient is receiving potassium supplements.
10. Monitor serum potassium levels with patients receiving potassium supplements or diuretics.
11. Place a cardiac monitor on patients with either hypokalemia or hyperkalemia as prescribed.
12. Assess patients for hypokalemia who have frequent nasopharyngeal suctioning or who have nasogastric suction.
13. Observe for signs and symptoms of hypokalemia. Serum potassium may not be an indicator of intracellular potassium levels. After cellular injury or death, potassium is released into extracellular fluid.

Patient Education

1. Teach the patient about the signs and symptoms of abnormal potassium levels.
2. Inform the patient why frequent blood tests are required to monitor potassium levels.
3. Inform the patient of dietary sources of potassium: bananas, oranges, meats, apricots, potatoes, and salt substitutes.

Signed Consent

Not required

SODIUM (Na)

The dominant electrolyte in the extracellular fluid is sodium. Sodium has a major role in regulation of body fluid volumes, muscular activity, nerve impulse conduction, and acid–base balance. Renal excretion of sodium is regulated chiefly by the hormone aldosterone. The presence of aldosterone enhances the reabsorption of sodium through an exchange of sodium and potassium ions.

Elevated serum sodium levels *(hypernatremia)* are caused by inadequate water intake, excessive excretion of water, increased aldosterone levels, and intake of excessive amounts of sodium.

Hyponatremia or a lowered sodium level is more frequent than hypernatremia. Hyponatremia can result from dysfunction of the renal tubular transport mechanism for sodium reabsorption which occurs in chronic renal failure, renal tubular acidosis and nephritis. Hyponatremia may also occur in the oliguric phase of acute renal failure as water retention is greater than sodium retention. Other causes of hyponatremia include diarrhea, Addison's disease, and diabetic acidosis.

Laboratory Results
Normal Range

Adult	136 to 145 mEq/L
Child	136 to 145 mEq/L

Nursing Implications
Procedure for Collection/Storage of Specimen

Venous blood is collected for specimen.

Possible Interfering Factors

None reported

Patient Care
1. Observe for abnormal sodium levels. An abnormal sodium level may result from abnormal body fluid volumes or abnormal sodium levels.
2. Maintain accurate intake and output records.
3. Measure daily weights at the same time each day, using the same scale, with the patient wearing similar weight clothes.
4. Evaluate the blood pressure readings in terms of fluid retention or depletion.
5. Provide proper diet and fluid allowances.
6. Assess for hypernatremia or hyponatremia.

Patient Education
1. Renal patients are likely to require alterations in dietary sodium and fluid. Patients who are retaining salt and water need to be instructed on sodium- and fluid-restricted diets. Patients who are placed on restricted sodium must be taught to read labels on frozen, canned, or packaged food products to note presence of sodium contained in the product. Patients who are excreting increased amounts of sodium need to receive instruction about increased sodium requirements.
2. Teach the patient that salt substitutes should not be used if potassium is restricted.
3. Inform the patient that sodium may be contained in cough medications, laxatives, or antacids.
4. Instruct the patient to inform nursing staff of fluid intake and urine output, or instruct the patient how to record intake and output.
5. Teach symptoms of fluid and sodium retention or depletion.

6. Since patients with chronic renal failure will be monitoring their own sodium–fluid status after discharge from hospitalization, instruct the patient on taking blood pressures.

7. Certain seasonings and condiments such as catsup, Accent (monosodium glutamate), pickles, olives, salad dressings, soy sauce, mustard, Worchestershire sauce, and bouillon may contain high amounts of sodium. Instruct the patient on foods to avoid or limit in the diet.

8. Artificial sweeteners may contain significant amounts of sodium in the form of sodium saccharin. Low-calorie diet drinks or substances may need to be restricted. Inform the patient of these restrictions.

NITROGENOUS WASTE PRODUCTS

A major function of the kidneys is to clean the blood of the nitrogenous breakdown products from protein metabolism. Creatinine and urea are the main nitrogenous waste products excreted by the kidneys.

CREATININE

Creatinine is a waste product formed from the breakdown of skeletal muscle. Production of creatinine is directly related to the muscle mass and is relatively constant from day to day. Since creatinine levels are not affected by diet, stress, steroids, or exercise, measurement of the blood levels of creatinine is one of the best indicators of renal function. With the muscle mass being less in a female, the serum creatinine level of women is slightly less than the serum creatinine level of men. Elevation of the serum creatinine level indicates renal dysfunction.

Laboratory Results
Normal Range

Adult	0.6 to 1.3 mg/dl
Child	0.3 to 1.2 mg/dl

Nursing Implications
Procedure for Collection/Storage of Specimen
Venous blood is collected for specimen.

Possible Interfering Factors
Increase test results
- bromsulphalein test (BSP)
- phenolsulfonphthalein test (PSP)
- ascorbic acid
- barbiturates
- chlordiazepoxide
- methyldopa

Patient Care

1. In patients with suspected renal damage, monitor the creatinine levels. A rise in creatinine levels does not occur until kidney functioning has been reduced by about 50%.
2. Patients may be disoriented or comatose when serum creatinine levels are above 12 mg/dl. Take precautions to avoid injury to the patient.
3. Elevated levels of creatinine can cause increased red blood cell breakdown. Monitor the hematocrit, provide rest periods, and observe for bleeding.
4. After renal transplantation, frequently monitor the serum creatinine levels. A rising creatinine level is one of the first indicators of organ rejection.
5. Monitor the serum creatinine levels regularly in patients who are receiving potentially nephrotoxic drug therapy.

Patient Education

1. Inform the patient of the necessity for frequent blood tests in determining renal function.
2. Inform the patient that protein intake is usually altered when blood levels of protein waste products are elevated. Protein intake is usually restricted to 20 to 80 g per dy in patients with renal dysfunction. Protein foods should contain all essential amino acids. Eggs, milk, meat, fish, and poultry contain all essential amino acids, but contain significant amounts of sodium, potassium and calcium.
3. Inform the patient and family that confusion is often a manifestation of accumulated waste products remaining in the blood.

Signed Consent

Not required

UREA NITROGEN (BUN or Blood Urea Nitrogen)

Urea is the main end product of protein metabolism. Since the kidneys remove urea from the blood, measurement of the level of urea in the blood provides an indicator of renal function. Renal dysfunction is the most common cause of elevated BUN levels; however, measurement of blood creatinine levels is a more precise indicator of renal function, as several factors affect the BUN level. A high-protein diet, use of steroids, stressful situations, fever, and sepsis increase the BUN level. A low-protein diet decreases the BUN level.

Laboratory Results
Normal Range

Adult	8 to 20 mg/dl
Child	8 to 18 mg/dl

Nursing Implications

Procedure for Collection/Storage of Specimen

Venous blood is collected for the specimen.

Possible Interfering Factors

Increase test results

- antibiotics
- antihypertensives
- blood transfusions
- diuretics
- radiopaque contrast media
- salicylates
- steroids
- acetohexamide
- chloral hydrate
- doxapram
- methysergide
- streptokinase (streptodornase)
- protein intake
- stress
- sepsis
- fever

Patient Care

1. Patients with elevated BUN levels may be mentally confused and disoriented. Assess the level of consciousness of the patient. Note normal signs and any alterations.
2. Excess urea can be excreted in saliva and perspiration. Provide good oral and skin hygiene.
3. Monitor stool color and perform guaiac test for occult blood, as ulceration of the gastrointestinal tract is frequently found with elevated BUN levels.
4. Administer antacids as prescribed to prevent GI ulceration.
5. Institute seizure precautions when the BUN is elevated.
6. Elevated BUN levels cause an increased breakdown of red blood cells. Monitor the hematocrit, provide rest periods, and observe for bleeding.

Patient Education

1. Inform the patient of the necessity for frequent blood tests in determining renal function.
2. Teach the patient that protein intake is usually restricted when blood levels of protein waste products are elevated. Protein intake is usually restricted to 20 to 80 g per dy in patients with renal dysfunction. Protein foods should contain all essential amino acids. Eggs, milk, meat,

fish, and poultry contain all essential amino acids, but also contain significant amounts of sodium, potassium, and calcium.

3. Inform the patient and family that confusion is often a manifestion of accumulated waste products remaining in the blood.

Signed Consent

Not required

URINE TESTS
COLLECTING URINE SPECIMENS

Urine tests provide valuable information regarding fluid, electrolyte, acid–base, and waste-product regulation. However, the value of urine tests is reduced if the specimens are not collected properly, as improper collection can cause false laboratory results. Strict techniques must be followed during collection of random, clean-catch, double-voided, and timed specimens.

RANDOM SPECIMENS

Random specimens can be collected in a clean container at any convenient time. The clean-catch technique is preferable for collection. Females should wash the perineal area prior to specimen collection. Since the first morning urine is concentrated, it contains more formed elements and is more useful for the microscopic examination of urine. The first morning specimen is less valuable in testing for metabolic substances, as the urine is less likely to contain these substances.

CLEAN-CATCH OR MIDSTREAM SPECIMENS

A clean-catch specimen is collected for a bacteriologic culture. Prior to specimen collection, both males and females clean the external genitalia with a cleansing solution. A male cleans the glans penis in a circular motion. A female separates the labia for the entire collection procedure and cleans the meatus with front-to-back motions. A cleansing sponge is used for each cleansing motion. The glans penis or meatus is rinsed with sterile water after the cleansing process. After the first portion of the urinary stream is voided into the toilet, a sterile collection container is used to collect the midstream portion of urine. The patient must be cautioned not to touch the inside of the collection container.

DOUBLE-VOIDED SPECIMENS

In testing for glucose or ketones in the urine of a patient with diabetes mellitus, double-voided specimens are collected. The patient first urinates and disposes of the urine, which may have been collecting in the bladder for a long period of time. After about 30 minutes, the patient urinates again into a clean collection container. The second voiding is tested for the presence of glucose and ketones.

TIMED SPECIMENS

Timed specimens involve collecting the total urine output over a specific time period. With timed specimens, the amount of substances excreted during the collection period can be quantified. Thus timed specimens provide more accurate assessments of kidney function than random specimens. Time periods range from 2 to 24 hours. Preservatives or refrigeration frequently are needed for the large collection containers. The timed collection is begun by voiding and discarding the first urine specimen. The first voiding marks the beginning of the collection period. All urine output is collected for the specified number of hours and poured into the collection container. The patient is instructed to void at the end of the time period, and this urine is added to the collection container. If any urine is discarded during the collection period, the collection process must be restarted.

The Perez reflex can be used for urine collection in children who are not toilet trained. The child is held over the collection container while the paravertebrae muscles are stroked. Application of suprapubic pressure is another technique that enhances voiding in the infant.

ROUTINE ANALYSIS

A routine urine test is the most important screening test for urinary tract disease. This laboratory test frequently provides the first indication of dysfunction of the urinary tract. The standard components of a routine urinalysis are determination of color, pH, specific gravity, glucose, ketones, protein, bilirubin, and microscopic examination of the urinary sediment.

COLOR

Several factors can alter the color of urine. Color alterations and associated pathologic conditions are provided in Table 3-1.

Laboratory Results
Normal Range

Pale yellow to golden yellow

Nursing Implications
Procedure for Collection/Storage of Specimen

Specimens should be refrigerated if there is a delay in the delivery to the laboratory.

TABLE 3-1. **ALTERATIONS IN URINE COLOR**

Pathologic Condition	Color
Hemorrhage, hemoglobinuria	Reddish to brown
Liver or biliary tract disease	Green, brown, or deep yellow
Urinary tract infections or fat globules in the urine (chyluria)	White or cloudy
Dehydration	Dark yellow to amber
Diabetes insipidus, diuretic phase of ARF	Nearly colorless
Porphyria	Burgundy red (with exposure to light)

TABLE 3-2. **URINE COLOR ALTERATIONS CAUSED BY DRUGS**

Drugs	Urine Color
Methocarbomol, furazolidone, iron, levodopa, methyldopa, metronidazole, nitrofurantoin	Brown to black
Anisindione, chlorzoxazone, pyridium, santonin, sulfasolozine	Orange
Phenindione, rifampin, phenazopyridine, ethoxazene	Orange red
Diphenylhydantoin, deferoxamine, phenolphthalein, phenothiazine, phensuximide, phenytoin	Red
Cascara, chlorpromazine, methyldopa	Dark on standing
Cascara, phenothiazine, phensuximide, phenytoin	Red-brown
Amitriptyline, methylene blue, triamterene	Blue green or blue
Riboflavin, quinacrine, primaquine, chloroquine, phenacetin	Deep or rusty yellow

Possible Interfering Factors

Numerous drugs can alter the color of urine. Table 3-2 lists the drugs and associated urine color.

Patient Care

1. Test red or smoky-colored urine for presence of blood or hemoglobin.
2. Test green, brown, or deep yellow urine for presence of bile pigments.
3. Collect a urine specimen for culture if indicated.

Patient Education

1. Warn patients of coloring effects of specific drugs.
2. Instruct the patient to report changes in urine color.

Signed Consent

Not required

ACETONE

The presence of two ketone bodies, acetone and aceto-acetic acid, can be detected in urine specimens. Laboratories, however, are replacing these individual tests by measuring the total level of ketone bodies in the urine. (For details related to this test, see page 257.)

ALBUMIN (Electrophoresis)

When proteinuria is detected, electrophoresis can be used to determine the amounts of specific proteins in the urine. Elevated albumin amounts are associated with glomerular abnormality. Decreased amounts of albumin are found in patients with tubular abnormalities.

Laboratory Results

Normal Range

Adult   about 1/3 of the urinary protein is albumin.

Nursing Implications
Procedure for Collection/Storage of Specimen
1. A 24-hr timed specimen is collected.
2. Contact laboratory to determine which preservative should be used.

Possible Interfering Factors
None reported

Patient Care
1. Observe for frothy urine; it may indicate protein excretion.
2. Observe the patient for signs of edema.

Patient Education
Instruct the patient and the family to save all urine and notify nursing staff of each voiding.

Signed Consent
Not required

BILIRUBIN
When red blood cells are destroyed, bilirubin is released into the blood-stream. This type of bilirubin (free or unconjugated) is not water soluble and cannot be excreted by the kidneys. Normally unconjugated bilirubin is processed by the liver to form conjugated bilirubin, which passes through the biliary tract to the intestines for excretion. With obstructions of the biliary tract, conjugated bilirubin is excreted in the urine. Liver obstruction resulting from chemical toxins or hepatitis can also cause bilirubin to appear in the urine.

Laboratory Results
Normal Range

    Adult and child   none present in urine

Nursing Implications
Procedure for Collection/Storage of Specimen
1. A random specimen is collected.
2. The specimen is sent to the laboratory immediately, as bilirubin decomposes rapidly.

Possible Interfering Factors
Increase test results
- chlorpromazine
- pyridium
- salicylate
- urobilin

Decrease test results
- urine that is not fresh

Patient Care

1. Observe for dark-colored urine; it may result from the presence of bilirubin.
2. Observe the color of the stools. Pale stools may be associated with increased bilirubin excretion in the urine.
3. Observe for jaundice and itching. Bile pigment deposits in the skin cause jaundice and pruritis. Give good skin care to patients with jaundice.
4. Screen urine for bilirubin, which may detect unsuspected hepatitis.
5. Monitor urine bilirubin levels as an indicator of recovery from hepatitis.

Patient Education

Instruct the patient to avoid alcohol. Caution should be exercised in use of alcohol and carbon tetrachloride, as these chemicals can cause liver damage.

Signed Consent

Not required

CASTS

Deposits of protein in the renal tubules trap cellular elements which leads to the formation of casts. The appearance of casts in the urine generally indicates renal disease. The identification of different types of casts assists in locating the site of renal damage. Hyaline casts do not contain trapped cellular elements and may be associated with exercise, fever, or renal glomerular damage. Fatty casts indicate renal parenchymal disease. Infections are signaled by the appearance of white blood cell casts. Waxy casts are present with acute tubular damage. Advanced renal failure is associated with dilated renal tubules. Casts formed in these dilated tubules are referred to as broad casts. A poor prognosis is indicated by broad casts.

Laboratory Results

Normal Range

Adult and child   a few hyaline casts may be present; otherwise no casts should appear in the urine.

Nursing Implications

Procedure for Collection/Storage of Specimen

1. A random specimen is collected.
2. The specimen should be sent to the laboratory immediately or refrigerated.

Possible Interfering Factors

Casts may disintegrate if the specimen is not examined or refrigerated within 4 hr of collection.

Patient Care

Assess for symptoms of renal disease if casts appear in the urine.

Patient Education

If renal disease is confirmed, instruct the patient regarding dietary changes and drug therapy.

Signed Consent

Not required

CREATININE CLEARANCE

Determination of the GFR is most frequently accomplished through measurement of the creatinine content in urine. Creatinine clearance tests are used to detect glomerular damage, follow glomerular disease, and evaluate effects of medical treatment. Normally creatinine is filtered but not reabsorbed or secreted by the kidneys; however elevated serum creatinine levels result in tubular secretion of creatinine. Creatinine clearance measurement does not always provide an accurate measurement of GFR. Creatinine clearance remains the test of choice for measuring GFR because of clinical and technical difficulties associated with inulin clearance tests.

Laboratory Results

Normal Range

Adult	100 to 120 ml/min
Child	95 to 150 ml/min

Nursing Implications

Procedure for Collection/Storage of Specimen

1. A timed specimen is collected (usually a 24-hr specimen).
2. Urine is refrigerated during the collection process.
3. Note the exact time of the first and last voidings.
4. A venous blood specimen for measuring plasma creatinine is collected during the test.

Possible Interfering Factors

- high protein diet
- coffee
- tea
- cola drinks
- vigorous exercise
- diuretics
- glycosuria
- metnuria
- ascorbic acid
- methyldopa
- levodopa

Patient Care

1. Instruct the patient to avoid consumption of meat, poultry, fish, cola drinks, coffee, or tea for 6 hr before and during the test.
2. Inform the patient that repeated urine collections may be needed to obtain accurate results.

Patient Education

1. Instruct the patient and family to save all urine and notify the nursing staff at each voiding.
2. Discuss dietary restrictions associated with the test with the patient.
3. Inform the patient and family that confusion is often a manifestation of accumulated waste products remaining in the blood.

Signed Consent

Not required

CRYSTALS

Normally the urine may contain crystals which are benign. However, crystals of uric acid, cystine, or sulfa drugs should be noted. In patients with histories of renal stone formation, the type of crystals should be identified.

Laboratory Results
Normal Range

Adult and child	calcium and phosphate crystals may normally appear in the urine

Nursing Implications
Procedure for Collection/Storage of Specimen

A random specimen is collected.

Possible Interfering Factors

None reported

Patient Care

1. Urinary alkaline agents may be prescribed for patients receiving drug therapy in order to prevent crystal formation. Urinary alkaline agents may be prescribed for patients with a history of cystine or uric acid stone formation. Give alkaline agents as prescribed.
2. Drugs to produce an acid urine may be prescribed for patients with a history of phosphate stones. Encourage fruit juices, such as cranberry juice, to produce an acidic urine.

Patient Education

1. Instruct the patient that dietary changes can alter the urine pH. A high protein diet results in acid urine formation. Vegetarian diets lead to alkaline urine formation.

2. Educate patients about prescribed drugs that alter urine pH.
3. Teach patients with a history of renal stone formation to monitor their urine pH.

Signed Consent
Not required

GLUCOSE

Urine is usually tested for the presence of glucose (glycosuria) to detect or monitor diabetes mellitus. Renal dysfunction of the tubular transport mechanism for glucose can also result in glucose spilling into the urine. Another cause for the detection of glucose in the urine is a low renal threshold. A low renal threshold for glucose is not associated with disease.

The urine of patients receiving hyperalimentation (total parenteral nutrition) should also be tested for the presence of glucose.

Laboratory Results
Normal Range

Adult and child	none present in urine

Nursing Implications
The specimen should be tested or sent to the laboratory immediately. If delivery to the laboratory is delayed, the specimen should be refrigerated.

Possible Interfering Factors

False negative

- Refrigeration will cause a false negative if the specimen is not allowed to warm up to room temperature prior to testing.

False positive

- bleaches in collection container
- cephalosporin
- chloral hydrate
- chloramphenicol
- corticosteroids
- ephedrine
- gluconates
- indomethacin
- isoniazid
- metaxalone
- nalidixic acid
- nitrofurantoin
- penicillin
- phenacetin
- probenecid

- salicylates
- streptomycin
- sulfonamides
- tetracycline
- thiazides
- vitamin C

Patient Care

1. Collect double-voided urines for testing glucose in patients with diabetes mellitus. Clinitest and Benedict's testing are not specific for glucose monitoring, as galactose, lactose, fructose, and maltose are detected by these testing agents.
2. Keep tablets and dipsticks to test urine glucose in a tightly-sealed container.
3. Anticipate that following a meal high in carbohydrates, some glucose may normally be detected in the urine.
4. Monitor for symptoms of urinary tract infection as glycosuria increases the frequency of this problem.

Patient Education

1. If diabetes mellitus is the cause of glycosuria, teach the patient about dietary alteration, insulin or hypoglycemic agents, and urine testing.
2. Teach the patient about symptoms of urinary tract infection.

Signed Consent

Not required

INULIN CLEARANCE

Inulin is a polyfructose that is filtered but not secreted or reabsorbed by the kidneys. Following an intravenous infusion of inulin, measurement of the amount of inulin in the urine provides a precise measurement of the glomerular filtration rate.

Laboratory Results
Normal Range

Adult   100 to 160 ml/min

Nursing Implications
Procedure for Collection/Storage of Specimen
Precise urine collection is a necessity.

Possible Interfering Factors
Increase test results

- fructose
- dextran
- glucose

- tagatose
- sorbose

Patient Care

1. Teach the patient that foods containing fructose, tagatose, and sorbose are excluded from the diet during the test period.
2. Insert an indwelling catheter for urine collection, as prescribed.

Patient Education

Explain the purpose and the procedure for the test to the patient.

Signed Consent

Not required

KETONES

The ketone bodies, beta-hydroxybutyric acid, acetoacetic acid, and acetone, appear in the urine with a dysfunction in carbohydrate metabolism or a low intake of carbohydrates. Uncontrolled diabetes mellitus is signaled by ketonuria, which results from utilization of fat and fatty acids instead of glucose for energy.

Laboratory Results

Normal Range

Adult and child   negative (no ketones present)

Nursing Implications

Procedure for Collection/Storage of Specimen

Random urine specimens are collected.

Possible Interfering Factors

Increase test results

- levodopa
- sodium sulfobromophthalein (Bromsulphalein)

Decrease test results

- urine that is not fresh

Patient Care

1. Notify the physician of presence of ketones in the urine.
2. When a patient with diabetes mellitus has acute illness, surgery, or increased urine glucose, test urine for ketones before each meal and at bedtime.
3. Anticipate that elevations in ketones are treated frequently with increased insulin dosages.

Patient Education

1. Teach the patient with diabetes mellitus about dietary alterations, insulin or oral hypoglycemic agents, and urine testing.

2. Inform the patient with diabetes mellitus to report the presence of urine ketones to the physician.

Signed Consent
Not required

OSMOLARITY
Osmolarity tests measure the number of particles in a solution. Testing urine osmolarity provides a more precise measurement of the kidneys' ability to concentrate urine than specific gravity measurement.

Laboratory Results
Normal Range

Random sample	40 to 1350 mOsm/kg
Adult and child 24 hr sample	500 to 800 mOsm/kg
Infant random sample	50 to 600 mOsm/kg

Nursing Implications
Procedure for Collection/Storage of Specimen

The test is performed on random and 24-hr specimens.

Possible Interfering Factors

None reported

Patient Care
In evaluating renal function, the urine osmolarity should be considered in relationship to the plasma osmolarity. An elevated plasma osmolarity with a low urine osmolarity indicates an inability of the kidneys to concentrate urine.

Patient Education
Instruct the patient and family to save all urine for 24-hr specimens and notify the nursing staff of each voiding.

Signed Consent
Not required

PARA-AMINOHIPPURIC ACID (PAH) CLEARANCE
PAH clearance tests measure the proximal tubular secretory capacity. This test involves infusing large amounts of PAH into the plasma. The plasma concentration of PAH exceeds the amount that can be filtered by the glomeruli over a specific time period. Since about 90% of PAH is filtered or secreted as blood flows through the kidneys, the concentration of PAH in the urine can be measured to assess the functioning of the proximal tubules.

Laboratory Results
Normal Range

Adult male	530 to 770 cc/min
Adult female	500 to 700 cc/min

Nursing Implications
Procedure for Collection/Storage of Specimen

Precise specimen collection is necessary.

Possible Interfering Factors

Increase test results

- sulfonamides
- procaine

Patient Care

PAH infusion must be precisely controlled in relationship to the maximum secretory capacity for PAH.

Patient Education

1. Explain the purpose and procedure of the test to the patient.
2. Explain to the patient that no solid foods should be consumed for 4 hr prior to the test.

Signed Consent

Not required

pH

The kidneys can alter the acidity or alkalinity of the urine. Fresh urine is normally acid. Causes of increased urine acidity include starvation and ketosis. An alkaline urine is associated with inability of the kidneys to secrete hydrogen and many bacterial infections of the urinary tract. A vegetarian dietary pattern can also cause an alkaline urine.

Laboratory Results
Normal Range

Adult and child	pH 4.6 to 8.0

Nursing Implications
Procedure for Collection/Storage of Specimen

1. A random specimen is collected.
2. The urine must be sent to the laboratory promptly or refrigerated. The pH of the urine will increase as the urine stands.

Possible Interfering Factors

A specimen not tested within 4 hr of collection may show an increased pH.

Patient Care

1. Administer medications as prescribed to produce acid or alkaline urine. Precipitates from crushing injury, blood transfusion reaction, salicylate intoxication, renal stones of cystine or uric acid, or sulfa drug therapy may cause blocking of the renal tubules. The urine should be kept alkaline to prevent this precipitation. A vegetarian diet can be used to achieve an alkaline urine. An acid urine is desired when treating certain blood infections, using methenamine and when treating renal phosphate stones.
2. Note that patients who are on weight-control diets that increase high-protein food intake can develop an acid urine.

Patient Education

1. Educate patients about dietary alterations if urine pH needs to be maintained at certain levels.
2. Educate patients about any drugs prescribed to alter their urine pH.
3. Teach patients with a history of renal-stone formation to monitor urine pH.

Signed Consent

Not required

POTASSIUM (K)

Measuring the amount of excreted potassium provides a measure of renal tubular function.

Laboratory Results
Normal Range

| Adult | 30 to 90 mmol/24 hrs |
| Child | 25 to 125 mmol/24hrs |

Nursing Implications
Procedure for Collection/Storage of Specimen

1. A 24-hr specimen is collected.
2. Contact the laboratory to determine which preservative should be used.

Possible Interfering Factors

• Intake of potassium

Patient Care

1. Assess for symptoms of hyperkalemia or hypokalemia.
2. If urinary excretion of potassium is limited, restrict patient's dietary intake as prescribed.
3. If the patient is on digitalis therapy and potassium is being excreted by diuresis, assess heart rate.

Patient Education

1. Instruct the patient and family to save all of the urine and notify nursing staff of each voiding.
2. Instruct the patient about potassium-restricted diet in patients with limited potassium excretion.
3. Educate the patient about effects of abnormal potassium excretion or retention.

Signed Consent

Not required

PROTEIN

The detection of protein in the urine (proteinuria) is associated with increased permeability of the glomeruli. Glomerulonephritis, nephritis, nephrotic syndrome, diabetic nephropathy, and polycystic kidney disease may cause proteinuria. Proteinuria is also a clinical manifestation in toxemia of pregnancy. Other causes of proteinuria are transient and include a high fever, vigorous exercise, and upright posture.

Laboratory Results

Normal Range

Adult and child	none to trace present in urine

Nursing Implications

Procedure for Collection/Storage of Specimen

1. A random specimen is collected.
2. A first morning urine specimen should be collected.

Possible Interfering Factors

- alkaline urine
- contrast media for intravenous pyelogram
- tolbutamide
- sulfa drugs
- para-aminosalicylic acid
- penicillin

Patient Care

1. In assessing urine specific gravity, consider that proteinuria may influence the results of the urine specific gravity. In a dilute urine, even a trace of proteinuria can indicate a significant urinary loss of protein.
2. With a significant finding of proteinuria, collect a 24-hr specimen to determine protein loss as prescribed.
3. With urine that has protein amounts greater than a trace, examine the urine for the specific type of protein present.
4. Monitor renal function if renal damage resulting from therapy with

penicillamine or gold salts is suspected. Proteinuria can indicate renal damage.

5. Observe for frothy urine, which may indicate protein excretion.
6. Edema often accompanies severe proteinuria; therefore perform nursing actions to prevent skin breakdown.

Patient Education

1. Instruct patients receiving penicillamine or gold salts how to monitor the urine for proteinuria.
2. Instruct the patient on aspects of skin care. A mild soap should be used. Patients on bedrest should change position frequently.

Signed Consent

Not required

TOTAL URINARY PROTEIN

This laboratory test determines the amount of protein excreted per day. Elevated levels of protein are associated with renal disease, infection of the prostate and epididymis, and toxemia during pregnancy.

Laboratory Results

Normal Range

Adult	none; however 5% to 15% of individuals normally excrete small amounts of protein

Nursing Implications

Procedure for Collection/Storage of Specimen

1. A 24-hr timed specimen is collected.
2. No preservative is used. The specimen is refrigerated during collection.

Possible Interfering Factors

Increase test results

- x-ray contrast media
- tolbutamide
- para-aminosalicylic acid
- pencillin

Patient Care

1. Frothy urine may indicate protein excretion.
2. Edema often accompanies severe proteinuria. Give good skin care.

Patient Education

Instruct the patient and the family to save all urine and notify nursing staff of each voiding.

Signed Consent

Not required

RED BLOOD CELLS

The presence of red blood cells in the urine indicates bleeding at some location in the urinary tract, from the glomeruli to urethra, or leakage of red blood cells through the glomerular membrane.

Laboratory Results
Normal Range

Adult and child	no more than two red blood cells per high power field

Nursing Implications
Procedure for Collection/Storage of Specimen

1. A random specimen is collected.
2. Send the specimen to the laboratory immediately or refrigerate, as red blood cells are destroyed if the urine stands at room temperature.

Possible Interfering Factors

Increase test results

- Menstrual blood may contaminate the specimen.

Patient Care
1. Monitor urine color.
2. Bedrest is frequently prescribed in the presence of hematuria.
3. The location of the bleeding may be determined by cytoscopy or urography.

Patient Education
Provide instruction about diagnostic techniques used to locate bleeding site.

Signed Consent
Not required

SEDIMENT

Urine specimens examined for sediment provide indications of urinary tract infections, glomerular damage, and renal tubular damage. The urine may normally contain cells, epithelial cells, one or two red blood cells, one or two white blood cells, an occasional hyaline cast, and crystals. Abnormal urine findings include more than two red or white blood cells, casts, and certain types of crystals.

SODIUM (Na)

Measuring the amount of sodium present in the urine provides an indication of renal function.

Laboratory Results
Normal Range

Adult	40 to 200 mmol/24 hrs
Child	50 to 225 mmol/24 hrs

Nursing Implications
Procedure for Collection/Storage of Specimen

1. A 24-hr urine specimen is collected.
2. Contact the laboratory to determine the preservative to be used.

Possible Interfering Factors

Intake of sodium

Patient Care

1. Teach the patient that dietary alterations will be required if sodium excretion is abnormally high or low.
2. Weigh the patient daily to determine whether there is fluid retention as a result of decreased sodium excretion.
3. Evaluate blood pressure readings carefully. Elevated blood pressures can result when the kidney is unable to excrete sodium.
4. Assess the patient for symptoms of hypernatremia or hyponatremia.

Patient Education

1. Instruct the patient and the family to save all of the urine and notify nursing staff at the time of each voiding.
2. Teach the patient who is retaining sodium about sodium- and fluid-restricted diets. Teach the patient who is excreting increased amounts of sodium about increasing sodium intake.
3. Remind the patient that salt substitutes should not be used if potassium is restricted.
4. Teach the patient the symptoms of sodium depletion or retention.
5. Since the patient with chronic renal failure may be monitoring his own sodium-fluid status after discharge from hospitalization, teach the patient how to take blood pressures.

Signed Consent

Not required

SPECIFIC GRAVITY

The urinary specific gravity measures the kidneys' ability to conserve water or concentrate the urine. The test measures the weight of dissolved substances in the urine in relationship to the amount of fluid in the urine. Normally the kidneys increase the specific gravity with a low-fluid intake, and decrease the specific gravity with a high-fluid intake. One of the first indications of renal tubular dysfunction is a decreased specific gravity. Another cause of a decreased specific gravity is diabetes insipidus. Increased specific gravity is associated with diabetes mellitus, dehydration, congestive heart failure, and hepatic disease.

Laboratory Results
Normal Range

Adult and child	1.001 to 1.035
Neonate	1.012

Nursing Implications
Procedure for Collection/Storage of Specimen

1. It is preferable that specimens be collected after overnight fasting.
2. A minimum of 20 ml must be collected if a urinometer is used in testing the specimen.

Possible Interfering Factors

Increase test results

- radiographic contrast media
- dextran

Patient Care

1. Note the results of urine specific gravity tests. In the absence of renal disease, the specific gravity is an indicator of the patient's state of hydration.
2. When measuring the specific gravity, have the specimen at room temperature.
3. Note that in renal disease the specific gravity may not vary from 1.010.

Patient Education
None

Signed Consent
Not required

UREA CLEARANCE
The urea clearance test is performed to measure the GFR. Since urea is passively reabsorbed and secreted by the renal tubules, measurement of the GFR with this test is less precise than creatinine and inulin clearance tests.

Laboratory Results
Normal Range

Adult (maximum clearance)	51 to 75 ml/min
Adult (standard clearance)	34 to 74 ml/min

Nursing Implications
Procedure for Collection/Storage of Specimen

1. Collection is performed after the patient has fasted through the night.

2. Collection procedure involves providing water and collecting urine and blood at specific times.

Possible Interfering Factors
Increase test results
- protein intake
- stress
- sepsis
- fever
- antihypertensives
- antibiotics
- blood transfusions
- diuretics
- radiopaque contrast media
- salicylates
- steroids
- acetohexamide
- chloral hydrate
- doxapram
- methysergide
- streptokinase (streptodornase)

Patient Care
Allow fruit juices for breakfast. No tea or coffee is allowed prior to the test.

Patient Education
1. Instruct the patient about dietary restrictions for the test.
2. Describe the procedure of collecting urine specimens at specific time intervals.

Signed Consent
Not required

URINE CLEARANCE TESTS
Urinary clearance tests measure the ability of the kidneys to remove or clear substances from the blood. The measurement of renal clearances of para-aminohippuric acid (PAH), inulin, urea, and creatinine provides information about renal function.

URINE CULTURE AND SENSITIVITY
Urine cultures detect the presence and cause of urinary tract infections.

Laboratory Results
Normal Range

Adult and child   urine is normally sterile; however less than 10,000 bacterial colonies/ml is considered to result from contamination.

Nursing Implications
Procedure for Collection/Storage of Specimen

1. A clean-catch or catheterized specimen is collected.
2. Specimens must be sent to the laboratory immediately.
3. Collect the specimen prior to beginning antibiotics.

Possible Interfering Factors

1. External contamination of specimen can cause false positive results.
2. False negative results can occur if antibiotics or sulfonamides have been administered.

Patient Care

1. If 10,000 to 100,000 colonies/ml are counted, have the culture repeated.
2. Avoid the use of intermittent or indwelling urinary catheters.

Patient Education

1. Instruct the patient on the technique of clean-catch collection.
2. Teach the patient symptoms of urinary tract infection, which should be reported to health care personnel.

Signed Consent

Not required

WHITE BLOOD CELLS

The appearance of white blood cells in the urine (pyuria) is a manifestation of infection in the urinary system.

Laboratory Results
Normal Range

Adult and child   no more than two white blood cells per high power field

Nursing Implications
Procedure for Collection/Storage of Specimen

1. A clean-catch specimen to reduce external contamination is preferred.
2. The specimen needs to be sent to the laboratory immediately or refrigerated.

Possible Interfering Factors

Increase test results

- contamination from the urethra and external genitalia

Patient Care
1. Avoid use of indwelling urinary catheters whenever possible.
2. If an indwelling urinary catheter is inserted, provide catheter care.
3. Be aware that many antibiotics are excreted by the kidneys. Dosages of the antibiotics may need to be reduced with renal dysfunction.

Patient Education
1. Teach the patient signs and symptoms of urinary tract infection.
2. Explain to the patient how to take the prescribed medications for urinary tract infection.

Signed Consent
Not required

DIAGNOSTIC TESTS
PLAIN ABDOMINAL FILM (KUB)
A plain abdominal film is an x-ray of the kidneys, ureters, and bladder (KUB). This procedure provides an x-ray film of the urinary system. Since this x-ray is noninvasive, it should precede other radiographic tests of the urinary system. The KUB is useful in assessing the size, shape, and position of the kidneys and revealing calcification in the urinary system.

Normal Results
Normal structure of kidneys, ureters, and bladder.

Nursing Implications
Preprocedure
Explain the purpose and the procedure for an abdominal x-ray to the patient.

During Procedure
The x-ray technician assists the patient to assume a supine position. In some cases an oblique position is used.

Postprocedure
No special care required

Signed Consent
Not required

RENAL ANGIOGRAPHY
During a renal angiogram contrast media is injected into the aorta near the renal arteries. This allows visualization of the renal vasculature. Renal angiography provides for identification of stenosed, absent, extra, or misplaced renal blood vessels. This test is used not only to diagnose renal artery stenosis and tumors but also to study renovascular hypertension.

Normal Results
Normal appearance of the renal vasculature.

Nursing Implications

Preprocedure

1. Explain the purpose and the procedure for renal angiogram to the patient.
2. Determine if the patient has any allergies to iodine or seafood. Report allergies to the physician.
3. Shave the inguinal area.
4. Maintain the patient at no fluids after midnight. Patients with decreased renal function may continue their normal fluid intake, as dehydration can cause renal shutdown.
5. Have the patient empty the bladder prior to the procedure.
6. Administer a preoperative sedative as prescribed.
7. Obtain preoperative assessment of peripheral pulses.

During the Procedure

1. Patient will lie supine on a hard table.
2. A local anesthetic is given by the physician.
3. Explain to the patient that a hot feeling may be perceived as the dye is injected.
4. Films will be taken.

Postprocedure

1. Apply a pressure dressing to the insertion site. Check the dressing for bleeding. If bleeding occurs, apply pressure and notify the physician.
2. Maintain bedrest for 12 to 24 hr.
3. Monitor vital signs frequently until stable.
4. Assess peripheral pulses distal to the insertion site for decreased circulation. Assess for numbness, tingling, and color of extremity.

Signed Consent

Required

RENAL BIOPSY

A renal biopsy is performed to obtain a sample of renal tissue for examination. During this procedure, a specially designed needle is inserted below the twelfth rib through the skin (percutaneous) or through surgical opening (open) in order to enter the kidney and obtain the tissue sample. This procedure is used for diagnosing renal disorders, determining drug therapy, determining severity of renal disease, and for assessing the function of a transplanted kidney.

Normal Results

Normal microscopic appearance of the renal tissues.

Nursing Implications

Preprocedure

1. Explain the purpose and procedure to the patient.
2. Hemoglobin, hematocrit, clotting studies, and type and crossmatch are

performed. Check to see that all laboratory results are charted. Alert the physician to any abnormalities.

3. The lower pole of the kidney is located by intravenous pyelography or x-ray of the abdomen.
4. Take and record baseline vital signs.
5. Administer a preoperative sedative if prescribed.

During the Procedure

1. Place the patient in a prone or sitting position.
2. Prepare the needle insertion site with a surgical scrub. A local anesthetic is given.
3. Ask the patient to hold his breath as the needle is inserted.

Postprocedure

1. Apply a pressure dressing to the insertion site.
2. Monitor vital signs frequently until stable.
3. Instruct the patient to lie on the side of the biopsy site for 30 min to prevent bleeding.
4. Monitor each voiding for clearing of hematuria. Gross hematuria should be reported to the physician immediately.
5. Maintain the patient on bedrest for 24 hr.
6. Collect urine for a culture and sensitivity.

Signed Consent

Required

CYSTOSCOPY

Cystoscopy is a procedure in which a small metal telescope is inserted into the bladder through the urethra. This procedure permits visualization of the bladder and ureteric openings. During the cystoscopy, separate urine specimens can be collected from each kidney. With the use of an operating cystoscope, foreign bodies or stones can be removed, tumors resected, or a transurethral resection of the prostate can be performed.

Normal Results

Normal appearance and structure of the bladder and ureteric openings.

Nursing Implications

Preprocedure

1. Explain the purpose and the procedure for a cystoscopy to the patient.
2. Maintain the patient NPO after midnight.
3. Administer intravenous or oral fluids for several hours prior to the cystoscopy as prescribed.
4. Administer a preoperative sedative if prescribed.

During the Procedure

1. Place the patient in the lithotomy position.
2. Local or general anesthesia is administered.

3. Instruct the patient to avoid moving.
4. Instruct the patient in deep breathing techniques. Deep breathing can relieve discomfort of cystoscope insertion.

Postprocedure

1. Maintain bedrest for a short time.
2. Assess the patient's urinary output and color of the urine. Urine may be tinged pink. The physician should be notified of bright red blood.
3. If not contraindicated, instruct the patient to drink large amounts of fluid.
4. Back pain and sensation of a full and burning bladder may occur. Instruct the patient to report these symptoms to you and to the physician.

Signed Consent

Required

INTRAVENOUS PYELOGRAPHY (Excretory Urography)

Intravenous pyelography (IVP) involves the intravenous injection of an iodine contrast medium, which is excreted by the kidneys. An IVP provides information concerning the location, size, shape, and function of the kidneys, as well as the state of the ureters and bladder. Intravenous pyelography can detect structural abnormalities of the urinary tract and obstruction sites.

Normal Results

Normal size, shape, and position of the kidneys, ureters, and bladder. The contrast media is excreted within a prescribed time.

Nursing Implications

Preprocedure

1. Explain the purpose and procedure of an IVP to the patient.
2. Explain that laxatives are administered on the evening prior to the test.
3. Allow no fluids after midnight; however, patients with decreased renal function may continue their normal fluid intake since dehydration can cause renal shutdown.
4. Determine if the patient is allergic to iodine.
5. Have the patient empty the bladder prior to an IVP.

During the Procedure

1. Contrast medium is injected. The patient may feel hot as dye is injected.
2. Films are taken during the procedure.
3. The patient will be asked to assume supine, prone, and oblique positions.
4. The procedure usually takes 1 to 2 hr. With delayed excretion, films may be taken at intervals during the following 24 to 48 hr.

Postprocedure

1. Provide food and fluids as soon as possible.
2. Continue to observe for reactions to the contrast medium.

Signed Consent

Not required

BIBLIOGRAPHY

Blumenfeld T, Hicks J, Hill J, Levitt M, Meites S, Natelson S, Rodgerson D, Smith E: Normal Values for Pediatric Clinical Chemistry. Columbus, Ohio, American Association of Clinical Chemists, 1974

Bold AM, Wilding P: Clinical Chemistry Companion. Oxford, Blackwell Scientific, 1978

Brown S, Mitchell F, Young D (eds): Chemical Diagnosis of Disease. Amsterdam, Elsevier/North-Holland Biomedical Press, 1979

Brundage DJ: Nursing Management of Renal Problems. St Louis, CV Mosby, 1980

French R: Guide to Diagnostic Procedures, 5th ed. New York, McGraw-Hill, 1980

Garb S: Laboratory Tests in Common Use, 6th ed. New York, Springer, 1976

Hekelman F, Ostendarp C: Nephrology Nursing: Perspectives of Care. New York, McGraw-Hill, 1979

Hekelman F, Ostendarp C: Nursing approaches to conservative management of renal disease. Nurs Clin North Am 10:431, 1975

Kaplan A, Szabo L: Clinical Chemistry: Interpretation and Techniques. Philadelphia, Lea & Febiger, 1979

Kee JL: Clinical implications of laboratory studies in critical care. Crit Care Quart No. 2, 3:1, 1979

Koushanpour E: Renal Physiology: Principles and Functions. Philadelphia, WB Saunders, 1976

Maude DL: Kidney Physiology and Kidney Disease. Philadelphia, JB Lippincott, 1977

Menzel LK: Clinical problems of electrolyte balance. Nurs Clin North Am No. 15, 3:559, 1980

Netter FH: The CIBA Collection of Medical Illustrations, Vol 6. Summit, New Jersey, CIBA Pharmaceutical, 1973

Roberts SL: Renal assessment: a nursing point of view. Heart and Lung 8:105, 1979

Robinson RL: Laboratory findings in the differential diagnosis of acute renal failure. Crit Care Quart No. 2, 3:87, 1979

Slawson M: Thirty-three drugs that discolor urine and/or stools. RN 43:40, 1980

Smith DR: General Urology, 9th ed. Los Altos, Calif, Lange Medical, 1978

Stark JL: BUN/Creatinine: your keys to kidney function. Nursing 80, No. 10, 5:33, 1980

Sunderman FW, Sunderman, FW Jr: Laboratory Diagnosis of Kidney Diseases. St Louis, Warren H. Green Inc, 1970

4

Tests Related to Pulmonary Function

Christina A. Ronshausen

OVERVIEW OF PHYSIOLOGY AND PATHOPHYSIOLOGY

The purpose of the pulmonary system is to transport oxygen to the cells, while carrying away carbon dioxide. Oxygen is used in energy production during cellular metabolism. If oxygen is not available, the cells go into anaerobic energy production with a resultant increase in lactic acid production and a decrease in cellular pH.

To have adequate oxygen available for energy production, the body needs the following:

- adequate ventilation (movement of air in and out of the lungs)
- adequate gas exchange at the lungs (external respiration)
- adequate gas exchange at the tissues (internal respiration)

Adequate ventilation is dependent upon an intact thoracic musculoskeletal system, patent conducting airways, functioning neurochemical regulation, and good integrity of lung tissue.

Adequate gas exchange in the lungs is affected by the following:

- ventilation to the lungs
- blood flow through the pulmonary capillary bed
- the thickness of the alveolar–capillary membrane
- the total surface area of the alveolar–capillary membrane
- relative gas gradients and the solubility of gases on each side of membrane

Any alteration in these components will produce pulmonary dysfunction. The presence of pulmonary dysfunction leads to decreased amounts of oxygen available for energy production.

Pulmonary dysfunction is classified as either obstructive or restrictive. Obstructive refers to those lung diseases which obstruct the flow of air through the tracheobronchial tree to the alveoli. Restrictive refers to conditions that restrict the movement of the thorax or the lungs. Some diseases may, however, produce both obstructive and restrictive effects on pulmonary functioning.

OBSTRUCTIVE PULMONARY DYSFUNCTION

Obstruction to the flow of air in the tracheobronchial tree is produced by:

- acute and chronic asthma
- acute and chronic bronchitis
- emphysema
- cystic fibrosis of the lung

Chronic asthma, chronic bronchitis, and emphysema are sometimes grouped together and called chronic obstructive pulmonary (or lung) disease (COPD or COLD). Some clinicians consider COPD as a separate entity and feel that patients can have one or a combination of these disorders.

COPD diseases are characterized as having persistent airway obstruction of nonspecific etiology, with slowing of the ability to forcibly exhale air from the lungs.

ASTHMA

Asthma is a disorder in which there is an unusual tendency for bronchospasm to occur in response to irritants. Bronchospasm leads to bronchoconstriction and increased secretion of mucus. The bronchospasm, bronchoconstriction, mucosal edema, and hypersecretion of mucus may be due to a reaction of the irritant (antigen) with the IgE antibody. This reaction causes a release of histamine and the slow-reacting substance of anaphylaxis (SRS-A).

The patient, during an asthma attack, has difficulty forcing air out of the narrowed airways, and some air is trapped distally. In an effort to get more air out, the patient endeavors to prolong expiration.

Because of the obstructed airflow, there is a mismatch of ventilated alveoli and blood perfusion. This mismatch results in decreased gas exchange.

- The *oxygen* level in the blood (P_aO_2) is decreased since carbon dioxide diffuses better than oxygen.

- The level of *carbon dioxide* in the blood (P_aCO_2) is usually normal.

BRONCHITIS

Bronchitis is a disorder in which there is chronic or excessive secretion of mucus and mucus plugs. This occurs as a result of airway response to an irritant. There is also an inflammatory swelling of the airways. The hypersecretion and pooling of mucus and the inflammatory swelling result in narrowing of the airways. This reaction does not, however, occur evenly throughout the lung. With the narrowed airways, the patient has difficulty getting air in and out of the lungs.

- With the resultant obstructed airflow and the mismatch of ventilation and perfusion, the patient has a lowered *oxygen* level in the blood.

EMPHYSEMA

The pathophysiologic process of emphysema has not been identified entirely. There is destruction of alveolar walls accompanied by enlargement of the air spaces. The destruction of the alveolar walls causes a loss of support (mesh-like effect) of the small airways. The loss of support permits collapse of these airways. With the destruction of the alveolar walls, there is also loss of some of the capillary bed resulting in a decreased area for gas exchange. The destruction of the alveolar walls is not uniform throughout the lung.

The collapse of the airways is more pronounced on exhalation. The patient has difficulty getting the air out so that a prolonged expiration will occur as a compensatory measure.

- With advancing disease, the collapsing of airways will lead to air trapping and an increase in lung volumes.

- With airway collapse and decreased area for gas exchange, the patient will have less *oxygen* in his blood.

- As the area for gas exchange decreases, there is less diffusion of carbon dioxide resulting in elevated *carbon dioxide* levels in the blood.

Alpha₁-antitrypsin

Approximately 1% of the patients with emphysema have been found to have an *alpha₁-antitrypsin* deficiency. The lack of this enzyme is thought to be a factor in the development of emphysema, especially in the young adult age group.

Alpha₁-antitrypsin is thought to inactivate the endoprotease released by dying cells. In the lung, these dying cells would be the macrophages which are in the alveoli, and are released in the presence of infection and inflammation to engulf the foreign organism or irritant.

- Without alpha₁-antitrypsin, the endoprotease of the dying cells could digest the alveolar walls leading to the development of emphysema.

CYSTIC FIBROSIS OF THE LUNG

Cystic fibrosis of the lung (CF) is one aspect of a larger disorder known as cystic fibrosis of the pancreas. In cystic fibrosis of the pancreas, there is an obstruction of the exocrine gland ducts owing to the viscous nature of its secretions. Areas of the body affected in addition to the pancreas are the lungs, the gastrointestinal tract, biliary system, salivary glands, paranasal sinuses, the uterine cervix, and the male genital tract.

In the lungs, the viscous nature of the secreted mucus makes it very difficult for the patient to eliminate the mucus. The mucus is a very rich media for bacterial growth. The child with CF is thus very susceptible to infections. With repeated infections, pathologic changes occur in the lungs.

Although the lungs are normal at birth, dilation and hypertrophy of the mucus glands occur. This leads to the development of mucus plugs in the distal airways, bronchiectasis, bronchitis, and bronchiolitis. Air trapping also occurs. Eventually some organisms of infection, such as *Pseudomonas,* colonize and can never be eradicated. Although antibody formation for the *Pseudomonas* antigens should occur normally, this does not occur in the child with CF.

- The sweat glands of the child with CF are normal; however, the production of *sodium* and *chloride* is four times the normal level.

- The amount of *sweat* produced is normal. The overproduction of sodium and chloride gives a salty taste to the skin.

- Testing of the chloride level on the skin is one of the diagnostic studies for cystic fibrosis.

HYPOXIA/HYPOXEMIA

Depending upon severity, obstructive lung diseases may result in a decreased level of *oxygen* in the blood and an increased level of *carbon dioxide.*

Oxyhemoglobin Mechanisms

Normally approximately 97% of oxygen is carried to the tissues of the body in combination with hemoglobin (oxyhemoglobin). The remaining 3% is dissolved in the fluid of the red blood cell. This dissolved oxygen acts as a driving force to combine oxygen with hemoglobin. The greater the driving force the greater the combination or saturation of hemoglobin with oxygen (S_aO_2). This saturation does not occur in a linear fashion (Fig. 4-1). The

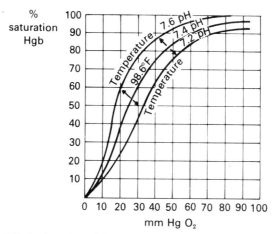

FIG. 4-1. *Shifts in the oxyhemoglobin dissociation curve. (Harper RW: A Guide to Respiratory Care: Physiology and Clinical Applications. Philadelphia, JB Lippincott, 1981)*

ability of the driving force (P_aO_2) to combine oxygen with hemoglobin is also affected by the body's pH.

- The lower the pH (*i.e.*, < 7.35) the less saturation will occur for the same amount of driving force. In other words, acidosis will cause the curve to shift to the right enabling the tissues to receive more oxygen.

- If the P_aO_2 is less than 60 mm Hg, the patient is said to be hypoxic.

Hypoxia causes many reactions in the body, some compensatory, some pathologic.

Compensatory Reactions

- Since the tissues in a person who is hypoxic need more oxygen, the heart rate and force of contraction intensify in order to increase cardiac output.

- The respiratory rate increases to provide more air for gas exchange.

- In order to shunt oxygenated blood to vital organs, peripheral vasoconstriction occurs.

- Hypoxia causes the kidneys to be stimulated to produce more erythropoietin. The hormone erythropoietin causes an increase in the production of *red blood cells* so that more oxygen can be carried to the tissues.

Pathophysiologic Reactions

Hypoxia causes some detrimental effects. The hypoxic cells go into anaerobic energy production. Anaerobic energy production is not as efficient as aerobic metabolism, so more lactic acid is produced. The additional lactic acid makes the cells and blood more acidotic. In acidotic states, more driving force (P_aO_2) is required to combine oxygen with hemoglobin.

- Hypoxia, in severe cases, can reduce the functioning of vital organs, especially the central nervous system and the renal system.

- Hypoxia can also have a detrimental effect on the lungs. Surfactant, used to keep the alveoli in the lungs open, needs oxygen present to be produced. If less surfactant is produced, alveoli will collapse. Less area for gas exchange then exists and less oxygen enters the blood. Thus the hypoxic state is worsened and the cycle continues.

RESTRICTIVE PULMONARY DYSFUNCTION

Restrictive lung disease refers to those disorders that restrict movement of the thorax or lungs. There are various ways of subclassifying the disorders. In this text they will be broadly subclassified as

- extrapulmonary disorders
- lung parenchymal disorders
- pleural disorders

EXTRAPULMONARY DISORDERS

Extrapulmonary disorders may be due to neurologic or neuromuscular dysfunction, thoracic defects, or obesity. Extrapulmonary implies that the lungs are normal in function.

ALVEOLAR HYPOVENTILATION OF NEUROLOGIC ORIGINS

Dysfunctions of neurologic or neuromuscular origin may produce *alveolar hypoventilation*. Head injuries, drug overdose, CO_2 narcosis, and Guillian–Barré syndrome may all cause *alveolar hypoventilation*.

- As a result of alveolar hypoventilation, lung volumes will be reduced and gas exchange may be significantly altered.
- Because of hypoventilation, the work of breathing is increased and the patient develops a rapid, shallow breathing pattern.

THORACIC DEFORMITIES

Thoracic deformities that restrict lung movement include kyphoscoliosis, congenital deformities, and chest trauma.

Kyphoscoliosis

Kyphoscoliosis is a combination of kyphosis and scoliosis. Kyphosis is a curvature of the thoracic spine with the convexity of the thickest part directed posteriorly. Scoliosis is a gradual lateral curvature of the thoracic spine with rotation of the vertebrae. Kyphoscoliosis may be due in part to posture, hereditary tendency, or disorders such as poliomyelitis.

The degree of affliction and interference with respiratory function varies. In severe cases, one side of the chest is retracted so as to cause extensive compression of that portion of the lung. The opposite side protrudes so as to cause overexpansion of the lung.

Since kyphoscoliosis combines two disorders, the effects are additive:

- There is increased resistance to expansion of both lungs.
- The total lung capacity and the vital capacity are reduced.
- These patients may have a rapid, shallow breathing pattern.
- There is a decrease in blood perfusion of the lung resulting in a discrep-

ancy of air and blood for gas exchange, causing decreased gas exchange in this area.

Funnel Chest and Pigeon Breast

Funnel chest and pigeon breast are two common congenital deformities of the chest. In funnel chest, also called pectus excavatum, the sternum is depressed or sunken in appearance. In mild cases, there usually is no pulmonary dysfunction. In more severe cases, there may be distortion or displacement of pulmonary structures. For example, if the bronchi are displaced, the patient may be more susceptible to respiratory infections owing to decreased ability in clearing the lungs of mucus.

Pigeon breast or pectus cavinatum is less common than funnel chest. The sternum and costal cartilages are projected forward and the sides of the chest appear somewhat flattened. This chest deformity rarely causes pulmonary dysfunction.

Chest Traumas

Chest traumas primarily consist of nonpenetrating, crushing, or compression injuries. Penetrating chest injuries will be discussed under pleural disorders.

Compression chest trauma usually results in single or multiple rib fractures and fractures of the sternum.

- The pain and muscle splinting that results from the fractures causes a rapid, shallow breathing pattern. The patient will also avoid coughing, increasing the chance of developing a respiratory infection.

When several ribs are fractured a *paradoxical movement* of the chest occurs. The side of the chest with the fractures will move in rather than out during inspiration. During expiration the affected side of the chest will bulge outward.

- Paradoxical movement causes shunting of air from one lung to the other (*i.e.*, the patient "inspires" part of the expired air). In addition, although the affected lung is poorly ventilated, it is being perfused with the blood.
- The result of this situation is an altered gas exchange and a resultant hypoxia.
- The patient tries to compensate by breathing faster.
- The CO_2 elimination is increased but the PO_2 is not altered significantly.

OBESITY

Obesity can adversely affect pulmonary function. The excess deposit of fat about the chest wall and abdomen may inhibit chest-wall expansion. Also the increased body size increases the demand for oxygen and increases carbon dioxide production. This places a tremendous demand on the pulmonary and cardiovascular systems.

Pickwickian Syndrome

The Pickwickian syndrome usually occurs in a person who is very obese, tends to be lethargic and drowsy, and has altered breathing patterns.

- The patient develops alveolar hypoventilation, polycythemia, hypoxemia, and hypercapnia.
- The lethargy and drowsiness are due to the elevated CO_2 levels.

LUNG PARENCHYMA DISORDERS

Lung parenchyma disorders include consolidation, abscess, cavitation, fibrosis, and atelectasis of the lung tissue.

CONSOLIDATION

Consolidation occurs when the alveoli and sometimes also the small airways become filled with cellular material. This process is usually due to infection or inflammation but may also occur with malignant processes. The location and size of the consolidation varies.

Pneumonia

Pneumonia is an inflammatory response to an identifiable agent. Pneumonia may be a primary process or develop secondary to another disease.

Most pneumonias are viral in origin but may be followed by a bacterial infection. This is possible because the viral infection destroys ciliated epithelial cells that interfere with the mucociliary escalator system, which is a defense mechanism. Interference with this defense mechanism allows for bacterial growth in the lung tissue.

The most frequent cause of viral pneumonias are influenza A and B. Gram-positive bacterial cocci that can produce pneumonia are *pneumococcus, Staphylococcus aureus,* and *Streptococcus pyogenes.* Some gram-negative cocci that can produce pneumonia are *Klebsiella bacillus, Pseudomonas,* and *Haemophilus.*

LUNG ABSCESS

An abscess of the lung parenchyma is pus within the lung tissue owing to necrosis. The necrosis of the lung tissue may be due to an inflammatory process caused by bacteria or fungi. An abscess may rupture. If the abscess ruptures into a bronchus the contents may be removed or it may spread to other parts of the lung.

Depending upon the size of the abscess, a cavity may be created and then replaced with scar tissue. Again depending initially upon the size of the abscess, then later upon the size of the cavity or scar tissue, the movement of the lung tissue in that area may be restricted.

FIBROSIS

Fibrosis of the lung refers to the presence of excessive amounts of connective tissue in the parenchyma. A variety of disorders that produce inflammation or necrosis may lead to the development of fibrosis. The extent of the fibrosis depends upon the degree of the primary process. Usually the fibrosis is localized and causes little interference in pulmonary function. Diffuse pulmonary fibrosis is more disabling and may be fatal.

Pneumoconiosis is an example of diffuse fibrosis caused by inhalation of specific inorganic and organic dusts. This usually occurs with certain occupations.

Inhalation of noxious gases may cause a chemical pneumonitis. Depending upon the type of exposure, the extent and concentration of exposure, total lung capacity, vital capacity, residual volume, and lung elasticity will be decreased.

ATELECTASIS

Atelectasis refers to the inadequate expansion of the alveoli. The alveoli become airless and collapse. Atelectasis may occur secondary to airway obstruction, compression, or inadequate quantities of surfactant to keep the alveoli open.

Absorption Atelectasis

When an airway obstruction occurs, the air within the alveoli is absorbed and the alveoli collapse. This is termed absorption atelectasis. The airway obstruction may be due to a mucus plug or surrounding structures such as a neoplasm impinging upon the airway. Some collateral ventilation through the pores of Kohn helps to keep the alveoli open.

Compression Atelectasis

Compression atelectasis results when an outside force drives the air out of the alveoli and collapses the alveoli. These outside forces may be pleural effusion, pneumothorax, or abdominal distention.

Surfactant Impairment

Certain conditions can impair the production of surfactant. Surfactant, which is produced in the alveoli, decreases the surface tension of the water lining the alveoli and allows the alveoli to remain open. Without surfactant, the surface tension of the water lining would cause the alveoli to collapse.

Infants born prior to 37 weeks gestation, infants born to diabetic mothers, infants with signs of fetal distress or perinatal asphyxia (especially the second born of twins) have a deficiency of phospholipid, which is used in the production of surfactant. Without the surfactant, atelectasis occurs. The lungs become stiff and inelastic, and profound hypoxia occurs.

PULMONARY EDEMA

Pulmonary edema occurs when the hydrostatic pressure within the pulmonary capillary bed exceeds the colloidal osmotic pressure. This change in pressures causes fluid to escape from the capillaries into the interstitial spaces. For a period of time, the lymph flow compensates for this shift in fluid; however, when the lymph flow cannot carry away the extra fluid in the interstitial spaces, the fluid then escapes into the alveoli.

- The additional fluid lining the alveoli will interfere with gas exchange, especially oxygen.
- There is also an increased tendency to develop atelectasis in the affected alveoli.
- The excess fluid in the interstitial spaces and the alveoli decreases the elasticity of the lung thus increasing the work of breathing.
- Also the tidal volume will be decreased.

Pulmonary edema may occur as a result of hypervolemia owing to intravenous therapy or left ventricular failure.

PULMONARY TUBERCULOSIS

Pulmonary tuberculosis results from the inhalation of mycobacteria into the lungs. The patient's resistance and the extent of exposure to the mycobacteria will influence the extent of the development of tuberculosis.

A granulomatous reaction occurs after exposure to the mycobacteria. This reaction causes consolidation of alveoli. The alveolar consolidation leads to infection and cavitation formation in the lung parenchyma. The cavitation becomes fibrotic and contains calcium deposits. These calcium deposits allow visualization of the tuberculosis process on a chest x-ray film. The consolidation can spread throughout a lobe of a lung.

The tubercle bacilli can also spread through the lymph system to lymph nodes. In a massive infection, a blood vessel is eroded and allows the tubercle bacilli to go into the blood. The bacilli can then travel in the blood to various organs of the body and can cause an infection in those organs.

PLEURAL DISORDERS

Disorders of the pleura and pleural space may result from the accumulation of air, fluid, blood, or purulent material in the pleural cavity. Pleural disorders can interfere with the expansion of the lung and the alveoli.

PLEURAL EFFUSION

Pleural effusion refers to the collection of fluid in the pleural cavity. This is a secondary process resulting from inflammation, malignancy, impaired lymphatic absorption, liver, renal, or heart disease. When a pleural effusion contains pus, this condition is known as *empyema.*

A *hemothorax* refers to the presence of frank blood in the pleural cavity. This is usually due to a penetrating type of chest injury.

PNEUMOTHORAX

A pneumothorax is the presence of air in the pleural cavity. A pneumothorax may be classified as traumatic, spontaneous, or therapeutic.

- In a *traumatic pneumothorax,* air enters the pleural space and collapses the lung to some extent. Mediastinal shift may occur toward the affected side.

- A *spontaneous pneumothorax* occurs without warning. There may or may not be an underlying pulmonary disease as the causative factor. Emphysema, pneumonia, or a neoplasm may cause a spontaneous pneumothorax.

- A *therapeutic pneumothorax* was once done in the treatment of tuberculosis but is not done presently.

ACID–BASE REGULATION
pH REGULATION

For cellular metabolism to occur at an optimal level, the pH of the extracellular fluid must be maintained with the narrow range of 7.35 to 7.45. In order to maintain this normal range, four physiologic processes occur.

1. Buffer Systems

   The first of these processes is the chemical buffering of the hydrogen ion (H^+) by both the extracellular and intracellular buffer systems. The hemoglobin in the red blood cells, the plasma proteins, and the carbonic acid–bicarbonate ($H_2CO_3 - HCO_3^-$) buffer system are the most important of these systems.

2. Hydrogen Ion Movement

   The second process is the movement of H^+ into or out of the cell depending upon the level of the H^+ ions. As the H^+ moves into the cell, potassium (K^+) moves out in order to maintain electrical neutrality.

3. Respiratory Compensation

   The third process is respiratory compensation, in which respiration either increases or decreases in order to blow off or retain carbon dioxide to maintain a normal pH. The CO_2 that will be blown off by the lungs is carried in the blood to the lungs in combination with hemoglobin.

4. Renal Compensation

   The fourth process is renal compensation. This process is the slowest of the four processes to occur. During renal compensation, hydrogen ions and bicarbonate ions are either eliminated or conserved to maintain the pH in the normal range.

The following equation illustrates the carbonic acid–bicarbonate buffer system dynamics and the interaction of the other physiologic processes.

$$CO_2 + H_2O \rightleftharpoons H_2CO_3 \rightleftharpoons H^+ + HCO_3^-$$

(This reaction can occur in either direction.)

Respiratory Component

The $CO_2 + H_2O$ side of the equation represents the respiratory component of the system.

- The CO_2 is actually the pCO_2 of the blood (*i.e.*, the partial pressure of CO_2 in the blood).

- The pCO_2 is an indicator of the amount of CO_2 blown off by the lungs and is thus an indicator of the functioning of the lungs.

- As the amount of CO_2 blown off decreases, the pCO_2 increases.

- This increase in pCO_2 stimulates the respiratory center and the buffer systems.

Renal–Metabolic Component

The $H_2CO_3 \rightleftharpoons H^+ + HCO_3^-$ side of the equation represents the renal–metabolic component of the system. The renal glomerular filtration, renal tubular reabsorption, and secretion processes regulate the H^+ and HCO_3^- elimination or conservation.

- The H^+ is excreted primarily in the form of NH_4 (ammonium ions).

- Approximately one-third of the H^+ ions are excreted in the form of H_2SO_4 (sulfuric acid) and H_3PO_4 (phosphoric acid).

- The bicarbonate is excreted or eliminated either with potassium or sodium or in exchange for chloride.
- Measurement of base excess or deficit indicates the amount of alkaline buffer substances in the blood. This measurement serves to indicate the effectiveness of the buffer system. A patient with metabolic acidosis will demonstrate a base deficit; with metabolic alkalosis, a base excess.

BLOOD TESTS
ALPHA$_1$-ANTITRYPSIN TEST

This test measures the presence of the enzyme alpha$_1$-antitrypsin in the blood. The level of this enzyme determines the presence of inflammation, tissue necrosis, and infection. The lack of alpha$_1$-antitrypsin may be a factor in the development of emphysema.

Alpha$_1$-antitrypsin inactivates the endoprotease released by dying cells. In the lung, these dying cells are the macrophages in the alveoli, which engulf organisms and foreign matter. Without alpha$_1$-antitrypsin, the endoprotease may digest the alveolar walls leading to the development of emphysema.

Elevated levels of the enzyme may occur in inflammation, cancer, and the use of oral contraceptives. Decreased levels may occur in emphysema in young adults, hepatic disease in children, and nephrotic syndrome.

Laboratory Results

Normal Range

    Adults and children   150 to 400 mg/dl

Nursing Implications

Procedure for Collection/Storage of the Specimen

Approximately 5 ml of venous blood is needed.

Possible Interfering Factors

Pregnancy may increase the level by 100%.

Patient Care

1. If the patient has elevated cholesterol or triglyceride levels, keep the patient NPO except for water prior to the test.
2. Assess the patient for any history, signs, or symptoms of pulmonary, hepatic, or renal disease.
3. Determine if the female patient is pregnant.
4. Check the patient's laboratory reports for elevated cholesterol—triglyceride levels.
5. Inquire as to family history of emphysema.

Patient Instruction

If the patient is found to have the deficiency of alpha$_1$-antitrypsin, begin educating the patient regarding the following:

- avoidance, if possible, of sources of air pollution
- avoidance of or stop smoking
- treatment modality, self-care of emphysema

Signed Consent

Not required

ARTERIAL BLOOD GASES (ABGs)

Measurement of arterial blood gases (ABGs) indicates the effectiveness of pulmonary function. ABGs is the best method for assessing the efficiency of ventilation and external respiration. ABGs can indicate ventilatory efficiency, the ability of hemoglobin to carry oxygen and carbon dioxide, the status of the buffer system, and the partial presence of oxygen and carbon dioxide dissolved in plasma.

Measurement of arterial blood gases is indicated in the management and evaluation of acutely and critically ill patients, patients being mechanically ventilated, and patients with acute or chronic pulmonary disorders.

Information obtained by arterial blood gases includes the following:

- pH indicates the acid–base state of the body; is dependent upon the CO_2 level in the blood; indicates the effectiveness of the buffer system

- P_aCO_2 the carbon dioxide tension of the blood; a direct indicator of pulmonary functioning

- P_aO_2 the oxygen tension of the blood, but not the oxygen state of the tissues; is the most important determinant of the amount of oxygen that combines with hemoglobin

- HCO_3 the amount of bicarbonate buffer in the blood

- S_aO_2 the saturation of hemoglobin with oxygen compared to hemoglobin's maximum capacity for binding with oxygen

EVALUATION OF ACID–BASE STATUS

Several factors are assessed to determine a patient's acid–base status. For the best results, several ABG measurements should be evaluated to arrive at a proper interpretation:

- pH measurement

  This reflects the hydrogen ion concentration in the blood. Acidosis is present if the pH is less than 7.35; alkalosis is present if the pH is more than 7.45.

- Carbon dioxide measurement

  The pCO_2 measures the partial pressure of the carbon dioxide molecules in the blood. The lungs are the major organ of excretion of carbon dioxide. If the level of CO_2 in the blood is elevated, the rate of respiration will increase in an effort to blow off the CO_2 and lower the acid level in the blood.

- Plasma bicarbonate measurement

  The bicarbonate in the blood represents the renal regulated or metabolic component of the acid–base system.

Laboratory Results
Normal Values

pH	7.35 to 7.45
pCO_2	35 to 45 mmHg (torr)
pO_2	80 to 100 mmHg (torr)
HCO_3	18 to 25 mEq/liter
S_aO_2	97%

Abnormal Values (according to classification)

	pH	pCO_2	HCO_3
acute respiratory acidosis	↓	↑	WNL
acute respiratory alkalosis	↑	↓	WNL
acute metabolic acidosis	↓	WNL	↓
acute metabolic alkalosis	↑	WNL	↑
respiratory acidosis with compensation	WNL*	↑	↑
respiratory alkalosis with compensation	WNL	↓	↓
metabolic acidosis with compensation	WNL	↓	↓
metabolic alkalosis with compensation	WNL	↑	↑

Nursing Implications
Procedure for Collection/Storage of Specimen
For details related to this test, see page 47.

Possible Interfering Factors

	Elevation	*Decreased*
pH	hyperventilation fever excessive alkali ingestion excessive vomiting, diarrhea high altitude	impaired liver function severe diarrhea diabetic acidosis some kidney disorders, hypoventilation some cardiac disorders
CO_2	congenital heart defects excessive vomiting, diarrhea hypoventilation fever	hyperventilation high altitude salicylate ingestion
O_2	supplemental oxygen therapy	congenital heart defects hypoventilation oxygen toxicity

*within normal levels

Patient Care

1. Observe the patient for changes in organ functioning (*e.g.*, tachycardia, decreased renal functioning).
2. Assess the patient's response to the acid–base disturbances.
   - respiratory acidosis—hypoventilation, sensorium changes, somnolence, semi-comatose, comatose, tachycardia arrhythmias
   - respiratory alkalosis—tachypnea, sensorium changes, numbness, tingling of hands and face
   - metabolic acidosis—headache, nausea, vomiting, diarrhea, sensorium changes, tremors, convulsions
   - metabolic alkalosis—nausea, vomiting, diarrhea, sensorium changes, tremors, convulsions
3. If the patient's ABGs reveal hypoxemia, alert the physician immediately and seek an order for institution of oxygen therapy.
4. Observe the patient's response to therapy.
5. Note whether the patient is receiving oxygen therapy.
6. Take a baseline temperature and note temperature at the time of blood gas collection.
7. Note whether the patient is receiving any drug therapy or demonstrates any physical conditions (*e.g.*, exercise, hyperventilation) that may alter the results of the tests.
8. Note any sign of bleeding or hematoma formation at the arterial puncture site.

Patient Education

1. Explain the purpose and the procedure of the test to the patient.
2. Instruct the patient in his care according to the problem identified by the laboratory reports.

Signed Consent

Not required

CARBOXYHEMOGLOBIN

This test measures the amount of carboxyhemoglobin in the blood. Carboxyhemoglobin is the combination of carbon monoxide and hemoglobin in the red blood cell. Carbon monoxide (CO) is a by-product of red blood cell destruction. A heavy exposure to smoke, such as from cigarettes and exhaust fumes from automobiles, increases the exposure to carbon monoxide. The affinity of carbon monoxide to hemoglobin is much greater than carbon dioxide to hemoglobin. This greater affinity results in less hemoglobin bonds available to combine with oxygen. The patient then becomes hypoxic. The degree of the hypoxia is dependent upon the amount of exposure to carbon monoxide.

Carbon monoxide poisoning can adversely affect the patient's arterial blood gas levels. The P_aO_2 will remain normal but the saturation of hemoglobin (S_aO_2) will be greatly reduced. The dissociation of carbon monoxide from hemoglobin is extremely slow so that the acute decrease in blood oxygen is not readily reversed.

Laboratory Results
Normal Value

1% of the hemoglobin bonds is attached to carbon monoxide

Abnormal Values

Heavy smokers ≥ 5% carboxyhemoglobin levels

Carbon monoxide poisoning ≥ 25% carboxyhemoglobin levels

Nursing Implications
Procedure for Collection/Storage of Specimen

Obtain a 5 ml sample of heparinized venous or arterial blood.

Possible Interfering Factors

None reported

Patient Care
1. Obtain immediately a history of carbon monoxide poisoning to facilitate appropriate treatment.
2. Observe the patient for signs and symptoms of hypoxia.
3. Be aware that patients with heavy carbon monoxide exposure may appear to be intoxicated.

Patient Education
Institute patient education based on the laboratory results and the presence and extent of central nervous system damage that may be present.

Signed Consent
Not required

COLD AGGLUTININS
Approximately 55% of patients with primary atypical pneumonia have demonstrated the presence of antibodies. These antibodies are also found in patients having pulmonary embolism and viral pneumonia, influenza A and B, and mycoplasma pneumonia.

Laboratory Results
Normal Value

Absence of antibodies in the blood

Positive Results

A four-fold rise in titer from early in the illness until convalescence.

In atypical pneumonia, the titer will rise 8 to 10 dy after onset of the illness, peak in 12 to 25 dy and fall approximately 30 dy after the onset of the illness.

Nursing Implications

(For details related to this test, see page 325.)

FUNGAL ANTIBODY TEST

The fungal antibody test is used to determine the presence of fungal precipitin antibodies in the blood. These antibodies occur in antigen–antibody reactions of the body after exposure to the fungi *Blastomyces dermatitidis, Histoplasma capsulatum,* and *Coccidioides immitis.* These fungi spores are inhaled from the dust, soil, and bird droppings causing the respiratory diseases blastomycosis, histoplasmosis, and coccidiomycosis. The antibodies occur in the blood approximately 1 to 4 wk after exposure, then disappear from the blood. Fungal skin tests and chest x-rays should be performed after a positive fungal antibody test.

Laboratory Results

Normal Values

Absence of the antibodies in the blood.

Nursing Implications

Procedure for Storage/Collection of the Specimen

Several milliliters of venous blood are collected.

Possible Interfering Factors

1. The fungal antibodies may be present in the blood of normal people.
2. In testing for blastomycosis, a cross reaction with histoplasmosis may occur.

Patient Care

1. Assess the patient for travel to southwest U.S. and Mississippi River areas, or for urban areas with large numbers of pigeons.
2. Assess patient for signs/symptoms of fungal disease.

Patient Education

No special instructions

Signed Consent

Not required

RED BLOOD CELL COUNT

Inadequate numbers of red blood cells (RBCs) or hemoglobin can produce hypoxia or hypercapnia. Immature or altered structures of the red blood cells can precipitate hypoxia in tissues such as in sickle cell anemia.

Some pulmonary disorders, such as chronic obstructive pulmonary disease, can cause chronic hypoxia. As a compensatory measure, the body will greatly increase the number of red blood cells. This condition is known as polycythemia. By increasing the number of red blood cells, the body is attempting to increase the oxygen-carrying capacity of the blood.

Anemia may occur in some bacterial infections such as hemolytic streptococcus owing to the destruction of red blood cells. Tuberculosis may cause anemia as a result of depletion of the bone marrow. (For details related to this test, see page 30.)

WHITE BLOOD CELL COUNT

A white blood cell count (WBC), as well as a differential, may be helpful in diagnosing pulmonary infections, inflammations, and allergies. Acute pulmonary infections may cause a sharp rise in the white blood cells, especially the polymorphonuclear leukocytes. Chronic infections, such as chronic bronchitis, may cause only a slight rise in the white blood cells (mononuclear leukocytes). Allergic disorders, such as asthma, may cause an elevation in the eosinophils.

(For details related to this test, see page 22.)

DIAGNOSTIC TESTS
BRONCHOGRAPHY

Bronchography is a diagnostic test that uses a contrast medium. The media is instilled into the tracheobronchial tree in order to visualize the bronchi. Narrowing, obstruction, or dilation of the bronchi can be visualized on a bronchogram. Bronchography causes some patients discomfort, and increases airway resistance and hypoxia.

Normal Results
Normal structure of the tracheobronchial tree

Nursing Implications
Preprocedure
1. Explain the procedure and its purpose to the patient.
2. Instruct the patient to perform good oral hygiene the evening before and the morning of the procedure.
3. Keep the patient NPO for 6 to 12 hr prior to the procedure as prescribed by the physician.
4. Assist the patient to perform postural drainage the morning of the procedure if prescribed by the physician.
5. Instruct the patient to remove and safely store removable dental structures.
6. Inquire if the patient has any loose teeth, capped teeth, dental bridges, or oral inflammations. Record any findings. Report the presence of oral inflammations to the physician.
7. Administer sedation as presented by the physician.

During the Procedure
1. Encourage the patient to relax during intubation to decrease patient discomfort.
2. Reassure the patient that breathing will not be obstructed.
3. Instruct the patient to breathe through the mouth.
4. Tell the patient when the throat will be anesthetized. This local anesthesia decreases gagging and increases patient comfort. Have the pa-

tient spit out the anesthesia rather than swallow it. Although it is rare, the local anesthetic can cause anaphylactic shock.

Postprocedure
1. Keep the patient NPO until the gag reflex has returned. The gag reflex will return in approximately 2 to 6 hr.
2. Observe the patient for side effects of the anesthesia, such as palpitations, rapid and bounding pulse, elevated blood pressure, or rapid, deep breathing.
3. Observe the patient for signs or symptoms of laryngospasm, or laryngeal edema.

Signed Consent
Required

BRONCHOSCOPY
Bronchoscopy allows inspection of lung abnormalities in the tracheobronchial tree and some of the bronchopulmonary segments. In bronchoscopy, a rigid or flexible scope is inserted into the trachea and bronchi. The flexible scope has a light at its tip to permit increased visualization. Samples of lung tissue can be obtained by biopsy for cytology examination. Bronchial washings can also facilitate the collection of cells for analysis. Therapeutic bronchoscopy can be done on patients who have very thick secretions and need assistance in removing the secretions. Therapeutic bronchoscopy is used also in the removal of foreign objects from the tracheobronchial tree.

Normal Results
Normal appearance of tracheobronchial structures

Nursing Implications
Preprocedure
1. Explain the procedure and its purpose to the patient.
2. Keep the patient NPO for 6 to 12 hr prior to the procedure.
3. Inform the patient that arterial blood gas samples and pulmonary screening tests may be done prior to this test.
4. Instruct the patient to perform good oral hygiene the evening before and the morning of the procedure.
5. Assist the patient to perform postural drainage the morning of the procedure if prescribed by the physician.
6. Instruct the patient to remove and safely store removable dental structures.
7. Inquire if the patient has any loose teeth, capped teeth, dental bridges, or oral inflammations. Record any findings.
8. Administer sedation as prescribed by the physician.
9. Inform the patient that the procedure will be done in a darkened room.
10. A general anesthetic may be used during the procedure. Inform the patient as necessary.

During the Procedure

1. Assist the patient into a comfortable position on his back with the neck hyperextended. A pillow can be placed under the neck to achieve hyperextension.
2. Encourage the patient to relax during intubation to decrease the patient discomfort.
3. Encourage the patient to keep the arms to the sides and to refrain from clenching the fists.
4. Encourage the patient to breathe through the mouth.
5. Assure the patient that breathing will not be obstructed.
6. Tell the patient when the throat will be anesthesized. This local anesthesia decreases gagging and increases patient comfort. Have the patient spit out the anesthesia rather than swallowing it. On rare occasions, the local anesthetic can cause anaphylactic shock.

Postprocedure

1. Position the patient to prevent aspiration.
2. Instruct the conscious patient to allow saliva to run out the side of the mouth rather than try to swallow it.
3. Keep the patient NPO until the gag reflex has returned. The gag reflex will return in approximately 2 to 6 hr.
4. Save all sputum expectorated for laboratory examination. Anticipate copious amounts of sputum as a result of trauma caused by passing the scope.
5. Observe the patient for side effects of anesthesia such as palpitations, rapid bounding pulse, elevated blood pressure, or hyperventilation.
6. Observe the patient for signs of respiratory distress owing to a laryngospasm.
7. Observe for signs of hemorrhage if biopsy was performed. A slight blood-streaked sputum is to be expected for 1 or 2 days. Excessive bleeding (frank blood in sputum) should be reported.
8. Observe the patient for signs of subcutaneous emphysema which could indicate perforation of the trachea or bronchus.
9. Assure the patient that a sore throat is to be expected. Provide appropriate care to decrease discomfort (*e.g.,* an ice collar).

Signed Consent

Required

CHEST X-RAY

The chest x-ray is used to examine the soft tissue and bony structures of the thorax. The chest x-ray is very important in the diagnosis of pulmonary disease. This study also provides information about the heart, ribs, spine, and a portion of the gastrointestinal tract. Chest x-ray films provide a record of absence or presence of disease. Serial x-rays help to determine the onset and progress of diseases of the chest.

Indications for a chest x-ray include screening of large selected populations for pulmonary lesions such as tuberculosis, as part of routine physical examinations, as part of routine hospital admission data base, and in the diagnosis of diseases of the chest.

CHEST TOMOGRAPHY

A chest tomography is used to examine in greater detail a small area of the thorax. Lesions may be obscured or poorly visualized on a standard chest x-ray film owing to overlapping thoracic structures. Tomograms consist of a series of x-rays focused at varying depths. Each x-ray film gives a sharp image of the structures at that depth. Tomograms may show the size and shape of the lesion, the presence of cavities or calcifications, and the surrounding vascular patterns.

Normal Results

A normal chest x-ray film reveals normal structure of the soft tissue of the lung, pleura, bony thorax, heart, and mediastinum.

Nursing Implications
Preprocedure

1. Explain the procedure and the purpose to the patient. The procedure should take only a few minutes.
2. Determine if the female patient may be pregnant by asking the date of the last menstrual period. If the pregnant patient is in the first trimester of pregnancy, the chest x-ray should not be done. Pregnant patients in the second and third trimester should wear a lead apron over the abdomen and pelvic areas during the procedure.
3. Ask the patient to remove all clothing above the waist and to put on a hospital gown.
4. The patient should remove all jewelry and other metal objects about the neck.

During the Procedure

1. Assist the patient into a standing position facing the x-ray film. If the patient is on bedrest, assist the patient into a sitting position if possible. A sitting position facilitates maximal lung expansion while the x-ray film is being taken and allows for better visualization of the structures of the thorax.
2. Encourage the patient to take a deep breath and exhale, then take a deep breath and hold it while the x-ray film is being taken.

Postprocedure

Assist the patient if necessary to put on personal clothing.

Signed Consent

Not required

PULMONARY FUNCTION TESTS

Pulmonary function tests are used to determine the presence, nature, and extent of pulmonary disease. Pulmonary dysfunction may be caused by obstructive or restrictive diseases. Functioning of the pulmonary system is dependent upon the integrity of the tracheobronchial tree, the parenchyma (alveoli) and the vascular system. Pulmonary function tests will indicate abnormalities in these structures. The tests may indicate pulmonary dysfunction prior to abnormalities being noted by physical examination or x-rays. The pulmonary function tests do not indicate the etiology of the dysfunction.

Indications for performing pulmonary function tests are the following:

- early detection of pulmonary or cardiopulmonary disease
- diagnosis of dyspnea
- epidemiologic studies of pulmonary diseases
- to follow the progress of a pulmonary disease

Pulmonary function tests are divided into three categories: conventional, specialized, and preoperative screening tests. Conventional pulmonary function tests include spirometry, static lung volumes, diffusing capacity determinations, and arterial blood gas studies. Specialized pulmonary function tests involve the study of closing volumes, body plethysmograph, CO_2 response, respiratory stress testing, exercise arterial blood gas studies, and maximal voluntary ventilation. Preoperative screening is usually limited to the use of the spirometry.

SPIROMETRY

The spirometer is the instrument most commonly used to measure tidal volume (V_T), forced vital capacity (FVC), and forced expiratory volume (FEV). A spirometer consists of a bell suspended in a container of water. The bell rises and falls as the patient inhales and exhales into a tube connected to the spirometer. A stylus marks on paper the movement of the bell.

The spirometry determines the effectiveness of the various structures and forces involved in the movement of the lungs and chest during breathing. The results can indicate the presence and degree of obstruction to airflow in the airways and the restrictions in the amount of air that can be inspired.

The *tidal volume* (V_T or TV) is the amount of air inspired during each breath in quiet, normal breathing. Only part of the tidal volume is involved in gas exchange in the lungs, since part of the lung structure only conducts the air to the alveoli.

The *forced vital capacity* (FVC) is the amount of air that is forcibly exhaled after a full inspiration. It is also the time required to exhale all the air possible and is designated as forced expiratory volume (FEV).

The amount of air that can be forcibly exhaled in one second is designated as FEV_1. The FEV_1 and FVC are measured and compared to determine the presence of obstructive or restrictive lung disease. In obstructive lung disease, the patient is unable to forcibly exhale the air, thus resulting in a prolonged expiration. Therefore both the FVC and FEV in one second (FEV_1) are decreased. In restrictive lung diseases, the patient cannot expand the chest fully, resulting in a decreased FVC value. The patient has no difficulty, however, in exhaling the air forcibly (FEV_1 is normal) (Fig. 4-2).

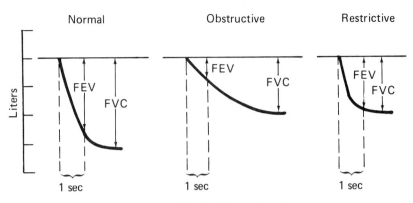

FIG. 4-2. *Spirometric values.*

Normal Results

Results are dependent upon sex, age, and height ± 20% of predicted value (Fig. 4-3).

Nursing Implications

Preprocedure

1. Explain the procedure and its purpose to the patient. The test will take approximately 15 to 30 min to complete.
2. Assess the patient's respiratory status.
3. Emphasize to the patient the need for maximum cooperation during the test in order to achieve valid results.
4. Explain to the patient that if dyspnea or fatigue occur, the test will be stopped to allow the patient to recover.

During the Procedure

1. Place nose slips on the patient's nose.
2. Instruct the patient to seal the lips tightly around the mouthpiece.
3. Instruct the patient to breathe normally for 1 minute. During this time the patient should become accustomed to the equipment.
4. Instruct the patient to take as deep a breath as possible, hold the breath for a short period then exhale as hard as possible, for as long as possible. This procedure may be repeated two or three times to see the patient's best effort; the information should then be used for calculation of results.

Postprocedure

Assess the patient's response to the test. Note that the patient may develop bronchospasm.

Signed Consent

Not required

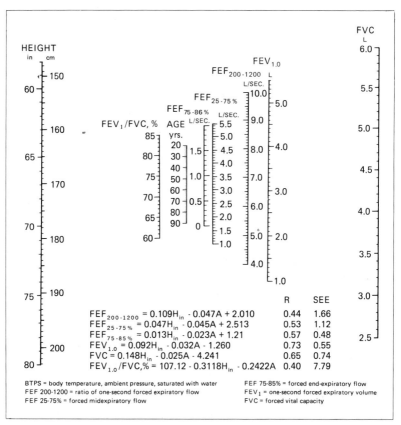

A — Prediction nomogram for normal men (BTPS).

FIG. 4-3. *Values for FEV_1/FVC, FEV_1, FVC, and miscellaneous expiratory flow rates in normal men (A) and normal women (B). The normal values are found by laying a straightedge between the subject's height and age and reading the values from the appropriate scales. (Morris JF: Spirometry in the evaluation of pulmonary function. West J Med 125:110, August 1976)*

(Illustration continued on opposite page)

STATIC LUNG VOLUMES

Static lung volumes are usually measured during the spirometry procedure. The lung volumes are subdivisions of the lung that can be represented graphically. These subdivisions are not anatomical subdivisions but represent various levels of air in the lung that can be measured after doing various breathing exercises. Combinations of two or more lung volumes are called capacities. Alteration in lung volumes or capacities may indicate pulmonary dysfunction. The lung volumes and capacities measured with spirometry are the following:

- Total lung capacity (TC)—the volume of air in the lung after a maximal inspiration

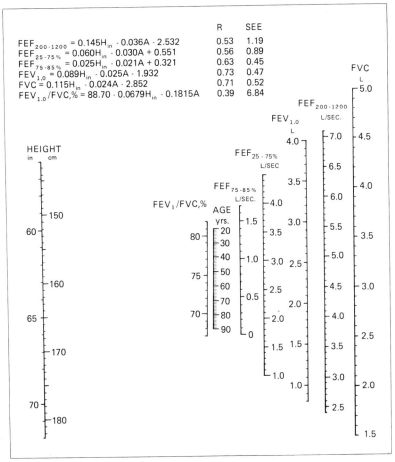

$$FEF_{200-1200} = 0.145H_{in} - 0.036A - 2.532 \quad 0.53 \quad 1.19$$
$$FEF_{25-75\%} = 0.060H_{in} - 0.030A + 0.551 \quad 0.56 \quad 0.89$$
$$FEF_{75-85\%} = 0.025H_{in} - 0.021A + 0.321 \quad 0.63 \quad 0.45$$
$$FEV_{1.0} = 0.089H_{in} - 0.025A - 1.932 \quad 0.73 \quad 0.47$$
$$FVC = 0.115H_{in} - 0.024A - 2.852 \quad 0.71 \quad 0.52$$
$$FEV_{1.0}/FVC,\% = 88.70 - 0.0679H_{in} - 0.1815A \quad 0.39 \quad 6.84$$

B   Prediction nomogram for normal women (BTPS)

FIG 4-3 *(Continued)*

- Tidal volume (V_T or TV)—the amount of air inspired during each breath in quiet normal breathing
- Inspiratory vital capacity (IVC)—the maximal amount of air that can be inhaled after a maximal expiration
- Functional residual capacity (FRC)—the amount of air left in the lungs after a normal expiration
- Expiratory reserve volume (ERV)—the maximal amount of air that can be expired after a normal expiration
- Residual volume (RV)—the amount of air left in the lungs after a maximal expiration
- Functional vital capacity (FVC)—the maximal amount of air that can be forcefully exhaled after a maximal inspiration (Fig. 4-4)

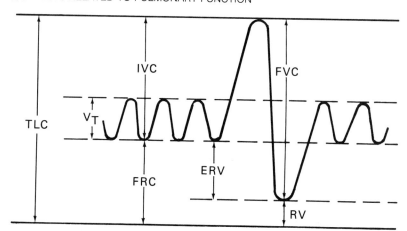

FIG. 4-4. *Representation of lung volumes and capacities.*

Normal Results

Results are dependent upon sex, weight, height, age, activity, and body demands for oxygen.

Nursing Implications

(For details related to this test, see page 151.)

Signed Consent

Not required

MISCELLANEOUS TESTS
SPUTUM SPECIMEN

Sputum is mucus containing material that is brought up from the lungs. Sputum is not the same as saliva or postnasal secretions. Sputum specimens are obtained to determine the cause of a respiratory infection. The sputum is examined to determine the presence of pathogenic or nonpathogenic organisms. The sputum specimen may also be cultured to grow colonies of the pathogenic organisms.

SPUTUM SENSITIVITY STUDIES

Sensitivity studies may be done to identify the specific antimicrobial drug that will be most effective. The procedure for collecting sputum specimens to identify the patient's bacteria is the same as for any sputum culture.

SPUTUM SPECIMENS FOR CYTOLOGY

Sputum specimens, which are collected for cytology, are examined for the presence of abnormal, cancerous cells. As old and diseased cells are "exfoliated" into the airways, the mucus produced in the airways collects these cells and is swallowed or expectorated by the patient. The sputum is thus examined for the presence of these cells, which will aid in diagnosing benign or malignant respiratory conditions.

More than one specimen may need to be collected or the culture may be negative. This is due to the irregularity of distribution of the cells in the sputum.

Laboratory Results

	Normal	Abnormal
Color	translucent	pink, yellow, green, bloody (rusty)
Consistency	viscous, tenacious	frothy, purulent, watery
Odor	absent	sweet, foul

Nursing Implications
Procedure for Collection/Storage of Specimen
1. It is imperative that the specimen is obtained before antimicrobial therapy is initiated, unless the examination is being done to evaluate the effectiveness of therapy.
2. Collect the specimen in an aseptic container. In patients who are unable to cough up sputum, the use of a heated, hypertonic saline solution may be administered by aerosol therapy to induce bronchial secretions. Sputum specimens can also be collected by aspiration from the tracheobronchial tree with trachial suctioning.
3. When tuberculosis is suspected, collect sputum specimens in the early morning on three or more consecutive days. Since the tuberculosis organism, *Mycobacterium tuberculosis*, is acid-fast, the test for tuberculosis in the sputum is called an AFB. AFB refers to the acid-fast bacillus.
4. Take the specimen to the laboratory as soon as possible after collection to assure that the organisms in the container are viable. If this is not possible, refrigerate the specimen.
5. Collect at least 1 tsp full of sputum for examination.
6. If the specimen is for culture and sensitivity, keep the container sterile.
7. Keep the container covered because the odor and sight of the specimen is offensive. This will also prevent the spread of microorganisms.

Possible Interfering Factors
Mixture with saliva or post-nasal secretions.

Patient Care
Observe the patient who is receiving an aerosol therapy for signs of bronchospasm.

Patient Education
1. Explain the procedure and its purpose to the patient.
2. Explain to the patient the importance of obtaining a specimen of sputum from the lungs.
3. Have the patient rinse out the mouth just prior to collecting the specimen to avoid collecting food particles. Instruct the patient to avoid the use of an antiseptic solution or toothpaste as these will decrease the viability of the organisms.

4. Instruct the patient to take several deep breaths and then cough forcibly.
5. Instruct the patient to furnish the specimen in the early morning when there is the most secretion in the tracheobronchial tree as a result of pooling during sleep.

Signed Consent

Not required

SWEAT TEST

This test measures the amount of sodium and chloride on the skin. In children suspected of having cystic fibrosis, the sodium and chloride levels will be elevated. (The sweat glands are not able to conserve salt.) Although the sodium and chloride levels excreted will be elevated in cystic fibrosis, the amount of sweat is not increased.

Normal Results
Dependent upon age and sex

Positive for Cystic Fibrosis

Chloride	60 mEq/dl
Sodium	10 mEq/dl greater than level of chloride

Nursing Implications
Procedure for Collection/Storage of Specimen

1. Wash area of skin to be tested with distilled water prior to the test. The back, chest, forehead, or forearm may be used.
2. Weigh ashless filter paper prior to placing it on the skin.
3. Place the weighed filter paper on the skin, cover with plastic, and secure with tape.
4. Apply thermal or pharmacologic stimuli as prescribed for the time span specified.
5. After the specified time has elapsed, remove the cover and weigh the filter paper.
6. Avoid handling the filter paper without instruments.

Possible Interfering Factors
Diet high in salt content

Patient Care

1. Assess the patient's recent intake of salt.
2. Determine the patient's tolerance to heat, which may aid in the diagnosis of cystic fibrosis.
3. Inquire as to recent illnesses, especially liver or renal disease.

Patient Education

If results are positive
1. Begin instruction in the care of the patient with cystic fibrosis
2. Refer the parents for genetic counseling

BIBLIOGRAPHY

Boyce B, King TKC: Blood-gas and acid-base concepts in respiratory care. Programmed instruction. Am J Nurs 76, No. 6:Pt 1:1–30, 1976

Burton GG, Gee GN, Hodgkin JE: Respiratory Care: A Guide to Clinical Practice. Philadelphia, JB Lippincott, 1977

Cameron TJ: Fiberoptic bronchoscopy. Am J Nurs 81, No. 8:1462–1464, 1981

Cherniack RM: Respiration in Health and Disease, 2nd ed. Philadelphia, WB Saunders, 1972

Cohen S: Pulmonary function tests in patient care. Programmed instruction. Am J Nurs 80, No. 6:1135–1161, 1980

Del Bueno DJ: A quick review on using blood-gas determinants. RN 41, 3:68–70, 1978

Fishbach FT: A Manual of Laboratory Diagnostic Tests. Philadelphia, JB Lippincott, 1980

Foley M et al: Pulmonary function screening tests in industry. Am J Nurs 77, No. 9:1480–1484, 1977

Hudgel DW, Madson LA: Acute and chronic asthma: A guide to intervention. Am J Nurs 80, No. 10:1791–1795, 1980

Kueppers F, Black LF: α_1—Antitrypsin and its deficiency. Am Rev Respir Dis 110:176–189, 1974

Lee CA, Stroot R, Schaper CA: What to do when acid-base problems hang in the balance. Nursing 75, Vol 5, No. 8:32-37, 1975

Marchisndo K: The very fine art of collecting culture specimens. Nursing 79, Vol 9, No. 4:34–43, 1979

Marici FN: The flexible fiberoptic bronchoscope. Am J Nurs 73, No. 10:1776–1778, 1973

Miller M, Sherman RL: Metabolic acid-base disorders, Part I. Programmed instruction. Am. J. Nurs 77, No. 10:Pt 1:1–32, 1977

Oakes A, Morrow H: Understanding blood gases. In Assessing Vital Functions Accurately, Nursing Skillbook, pp 69–78. Horsham, PA, Intermed Communications, 1977

Price SA, Wilson LM: Pathophysiology: Clinical Concepts of Disease Processes. New York, McGraw-Hill, 1978

Promisloff RA: A spirometry update. Nursing 78, Vol 8, No. 11:90, 92, 1978

Sackner MA: Bronchofiberoscopy. Am Rev Respir Dis 111:62–88, 1975

Shapiro BA, Harrison RA, Trout, CA: Clinical Application of Respiratory Care, 2nd ed. Chicago, Year Book, 1979

Shrake K: The abc's of abg's or how to interpret a blood gas value. Nursing 79, Vol. 9, No. 9:26–33, 1979

Tinker JH: Understanding chest x-rays. Am J Nurs 76, No. 1:54–58, 1976

Traver GA: The nurse's role in clinical testing of lung function. Nurs Clin North Am 9, No. 1:101–110, 1974

Wade JF: Respiratory Care Nursing, 2nd ed. St Louis, CV Mosby, 1977

Waldron MW: Oxygen transport. Am J Nurs 79, No. 2:272–275, 1979

West JB: Respiratory Physiology—the Essentials. Baltimore, Williams & Wilkins, 1974

Widmann FK: Clinical Interpretation of Laboratory Tests, 8th ed. Philadelphia, FA Davis, 1979

Worthington L: What those blood gases can tell you. RN 42, 10:23–27, 1979

5

Tests Related To Digestive Function

Barbara G. Mason

*(Formerly, Australian Antigen; Hepatitis Associated Antigen [HAA])

OVERVIEW OF PHYSIOLOGY AND PATHOPHYSIOLOGY

The function of the digestive system is to provide the body with a continual supply of fluids, nutrients, and electrolytes and to eliminate the waste residue of digestion. The system consists of a hollow muscular tube, called the gastrointestinal tract, that extends from the mouth to the anus and several accessory organs that contribute to the digestive process. The principal accessory organs which contribute to the digestive process are the salivary glands, the liver, the gallbladder, and the pancreas.

THE DIGESTIVE PROCESS

The digestive process is made up of several phases that include the following:

- the *mechanical breakdown* of large food particles into smaller ones
- the *secretion* of mucus, enzymes, electrolytes, hormones, and other *digestive juices*
- the orderly *mixing and movement* of food and secretions through the tract at a rate consistent with digestion and absorption
- the *digestion* of large complex substances into smaller simpler ones
- the *absorption* of the end products of digestion into the blood stream
- the *elimination* of undigested and unabsorbed food and other waste products

Dysfunction can occur anywhere in the digestive tract and can involve any of the phases of the digestive process. Factors that produce dysfunction are obstructions, infections, inflammations, trauma, neurologic disturbances, neoplasms, and emotional disturbances. Many dysfunctions are interrelated or evolve as complications of other dysfunctions.

MASTICATION

The first phase of the digestive process is the mechanical breakdown of large food particles into smaller ones. This occurs in the mouth and is termed mastication. Mastication is dependent upon the condition of the teeth, gums, and mucus membranes; the mobility of the tongue; and jaw articulation.

- The efficiency of mastication is altered by disorders such as dental caries, abscesses around the roots of the teeth, periodontal disease, ill-fitting dentures, and inflammations and neoplasms of the tongue and buccal mucosa.
- Interference with the functioning of the twelfth cranial (hypoglossal) nerve will mean interference with tongue mobility and the ability of the tongue to move food to the teeth for mechanical breakdown.
- Trauma to the jaw may cause limitation of movement. In cases such as fractures, the jaw may have to be completely immobilized by wiring.

SECRETIONS

Secretory glands are present throughout the gastrointestinal tract. All of the accessory organs participate in the secretory phase of the digestive process. The secretory glands have two primary functions: (1) to provide mucus for the lubrication and protection of the walls of the entire tract, and (2) to produce digestive juices that break down the foods for absorption.

The digestive juices consist primarily of enzymes and electrolytes and are secreted from the mouth to the ileus in response to the stimulation of food.

- Dysfunction during the secretory phase can result from under- or over-production of digestive juices and lubricants and from the ingestion of irritants.
- Hypersecretion may be the result of infectious diseases or local irritants.
- Faulty lubrication can affect motility and absorption.
- Irritants such as alcohol, salicylates, and foods contaminated with bacteria may cause damage to mucus-secreting cells.

MOTILITY

Motility in the gastrointestinal tract refers to the orderly mixing and movement of food and secretions at a rate that is consistent with digestion and absorption. There are two kinds of movement in the gastrointestinal tract: peristalsis and segmentation contraction. Peristalsis is a forward-propelling movement. Segmentation contraction is a mixing and churning movement that facilitates digestion and absorption.

- Disturbances in movement or motility can be related to mechanical obstruction, neuromuscular dysfunction, inflammation, diseases of the colonic mucosa, and emotional factors.

ABSORPTION

Most foods cannot be absorbed in their natural form through the walls of the gastrointestinal tract. They must be broken down into small simple chemical formations. This is the digestive phase. Various digestive enzymes and juices are secreted in the mouth, stomach, pancreas, liver, and small intestine (Table 5-1). They selectively react with the fats, proteins, and carbohydrates to break them down into simple nutrients.

- Disorders that prevent or interfere with digestive secretions, such as pancreatitis and stones in the common bile duct, lead to poor digestion and consequently to poor or no absorption.

Small Intestine

Ninety percent of absorption occurs in the small intestine. Millions of little projections called villi vastly increase the absorptive surface of the small intestine. Absorption occurs by active transport and diffusion through the gastrointestinal mucosa into the portal bloodstream.

- Dysfunction with absorption, or malabsorption, can be due to disease processes such as celiac disease and idiopathic steatorrhea that destroy or cause the villi to atrophy.
- Dysfunction may be due to disorders that require resections of portions of the small intestine as is sometimes necessary with chronic regional enteritis.

TABLE 5-I. **PRINCIPAL DIGESTIVE ENZYMES AND JUICES**

Source	Enzyme/Digestive Juice	Action
Salivary glands	Ptyalin (salivary amylase)	Starch digestion
Stomach	Hydrochloric acid	Starch digestion
	Pepsin	Protein digestion
	Intrinsic factor	Vitamin B_{12} absorption
	Gastric lipase	Fat digestion
Duodenum	Enterokinase	Trypsinogen digestion
Pancreas	Trypsin	Protein digestion
	Pancreatic lipase	Fat digestion
		Starch digestion
Liver	Bile and bile salts	Emulsifies fats, facilitates the absorption of fat-soluble vitamins A, D, E, and K
Small intestine	Enteric amylase	Starch digestion
	Maltase	Glucose production
	Lactase	Glucose galactose production
	Sucrase	Glucose fructose production
	Enteric lipase	Fat breakdown
	Aminopeptidase	Polypeptide breakdown
	Dipeptidase	Splits dipeptides into amino acids
	Nucleotidase	Splits nucleotides

- Malabsorption can also occur as a result of dysfunction in any of the other phases of the digestive process such as hypermotility, obstruction, and reduced enzyme secretions.
- Diarrhea, an obstructed bile duct, and reduced secretions of amylase, lipase, or trypsin can all be responsible for malabsorption.

Large Intestine

Absorption in the large intestine occurs in the proximal half of the colon. Water, sodium, and chloride are absorbed in this area.

- Dysfunction of the large intestine is usually related to motility in the form of atony, obstruction, hypermotility, and spasm.
- Some of these problems are directly related to infectious disease processes (diverticulitis, appendicitis), others to neuromuscular disorders (paralytic ileus), and others to immune system dysfunction (ulcerative colitis).

ACCESSORY ORGANS OF DIGESTION
LIVER

The accessory organs are most important in the digestive and metabolic processes of the body. The liver plays an essential role in the metabolism of carbohydrates, fats, and proteins after they are absorbed from the intestines.

- Carbohydrates are converted into glycogen, stored in the liver, and then released as glucose to meet body requirements.

- Protein metabolism involves synthesizing essential proteins such as albumin (a protein necessary for the maintenance of colloidal osmotic pressure). It also synthesizes prothrombin, fibrinogen, and other clotting factors. The liver begins the breakdown of amino acids, releasing ammonia and converting it into urea to be excreted by the kidneys.
- In fat metabolism, the liver is responsible for the production of phospholipids, lipoproteins, and cholesterol.

Two other major functions of the liver are the detoxification of endogenous and exogenous substances, and the metabolism of bilirubin and the production of bile. Bile is important for the emulsification of fats and the fat soluble vitamins so that they can be absorbed. The principal function of the gallbladder is the storage and concentration of bile.

PANCREAS

The pancreas is made up of two basic types of cells having entirely different functions.

The exocrine cells (acini) produce the principal components of pancreatic juice: lipase, amylase, and trypsin. These enzymes digest fats, starches, and proteins respectively. The pancreatic ducts join the common bile duct, and both empty into the duodenum where most of the digestion and absorption occur.

The other type of cells, the endocrine cells, are the alpha and beta cells of the islets of Langerhans. These cells produce the hormones insulin and glucagon. (For details related to this chapter, see page 230.)

DIAGNOSTIC FEATURES

The diagnosis of disorders of the digestive system is often very difficult because many disorders have similar signs and symptoms.

- Anorexia, nausea, vomiting, bowel changes such as constipation and diarrhea, and abdominal pain may occur with almost any dysfunction of the digestive system.
- These symptoms may also occur as manifestations of disorders in other systems. Patients with renal disease, congestive heart failure, rheumatoid arthritis, emphysema, diabetes, and various drug reactions may exhibit some of these same gastrointestinal signs and symptoms.
- Emotional disturbances such as anxiety states and alterations of mood often are expressed in terms of functional indigestion or functional disturbances of the bowels.

The diagnosis of most digestive disturbances cannot be made on the basis of the history and physical examination alone. The various laboratory and diagnostic tests have to be an essential component of the diagnostic procedures.

BLOOD TESTS
BROMSULPHALEIN (BSP) RETENTION TEST

Bromsulphalein test is a general screening test for overall liver function. It tests the ability of the liver cells to remove a dye that has been injected into the circulatory system and excreted into the bile. Removal of the dye depends on functioning liver cells, hepatic blood flow, and lack of obstruction. The test is useful for detecting early liver disease and for following the progress of known liver disease such as cirrhosis. Increased levels of retention are seen in liver cell damage, bile duct obstruction, acute and chronic hepatitis, cirrhosis of the liver, cancer of the liver, heart failure, shock, and acute hemorrhage. Bromsulphalein dye is very irritating to veins and can cause thrombophlebitis. The test should be used only when specifically indicated as being necessary.

Laboratory Results
Normal

5% retention in 45 min

Nursing Implications
Procedure for Collection/Storage of Specimen

1. The patient should be in a fasting state. The removal rate is more rapid after meals because of increased blood flow.
2. Dye should be given by a physician (5 mg/kg body weight) intravenously. Note the time when the injection is completed.
3. A venous sample should be taken from the opposite arm 45 min after injection of the dye.
4. Avoid hemolysis of the blood sample by not shaking the specimen.

Possible Interfering Factors

There are many drugs that may artificially elevate the results of this test, such as the following:

- acetohexamide (Dymelor)
- anabolic/androgenic steroids
- antifungal agents
- barbiturates
- cardiotonic glycosides (digoxin)
- aureomycin
- clofibrate (Atromid-S)
- dehydrocholic acid (Decholin)
- diphenylhydantoin (Dilantin)
- estrogens
- heparin
- indomethacin (Indocin)
- kanamycin (Kantrex)
- meperidine (Demerol)
- methadone
- methyldopa (Aldomet)
- MAO inhibitors

- morphine
- nicotinic acid
- oxacillin (Bactocill)
- phenazopyridine (Pyridium)
- phenolphthalein
- PSP (phenolsulfonphthalein)
- probenecid (Benemid)
- procainamide (Pronestyl)
- oral contraceptives
- radiopaque contrast media

Patient Care and Education

1. Explain the purpose of the test and procedure.
2. Weigh the patient before the test.
3. The patient must fast for 8 to 12 hr before the test and during the test. Water is permitted. Coffee and tea without sugar and cream may be given.
4. The patient should not receive any other dyes for 2 dy prior to the test.
5. The dye is very irritating to the tissues. The dye could cause sloughing. Check to see if any dye has leaked into the tissue. Observe local injection site for signs of thrombophlebitis.
6. BSP may be hazardous in patients with asthma.
7. Some patients may have an allergic reaction. Observe patients closely for urticaria, nausea, vomiting, dizziness, lowered blood pressure, tachycardia, and dyspnea.
8. BSP should be kept at room temperature.

Signed Consent

Not required

FLOCCULATION TESTS (Cephalin Flocculation—Thymol Turbidity)

Both of these tests are now being replaced by the more specific enzyme tests such as serum determinations of alkaline phosphatase, SGOT, and SGPT. In the cephalin flocculation test, serum is mixed with a colloidal suspension of cephalin and cholesterol. The blood of patients with liver disease will flocculate or clump the suspension. The thymol turbidity test mixes patient's serum with an aqueous solution of thymol. If liver damage is present, the solution will become turbid or cloudy. The tests are used to diagnose liver damage and to differentiate liver disease from biliary obstruction. With both tests, often it is possible to detect cell damage before jaundice appears. However, a positive test is not always conclusive for liver damage since rheumatoid arthritis and malaria also may show positive reactions. Other conditions that may show increased levels are the following:

- acute hepatitis
- multiple myeloma
- sarcoidosis
- coccidiosis
- tuberculosis
- lymphogranuloma venereum
- cirrhosis
- lupus erythematosus
- Hodgkin's disease
- subacute endocarditis
- histoplasmosis

Negative results may be seen with liver abscess and neoplasms.

Laboratory Results
Normal Range

Adults and children

    Thymol turbidity: 0–4 u

    Cephalin flocculation: 0–2 u (after 48 hr)

Nursing Implications
Procedure for Collection/Storage of Specimen

1. The ingestion of fatty foods may interfere with thymol turbidity and give a false positive reaction.
2. If the patient is taking methyldopa (Aldomet), either a false negative or a false positive reaction may be seen.
3. False positive reactions on the cephalin flocculation test may be seen with the following drugs:
   - ampicillin
   - kanamycin
   - oxacillin
   - penicillamine
   - adrenocorticotropic hormones
   - insulin
   - procainamide (Pronestyl)
   - tolbutamide (Orinase)
   - TAO (troliandomycin)
   - nicotinic acid
   - indomethacin (Indocin)
4. False negative reactions on the thymol turbidity test may be seen with patients receiving heparin therapy.

Patient Care and Education

1. There are no food or drink restrictions for the cephalin flocculation test.
2. For the thymol turbidity test, have the patient avoid foods and beverages containing fat (including milk) for at least 12 hr before the sample is drawn. The patient may have water.

Signed Consent

Not required

HEPATITIS B SURFACE ANTIGEN (HB$_s$Ag)*

This is the diagnostic test to detect the Hepatitis B surface antigen (HB$_s$Ag). A positive test for HB$_s$Ag indicates that the patient has Type B (serum) hepatitis. A negative test is really inconclusive since the antigen may have already disappeared (the antigen is only present in blood during the incubation period), or the patient may have Type A hepatitis. Persons with a positive test for HB$_s$Ag should never be permitted to donate blood or plasma.

Laboratory Results

Normal

Negative

Nursing Implications

Procedure for Collection/Storage of Specimen

1. Collect blood by venipuncture.
2. Send the specimen to the laboratory as soon as possible.
3. Handle all specimens as if they are contaminated. Take special precautions with needles and syringes. Use disposable equipment and place in proper containers.
4. The blood specimens should be prominently labeled as coming from a patient with suspected hepatitis so that adequate precautions can be observed.

Possible Interfering Factors

Patients with lymphocytic leukemia, chronic renal disease, renal dialysis, Down's syndrome, and Hodgkin's disease may have false positive results.

Patient Care and Education

1. There are no food or drink restrictions prior to or during the test.
2. If a patient is transfused with blood containing a positive HB$_s$Ag, he will have a 40% to 70% chance of contracting hepatitis B.
3. Patients undergoing hemodialysis have a particularly high incidence of hepatitis B because of the necessity of the frequent invasion of the patient's circulation.

---

*Formerly, Australian Antigen; Hepatitis Associated Antigen (HAA)

4. All blood donors should be properly screened using this test. Blood donations should not be accepted from alcoholics, narcotic addicts, or persons with questionable health status.
5. Use disposable needles for injections and intravenous administration and dispose in appropriate containers.
6. Observe patients for signs and symptoms of hepatitis (headache, fever, nausea, vomiting, and tenderness over liver. Jaundice and dark urine usually appear only in the later stages of the disease).

Signed Consent

Not required

HIPPURIC ACID TEST

This test is used to assess the detoxification functioning of the liver. Benzoic acid is converted to hippuric acid primarily in the liver and excreted in the urine. Sodium benzoate is administered either orally or intravenously and the urine analyzed for the amount of hippuric acid excreted in a given period of time. The intravenous method of administration is preferred over the oral method because it is independent of the rate of absorption from the intestinal tract and is a faster route of administration.

Laboratory Results

Normal Values

0.7 g/24 hr

Abnormal Values

less than 2.5 g/4 hr when sodium benzoate is given orally

less than 0.7 g/1 hr when sodium benzoate is given IV

Nursing Implications

Procedure for Collection/Storage of Specimen

Oral method

1. The patient is given a solution of 6 g sodium benzoate in 30 ml of water. Note the time of administration.
2. The patient fasts until the end of the test.
3. Discard the first urine sample and then collect all urine for the next 4 hr.
4. Keep the specimen cold during the collection hours.

Intravenous method

1. The patient should empty the bladder completely. Discard the urine.
2. Then give the patient a glass of water.
3. The patient is given 1.77 g of sodium benzoate in 20 ml distilled water over a period of 5 to 10 min. Note the time that the injection is completed.
4. A urine specimen should be collected 1 hr after the injection.

Possible Interfering Factors

None reported

Patient Care and Education
1. Explain to the patient the purpose of the test and the procedure.
2. Some physicians may prescribe a light breakfast of toast and coffee for the patient.

Signed Consent
Required

SERUM AMYLASE

Amylase is an enzyme that digests starches. This enzyme is secreted primarily by the pancreas and the salivary glands. It is also secreted in lesser amounts by the liver and the fallopian tubes. Elevation of serum amylase is most often associated with acute pancreatitis. Levels may also be elevated in such conditions as stones in the common bile duct, intestinal obstruction, and diseases of the salivary glands. Routine serum amylase tests may be prescribed the first few days after any surgery that may have injured the pancreas.

Increased levels of serum amylase may be seen in the following:

- acute pancreatitis
- chronic pancreatitis
- alcohol poisoning
- intestinal obstruction
- obstruction of the pancreatic ducts
- perforated peptic ulcer
- acute cholecystitis
- partial gastrectomy
- obstruction or inflammation of the salivary glands
- mumps
- ruptured tubal pregnancy
- advanced renal insufficiency

Decreased levels of serum amylase may be seen in:

- hepatitis
- cirrhosis of the liver
- marked destruction of the pancreas
- toxemia of pregnancy
- severe burns
- severe thyrotoxicosis

Laboratory Results
Normal Range

Adults and children (may be undetectable in the newborn)	60 to 200 Somogyi u/100 ml

Nursing Implications
Procedure for Collection/Storage of Specimen

1. Collect blood by venipuncture.
2. Caution should be taken not to contaminate the specimen by coughing, sneezing, or talking over the specimen since even tiny droplets of saliva can cause elevations of reading.
3. If the patient is having attacks of left upper quadrant pain, obtain a blood sample during an acute attack for possible diagnosis of pancreatitis.

Possible Interfering Factors

1. There is no special preparation of the patient.
2. Serum amylase examinations are usually followed in 6 to 10 hr by a urinary amylase determination. Amylase is excreted in the urine. Serum levels tend to remain high for a short period of time (sometimes only a few hours), while urine levels may be high for a week.
3. If the patient is suspected of having pancreatitis, serial determinations of serum will be done to evaluate the progress of the disease.
4. Acute alcohol ingestion or poisoning may cause an increased serum amylase.

Signed Consent
Not required

SERUM BILIRUBIN (van den Bergh Test)
Bilirubin is the end product of the breakdown of the red blood cell and its hemoglobin. Bilirubin is removed from the body by the liver and excreted in the bile through the biliary tract into the duodenum. Bilirubin is a heavily pigmented substance that does not have any active physiologic role in the body. It is important because the presence (or lack) of its pigment can indicate disorders of the liver, the biliary tract, and normal red blood cell destruction. Patients who have these disorders will have problems with bilirubin metabolism and excretion and thus will show such symptoms as clay-colored stools, mahogany-colored urine, and yellow skin.

Bilirubin exists in two forms in the body, indirect (or unconjugated) and direct (or conjugated). Indirect bilirubin is produced by the hemoglobin breakdown and immediately binds itself to plasma protein so that it can be absorbed by the liver. Once inside the liver, the bilirubin is removed from the protein and combines or conjugates with other substances that make it more soluble. The bilirubin is then known as conjugated or direct bilirubin. It is this soluble conjugated bilirubin that is excreted in the bile.

A routine examination will measure total bilirubin (a combination of direct and indirect). If this level is elevated, then a differentiation of the bilirubin will be made. An increase in indirect (unconjugated) bilirubin is more frequently associated with increased red blood cell destruction. An increase in direct (conjugated) bilirubin is most frequently associated with a blockage of the biliary tract and liver diseases. The van den Bergh test is the test done to differentiate direct (conjugated) from indirect (unconjugated) bilirubin.

Laboratory Results
Normal Range

Adults and children

Total:	0.2 to 0.9 mg/dl
Direct:	0.1 to 0.4 mg/dl
Indirect:	0.1 to 0.5 mg/dl

Neonate Normal Range

3 to 5 dy old

Total:	1 to 12 mg/dl
Direct:	0 to 1 mg/dl
Indirect:	1 to 11 mg/dl

Nursing Implications
Procedure for Collection/Storage of Specimen

1. Collect blood by venipuncture before breakfast. Use heel puncture technique for infants.
2. Protect the sample from bright light.
3. Avoid hemolysis by avoiding air bubbles and unnecessary shaking.
4. Store in the refrigerator if the specimen cannot be examined immediately.

Possible Interfering Factors

1. Serum bilirubin may be high if the patient has had food or drugs that give orange or yellow color to the serum.
2. There are many drugs that may temporarily modify liver function such as the following:
   - carotene
   - aspidium
   - erythromycin
   - caffeine
   - barbiturates
   - anabolic/androgenic steroids
   - gentamicin
   - indomethacin (Indocin)
   - isoniazid (INH)
   - sulfisoxazole
   - penicillin
   - lincomycin (Lincocin)
   - methyldopa (Aldomet)
   - phenothiazines (*i.e.,* Thorazine, Phenergan, Torecan, etc.)

- progestin–estrogen oral contraceptives
- vitamin A
- vitamin K

Patient Care and Education

1. Do not give patient foods with high orange or yellow content (carrots, pumpkin, squash, etc.) before the test.
2. Assess the patient for signs of hepatic disorders. Check for jaundice, edema, ascites, color of stools, dark urine, presence of bruising, pruritus, and general nutritional status.
3. Prepare the patient for further liver function tests and biliary tract procedures.
4. In newborns, signs of jaundice may indicate increased hemolysis of red blood cells or physiologic jaundice. If increased bilirubin levels reach a critical point, damage may be done to the central nervous system. The level of bilirubin is the deciding factor for performing exchange transfusions.

Signed Consent

Not required

SERUM CAROTENE

Serum carotene is used primarily as a screening test for fat malabsorption syndromes. Carotene is a fat-soluble vitamin found in green and yellow vegetables, especially carrots. It is a precursor of vitamin A. When fat is poorly absorbed, the absorption of the fat-soluble vitamins is impaired. A low carotene serum level is indicative of fat malabsorption syndrome. Diet will influence the amount of carotene in the blood.

Decreased levels of serum carotene may be found with the following:

- fat malabsorption syndrome
- steatorrhea
- celiac disease
- sprue
- obstructive jaundice
- cystic fibrosis
- hepatic disease
- poor dietary intake

Increased levels of serum carotene may be found with the following:

- myxedema
- diabetes mellitus
- hypothyroidism
- chronic nephritis
- hyperlipidemia
- excessive dietary intake, especially of carrots (hypervitaminosis A)

Laboratory Results
Normal Range

Adults	50 to 300 mcg/100 ml
Infants up to 2 yr	0 to 40 mcg/100 ml
Children 2 yr and over	40 to 130 mcg/100 ml

Nursing Implications
Procedure for Collection/Storage of Specimen

1. Collect blood by venipuncture.
2. Some physicians may want patient to fast.
3. Protect the sample from light.

Possible Interfering Factors

1. Mineral oil interferes with carotene absorption.
2. A fat-free diet eliminates 90% absorption of carotene.

Patient Care and Education

1. Food and fluid restrictions will depend on the physician's orders. The test may be done to determine carotene levels with a diet high in carotene, or it may be done to determine carotene levels without added dietary carotene. If carotene is restricted, the patient should be fasting and should receive no vitamin A or foods containing vitamin A or carotene for 24 to 48 hr prior to testing.
2. The patient may have water.

SERUM FOLIC ACID

Folic acid is one of the B group vitamins necessary for DNA and red blood cell production and maturation. It is synthesized by bacteria in the small intestine into compounds known as folates and stored in the liver. Since only small amounts of folate can be stored, folic acid deficiency usually accompanies malnutrition. The major dietary sources of folic acid are green leafy vegetables, fruits, eggs, milk, and liver. In addition to dietary inadequacies, folic acid deficiencies may be caused by excessive use due to hemolytic disorders and carcinomas, drugs which are folic acid antagonists, liver disease, and intestinal malabsorption. Intestinal malabsorption may be caused by diseases such as sprue, celiac disease, and idiopathic steatorrhea.

Laboratory Results
Normal Range

Adults and children   5 to 21 ng/ml

Nursing Implications
Procedure for Collection/Storage of Specimen
Collect the blood by venipuncture (10 ml).

Possible Interfering Factors

Drugs that may decrease values (folic acid antagonists) are the following:

- phenytoin sodium (Dilantin)
- estrogens
- oral contraceptives
- phenobarbital
- para-aminosalicylic acid (PAS)
- ampicillin
- chloramphenicol (Chloromycetin)
- erythromycin
- lincomycin
- penicillin
- tetracycline

Patient Care and Education

1. There are no food or drink restrictions for the test.
2. Elderly persons and others who do not eat fresh uncooked vegetables and fruits for whatever reason are more susceptible to folic acid deficiency.
3. Infants fed on milk diets almost exclusively are very susceptible to folic acid deficiency.
4. Folic acid requirements are increased in pregnancy (especially during the last trimester) and in patients with hemolytic anemias.
5. Patients receiving prolonged intravenous feeding or hyperalimentation also are very susceptible and should be given vitamin supplements.

Signed Consent

Not required

SERUM GASTRIN

Gastrin is a hormone secreted by the mucosa of the pyloric antrum of the stomach. It can also be produced by nonbeta cell tumors of the pancreas. In the stomach, gastrin is released in response to vagal stimulation by food substances such as protein and alcohol, the mechanical distention of the antrum, and alkaline pH. Gastrin is absorbed into the blood stream and carried back to the gastric glands where it acts as the primary stimulus for gastric acid secretions. Increased serum gastrin levels usually result in increased gastric acid secretions. A feedback inhibition mechanism occurs when the gastric acid secretions reach a pH of 2. The increased gastric acidity (mainly hydrochloric acid) inhibits the production of gastrin, thus protecting the stomach against further excessive acid secretions.

Serum gastrin levels will be slightly increased with gastric and duodenal ulcers and with gastric carcinoma. There is a marked increase of serum gastrin in patients with pernicious anemia owing to the lack of production of hydrochloric acid in the stomach. There is also a marked increase in patients with Zollinger–Ellison syndrome because gastrin is being secreted by an adenoma of the pancreas.

Laboratory Results
Normal Range

Fasting	50 to 155 pg gastrin/ml serum
Postprandial	80 to 170 pg gastrin/ml serum

Abnormal Range

500 pg gastrin/ml serum or above

Nursing Implications
Procedure for Collection/Storage of Specimen
1. The patient should be fasting. The amount of secretion will vary with stimulus by food.
2. Collect the blood by venipuncture (about 10 ml).
3. Keep the specimen cold and send it immediately to the laboratory.

Possible Interfering Factors

The intravenous infusions of calcium and secretin may cause increases in serum gastrin levels. Patients with Zollinger-Ellison syndrome will show definite increases with both of these substances.

Patient Care

Patients with increased serum gastrin levels may have to undergo further laboratory tests for gastric acid analysis. These are done to assess the patient's ability to secrete acid and to determine that amount.

Patient Education

The patient should be instructed to fast for 12 to 14 hr before the specimen is drawn. The patient may have water.

Signed Consent
Not required

SERUM IRON

Levels of serum iron are checked to make more definitive diagnoses of iron deficiency. Increased serum iron levels occur when there is an excessive intake of iron, when there is impairment in utilization, such as might be encountered with liver damage, or if there is an abnormal destruction of red blood cells. Decreased serum iron levels may occur when dietary intake of iron is low, when absorption is impaired, or when there is blood loss.

Iron is carried in the serum in combination with a protein called transferrin. About 30% of the total capacity of transferrin is bound to iron. The measurement of the capacity of transferrin to bind with iron is usually made in conjunction with the serum iron test. This test is called the total iron-binding capacity (TIBC). When the body has low serum iron levels, the TIBC is increased because there are more transferrin sites available for binding. When serum iron levels are high, the TIBC is decreased because the capacity of transferrin to bind any additional iron becomes saturated.

Serum iron may be increased with the following:

- acute liver disease
- acute viral hepatitis
- idiopathic hemochromatosis (excess iron deposition in the liver and elsewhere)
- excessive iron intake (blood transfusions, iron therapy)
- hemolytic anemias
- pyridoxine deficiency anemia
- thalassemia
- pernicious anemia
- aplastic anemia

Serum iron may be decreased with the following:

- iron-deficiency anemia
- acute and chronic blood loss
- chronic kidney disease
- chronic infections or diseases
- rheumatoid arthritis

Laboratory Results
Normal Range

Serum iron		
	Males	80 to 160 mcg/dl
	Females	50 to 150 mcg/dl
	Children	55 to 185 mcg/dl
	At birth	110 to 270 mcg/dl

Total iron-binding capacity (TIBC) 250 to 450 mcg/dl—adults and children

Nursing Implications
Procedure for Collection/Storage of Specimen

1. The blood sample is drawn by venipuncture (10 ml).
2. The equipment (including syringes) must be chemically clean.
3. Prevent hemolysis by not shaking specimen or by not using a container that is chilled.

Possible Interfering Factors

1. Drugs causing increased serum iron values are the following:
    - chloramphenicol (Chloromycetin)

- fluorides
- iron dextran complex
- oxalate
- oral contraceptives

2. Drugs causing decreased serum iron values are the following:
   - ACTH
   - hydroxyurea (Hydrea)
   - steroids

3. Serum iron may be decreased during the last half of pregnancy.
4. Transferrin may be elevated in children 2½ to 10 yr of age and in pregnant women during the third trimester.
5. A patient who has had recent treatment for anemia with vitamin B_{12} or folic acid may have low serum iron levels.
6. Hemolysis of samples may produce a falsely increased reading.

Patient Care and Education

1. There are no food or drink restrictions for this test.
2. Low serum iron levels in the adult generally indicate that blood has been lost from the body by hemorrhage or excessive menstruation. Chronic diarrhea, malabsorption syndromes such as celiac disease, the high intake of cereal products with the low intake of animal protein, and clay-eating may be causes of low serum iron in children.
3. The patient will probably have to be prepared for an examination of the bone marrow plus diagnostic procedures commonly employed in the study of gastrointestinal bleeding (x-rays, stool examinations, endoscopies).
4. Oral or parenteral iron preparations usually are administered to patients with low serum iron. Also, patients will need to be instructed to include in their diet foods high in iron content such as liver, lean red meats, and green leafy vegetables.

SERUM LIPASE

Lipase is an enzyme secreted by the pancreas. Its function is to change fats to fatty acid and glycerol. Lipase will appear in the bloodstream following damage to the pancreas or blockage of the pancreatic ducts. Serum lipase and serum amylase levels rise at the same rate, but serum lipase levels can remain elevated 7 to 14 days after amylase levels return to normal. The serum sample is incubated with an olive oil substrate for 24 hours. The results of the test are expressed in terms of the amount of sodium hydroxide (NaOH) required to neutralize the fatty acids produced by the action of the lipase in the serum on the olive oil.

Increased lipase levels are associated with:

- pancreatitis
- obstruction of the pancreatic duct
- severe renal disease

- perforated ulcer
- intestinal obstruction
- pancreatic carcinoma
- acute cholecystitis
- cirrhosis
- infectious hepatitis

  Lipase levels are normal in mumps.

Laboratory Results
Normal Range

1.0 to 1.5 u/ml

Nursing Implications
Procedure for Collection/Storage of Specimen

1. The patient should be fasting overnight, but may drink water. If it is not possible to obtain a fasting specimen, the nurse should note when the sample was drawn in relation to the patient's last meal.
2. Collect venous blood.
3. The sample requires 24 hr incubation in oil.

Possible Interfering Factors

1. Myocholine, urecholine, codeine, morphine, and meperidine (Demerol) may elevate lipase levels into abnormal range if taken within 24 hr before sample is drawn.
2. Elevation of lipase may not occur until 24 to 36 hr after the onset of illness.

Patient Care and Education
1. Explain the test and the procedure to the patient.
2. The patient should be fasting overnight.
3. Increased lipase usually is associated with obstruction of the pancreatic ducts and decreased calcium levels. Watch for signs of tetany including muscular twitching, jerking, and irritability.

Signed Consent
Not required

SERUM VITAMIN B$_{12}$
Two of the factors necessary for the normal maturation of red blood cells are the intrinsic factor (a mucoprotein substance produced by the gastric mucosa) and the extrinsic factor (vitamin B$_{12}$). Vitamin B$_{12}$ cannot be absorbed into the blood stream without the intrinsic factor. Vitamin B$_{12}$ is absorbed at the distal portion of the ileum and is stored in high concentrations in the liver. Deficiencies of vitamin B$_{12}$ may be found in patients who have inadequate absorption owing to the lack of intrinsic factor, malabsorption as a result of disorders of the small bowel, inadequate dietary intake, and met-

abolic disturbances that accompany hyperthyroidism, pregnancy, and certain malignancies.

Decreased levels of serum vitamin B_{12} may occur in the following:

- pernicious anemia
- total or partial gastrectomy
- ileal resection
- malabsorption (sprue, celiac disease, regional ileitis)
- alcoholism
- strict vegetarianism
- fish tapeworm infestation
- pregnancy

Increased levels of serum vitamin B_{12} may occur in the following:

- liver diseases (hepatitis, cirrhosis)
- leukemia
- leukocytosis
- polycythemia vera

Laboratory Results
Normal Range

Adults and children   130 to 785 pg/ml

Nursing Implications
Procedure for Collection/Storage of Specimen

Collect the blood by venipuncture (10 ml).

Possible Interfering Factors

None reported

Patient Care and Education
1. There are no food or drink restrictions for this test.
2. In addition to the blood studies, the patient should be prepared for additional diagnostic procedures for differential diagnosis. Possible examinations would include bone marrow aspiration, gastric analysis, Schilling test, and the therapeutic trial of injections of vitamin B_{12}.

Signed Consent
Not required

STOOL TESTS
COLLECTION OF STOOL SPECIMEN FOR FECAL ANALYSIS

The examination of feces is very important in diagnosing diseases and disorders of the gastrointestinal tract. Fecal analysis is usually indicated for patients with diarrhea, constipation, bleeding, or any unusual or persistent abdominal complaints. Specimens are usually examined macroscopically and microscopically for blood, mucus, pus, tissue fragments, food residue, bacteria, and parasites. Specimens also may be examined chemically for such substances as fat, starch, and urobilinogen.

Laboratory Results
Normal Range

Adults and children

25% to 30% solids

70% to 75% water

color—brown

pH 6.8 to 7.3

Contents include calcium, phosphate, carbohydrates, fat, nitrogen, protein, and small amounts of undigested food.

Nursing Implications
Procedure for Collection/Storage of Specimen

1. Feces should be collected in a dry, clean container, either a bedpan or a wide-mouth laboratory container. A plastic container is best so that the specimen does not become dehydrated.
2. The specimen should be free from urine. Do not use the stool that has been deposited in the toilet.
3. A fresh stool is the best specimen. If the stool cannot be examined immediately, place it in the refrigerator. Stools to be examined for parasites should be kept warm. For best results send all stools to the laboratory as soon as they are collected. Stools darken upon standing.
4. Diarrheal stools may be used as specimens.
5. The entire stool should be collected even though only a small amount may be needed for analysis. Stools need to be inspected macroscopically for amount, consistency, color, and odor as well as microscopically for microorganisms.
6. Label all stools with the patient's name, date, and time of collection and the reason for testing.

Possible Interfering Factors

1. Ingestion of meat may interfere with some tests by giving a false positive for occult blood.
2. Ingestion of barium, bismuth, and oil will alter the findings.
3. Some antibiotics will alter the findings. If possible, collect the sample before antibiotic therapy is started.
4. The color of the stool may be influenced by diet, food dyes, and drugs:
   - green—spinach, chlorophyll, indomethacin (Indocin)
   - greenish black—iron
   - black—charcoal, licorice, iron, bismuth
   - dark grey—bismuth

- dark brown—chocolate, cocoa, large quantities of meat
- light-colored—milk, infant's formula, small amounts of meat
- light yellow-brown—milk, infant's formula
- dark red—beets, bromsulphalein
- white or white speckled—antacids, barium

Patient Care and Education

1. Explain the purpose of the test and the procedure for collection to the patient. Tell the patient not to use toilet paper to collect the stool; most toilet papers contain bismuth which may interfere with the test.
2. Note the color, odor, consistency, shape, size, and presence of any unusual material in the feces. Unusual findings may be:

   Color
   - black tarry stools (upper GI bleeding)
   - bright red bleeding (ruptured hemorrhoids or anal disorders; hemorrhaging anywhere in GI tract)
   - clay-colored (bile obstruction)

   Odor
   - varies with pH of stool. pH is dependent primarily on bacterial fermentation and putrefaction. It may be affected also by ingestion of meat and vegetables.
   - pungent, sour smelling (increased protein content)
   - decreased odor with use of antibiotics

   Consistency
   - mucus mixed with stool (small intestinal inflammation/irritable bowel)
   - mucus on exterior of stool (large intestinal inflammation)
   - excessively hard (delayed transit time, constipation)
   - pus (rectal–anal fistulas and abscesses, chronic ulcerative colitis)

   Size and shape
   - pellets (chronic constipation, intestinal spasms)
   - ribbon or pencil-shaped (spastic colon or low stricture)
   - large caliber (dilatation of the colon, constipation)

3. If bleeding occurs, note if it is bright or dark and where the blood was found (toilet tissue, underwear, stool, toilet bowl). Does the patient complain of pain and is the pain relieved with the bowel movement?
4. Note any abnormal sensations associated with bowel movements, such as crawling, burning, and itching.
5. Note any change in normal bowel patterns, such as a change in color, consistency, and frequency of occurrence, and ask the patient to report any change.

Signed Consent

Not required

BLOOD IN STOOL

Blood in the feces may be an indication of serious bleeding anywhere in the gastrointestinal tract. Blood coming from lesions in the lower colon, rectum, or anus will be bright red and easily recognized. Blood coming from the area of the stomach may be digested and give the stool a black, tarry appearance (melena). Severe hemorrhaging anywhere along the GI tract can cause bright red stools (hematochezia). In many instances, blood seeping from the stomach or small intestines may be occult, meaning that it will not be seen upon inspection. Tests that determine occult blood in the feces use chemicals that react with the hemoglobin content and cause a color change. The most common tests are done using guaiac, benzidine, and orthotoluidine (Occultest).

Laboratory Results

Normal

Negative for blood

Nursing Implications

Procedure for Collection/Storage of Specimen

1. Usually any random sample may be used. Only a small amount is needed for testing.
2. The specimen does not need to be kept warm or examined immediately.
3. The Occultest and benzidine tests require that the patient be on a meat-free diet. The guaiac test does not require this.

Possible Interfering Factors

1. The patient may have a false positive reaction for occult blood if any of the following has been ingested:
   - medications containing iron
   - large quantities of meat, poultry, fish
   - bromides
   - colchicine
   - iodides
2. Some people on meat-free diets will show a positive test if their gums bleed when brushing their teeth.
3. The patient may have a false negative result if the patient has taken vitamin C in quantities greater than 500 mg/dy.

Patient Care and Education

1. Explain the purpose of the test and the procedure for collection to the patient.
2. When using the Occultest and benzidene tests, the patient may be placed on a meat-free diet for 3 dy prior to the test because the meat may give a false positive result. Poultry and fish should also be omitted from the diet.
3. Mark the lab requisitions if the patient has recently ingested bismuth, barium, mineral oil, laxatives, iron, or charcoal.

4. The nurse should note the color, consistency, odor, shape, and size of the bowel movements as well as look for the presence of mucus and blood in the stool. Note if the blood is bright red or dark colored and where it is found (toilet tissue, underwear, stool, toilet bowl).

Signed Consent

Not required

STOOL CULTURES FOR BACTERIA AND VIRUSES

Stool cultures are usually indicated whenever a patient has diarrhea or is suspected of having dysentery. Cultures are done to identify bacteria, viruses, and parasites. Normally there are approximately 50 different varieties of bacteria in the stool including several pathogenic varieties.

Laboratory Results

Varies with type of bacteria

Nursing Implications

Procedure for Collection/Storage of Specimen

1. Virus cultures—stools should be tested almost immediately after collection. If there is a delay, keep the specimen cold or frozen until it can be transported to the laboratory.
2. Bacterial cultures—stools should be examined immediately.
3. If the patient has diarrheal stools, dip a large cotton swab in the specimen and suspend the swab in a sterile test tube for delivery to the lab. Be sure to include any purulent appearing areas.
4. Specimens may also be collected on swabs at proctoscopy.
5. Swabs should be suspended in sterile test tubes with culture media. Take precautions to see that the swab does not touch the media. The purpose of the media is to provide moisture in the tube so that the swab will not dry out before arriving at the laboratory.
6. Usually at least three cultures are done if the clinical signs and symptoms of the patient indicates a bacterial involvement and the first two cultures were negative.
7. Indicate the suspected disease or pathogen on the specimen container. This will facilitate the use of the correct culture media once the specimen is in the laboratory.

Possible Interfering Factors

Antibiotics and the sulfonamides may give false negative reactions.

Patient Care and Education

1. Explain the purpose of the test and the procedure for collection to the patient.
2. If a positive diagnosis of an infectious disease is made, persons who have been in contact with the patient should have their stools tested. Three negative stool cultures will indicate the absence of disease. This precautionary measure will help prevent the spread of the infection.

Signed Consent

Not required

EXAMINATIONS FOR OVA AND PARASITES

Stool samples are collected and examined microscopically for identification of the presence of ova and parasites. Loose diarrheal stools are more likely to contain the trophozite stage of the intestinal amoebas and flagellates. Well-formed or semi-formed stools usually harbor the ova or cystic forms of parasites. Stools containing hookworm ova are usually positive for occult blood.

Laboratory Results

Normal

Adults and children a large percentage of the population normally harbors harmless parasites such as *Entamoeba coli* and certain flagellates

Nursing Implications

Procedure for Collection/Storage of Specimen

1. The sample should be taken to the laboratory as soon as the sample is collected. Collect the specimen in a plastic container to prevent dehydration.
2. Specimens to be examined for mobile trophozites should be kept at body temperature. The specimen should be examined within 30 min after collection while the organisms are still in an active stage.
3. Examinations for ova or cysts can be done on cold stools.
4. Proctoscopic scrapings or aspirations can be used to test for trophozites.
5. When purgatives are given for tapeworms, the treatment is not complete until the head (scolex) of the parasite is eliminated in the stool. All stools must be kept and examined until the scolex is identified as having been passed in the stool.
6. The cellophane tape test is used for pinworms (enterobiasis). The method of collection is as follows:
   a. Blot a strip of clear cellophane tape around the anal area to pick up the eggs. Then spread the tape on a glass slide and send to the laboratory.
   b. The test should be done in the morning before the patient has bathed or defecated—preferably before getting out of bed.
   c. In children, eggs can often be obtained from underneath the fingernails.
   d. The examination may need to be repeated on consecutive days.

Possible Interfering Factors

Barium, bismuth, mineral oil, and antibiotics may interfere with the results.

Patient Care and Education

1. There are no food or drink restrictions prior to the collection of the specimen.
2. Never give oily cathartics prior to the collection of the specimen.
3. Note any abnormal sensations associated with bowel movements such as crawling, burning, itching.
4. Emphasize measures of personal cleanliness such as
   - Wash hands after using the toilet and before eating.
   - Cut fingernails short (particularly children with pinworms).
   - Keep tight fitting cotton pants on infected children.
   - See that an infected person sleeps alone.
   - Handle bedding and underclothing carefully to prevent spread of infection.
5. Patients with positive reports of salmonella or shigella should be placed on enteric isolation if confined to the hospital.

Signed Consent

Not required

FECAL FAT

This test is one of the best screening tests for determining a malabsorption syndrome. Stool specimens are collected to see if fat is being digested. If the patient has pancreatic disease with a deficiency of the enzyme lipase or a biliary tract obstruction, sprue, or some other intestinal malabsorption condition, fat will not be digested. A condition known as steatorrhea or excess fat in the stools will exist. The stool will be frothy, foul smelling, grayish, and greasy. There will also be a great deal of foul-smelling flatus. The test consists of collecting stool specimens over a 3 dy period, drying the specimen, extracting the fat with an evaporative solvent, and then weighing the resultant fat.

Laboratory Results

Normal Range

Adults and children over 2 yr of age

With a daily intake of 75 to 100 g of fat, the 24 hr fecal fat content should be less than 6 g. Six or more of fat is evidence of steatorrhea.

Infants under 2 yrs of age

Fecal fat should be less than 15% of dietary fat intake.

Nursing Implications

Procedure for Collection/Storage of Specimen

1. Collect all of the stool specimens for 3 dy. Collect the entire stool and label according to the day.
2. The stool collection and examination should be done prior to barium x-ray examination.
3. Weigh the specimen container prior to collection of the stool.

Possible Interfering Factors

1. Ingestion of barium will make the test results invalid for 48 hr.
2. Mineral oil, laxatives, and enemas will interfere with testing and should not be administered.

Patient Care and Education

1. The patient may be placed either on a normal (75 to 100 g fat) diet, or a fat-restricted diet for 2 or 3 dy prior to collection. The diet will vary according to what the physician wants to analyze. Then stools should be collected for the next 3 dy.
2. Explain the purpose of the test and the procedure for the collection of the stool to the patient.
3. Avoid giving the patient castor oil or laxatives that would affect gastric motility and the dietary intake of fats.
4. Note the color, consistency, odor, and the size of the stool specimens.

Signed Consent

Not required

FECAL UROBILINOGEN

Fecal urobilinogen is responsible for giving the stool its brown color. Fecal urobilinogen is produced in the small intestine by the action of intestinal bacteria on the bilirubin in the bile. Increased amounts of fecal urobilinogen in the stool are found when there is an increased hemolysis of red blood cells. Decreased amounts of fecal urobilinogen in the stool are indicative of obstructive biliary disease. Stools will be clay colored with decreased levels of urobilinogens.

Laboratory Results

Normal Range

75 to 350 mg urobilinogen/100 g of stool

Nursing Implications

Procedure for Collection/Storage of Specimen

Feces should be collected according to the same procedure as outlined for fecal analysis. (For details related to this test, see page 180.)

Possible Interfering Factors

The test results may be altered by antibiotics and intestinal antibacterials such as sulfathalidine that interfere with the growth of the bacteria necessary for the production of urobilinogen.

Patient Care and Education

1. Explain the purpose of the test and the procedure for collection to the patient.
2. There are no food or drink restrictions prior to the test.
3. Note the color, odor, consistency, and the size of the bowel movements.

Signed Consent

Not required

URINE TESTS
URINE AMYLASE

Amylase is an enzyme that digests starch. It is produced in the pancreas, liver, salivary glands, and fallopian tubes. It is excreted in small amounts in the urine. Elevated levels of urine amylase are associated with acute pancreatitis, choledocholithiasis, and inflammations of the salivary glands. High serum levels cause increased excretion of amylase in the urine. The urine amylase test is more sensitive than the serum amylase test. The urine amylase levels remain high for about a week after the serum amylase levels have returned to normal.

Laboratory Results

Normal

Adults and children   under 260 Somogyi u/hr

Nursing Implications

Procedure for Collection/Storage of Specimen

1. A timed collection is required. Some institutions use 2-hr specimens; some use 12- or 24-hr specimens. A 2-hr specimen is usually collected.
2. Indicate to the laboratory the exact times of the beginning and the end of the collection period. The beginning of the collection period is the time when the patient empties his bladder and the specimen is discarded. All subsequent specimens are saved.
3. All urine is refrigerated or kept on ice until the entire specimen is sent to the lab.

Possible Interfering Factors

1. If the specimen is contaminated by fluorides, there may be a decrease in levels of urine amylase.
2. An increase in urine amylase levels may occur in patients with mumps, diseases of the salivary glands and ducts, and with some intestinal obstructions.
3. Drugs that might produce an elevation of urinary amylase are the following:
   - urecholine
   - codeine
   - meperidine
   - morphine
   - other narcotic drugs
   - ethyl and methyl alcohol in large amounts

Patient Care and Education

1. Instruct the patient about the purpose of the test and the procedure.
2. There are no food or drink restrictions prior to or during the test.
3. Encourage the patient to drink fluids during the test.

Signed Consent

Not required

URINE BILIRUBIN AND UROBILINOGEN

Bilirubin should not be present in urine. It is usually found in patients with jaundice and indicates the presence of liver cell disease or hepatic–biliary obstruction. Only conjugated or direct bilirubin will be found in the urine, as free or indirect bilirubin is not water soluble. Urinary bilirubin will be found whenever a disease process increases the amount of conjugated or direct bilirubin in the bloodstream. Bilirubin will give urine a brown or dark yellow color.

Normally there is a small amount of urobilinogen in the urine. Urobilinogen is produced in the intestinal tract by the action of enteric bacteria on bile. Most of the urobilinogen is excreted in the feces, but small amounts are returned to the circulation and excreted by the kidneys in the urine. Tests for urinary bilirubin and urobilinogen help to differentiate jaundice owing to liver cell damage or biliary tract obstruction from hemolytic jaundice.

Increased levels of urinary urobilinogen may be seen in the following:

- acute infectious and toxic hepatitis
- hemolytic jaundice and anemia
- cirrhosis
- pulmonary infarct
- pernicious anemia
- malaria
- congestive heart failure
- infectious mononucleosis

Decreased or absent levels of urinary urobilinogen may be found with the following:

- cholelithiasis
- severe inflammatory diseases
- cancer of the head of the pancreas
- severe diarrhea
- renal insufficiency

Laboratory Results

Normal Range

Adults and children	Bilirubin	none
Adults	Urobilinogen	0 to 4 mg/24 hr
Children	Urobilinogen	3 mg/24 hr

Nursing Implications

Procedure for Collection/Storage of Specimen

1. The test must be performed on a fresh urine sample.
2. Be sure to note the total time during which the sample is collected.

3. Make sure the total specimen is sent to the lab, since the volume of the specimen is critical in determining the accurate test results.
4. Have the patient empty the bladder at 2 PM and discard the sample. At 4 PM have the patient void again. Send this specimen to the lab. If the patient voids before 4 PM, send this specimen to the lab and cancel the 4 PM collection.
5. The specimen should be taken to the lab without delay. This is necessary because the bacteria in the urine will act on the urobilinogen, causing it to be oxidized into urobilin.
6. The sample should be kept in a brown bottle to protect it from light.
7. Sometimes the urine sample is strip tested (similar to Testape). However, this test is not accurate enough to detect decreases or absence of urobilinogen. If the urine is strip tested, follow manufacturer's directions.

Possible Interfering Factors

1. The test results may be altered by antibiotics and intestinal antibacterials such as sulfathalidine. These drugs inhibit the growth of bacteria in the intestinal tract and therefore interfere with the production of urobilinogen in the intestines.
2. False elevations may occur if the patient has recently received the following:
   • bromsulphalein (BSP)
   • chlorpromazine (Thorazine)
   • sulfonamides
   • P-aminosalicylic acid (PAS)
   • bananas
   • cascara
   • diatrizoate sodium (Hypaque)
   • procaine (Novocaine)
   • phenazopyridine (Pyridium)

Patient Care and Education
1. There are no food or drink restrictions prior to or during the test.
2. Bilirubin can be grossly detected in the urine by shaking the specimen and noting if yellow foam occurs.

Signed Consent
Not required

DIAGNOSTIC TESTS
BARIUM ENEMA

The barium enema uses x-ray and fluoroscope to visualize the entire large intestine. The patient is given an enema of barium sulfate solution which makes the colon radiopaque. This procedure is used for diagnosing the presence of malignancies, benign polyp growths, diverticulosis, obstructions, and ulcerative colitis. The preparation may be too exhausting for acutely ill patients.

Normal Results

Normal anatomical appearance of the large intestine

Nursing Implications

Preprocedure

1. Explain the purpose of the test and procedure. Inform the patient that an enema of barium sulfate will be given and that the patient will have to try to hold the enema solution until films are made. Many patients find this procedure very embarrassing, especially if they cannot retain the solution. Relieve the patient's anxiety with discussion and reassurance.
2. Give the patient a clear liquid supper. Hold food and fluids after midnight until the study is completed. Observe elderly or debilitated patients for adverse effects of the enemas, such as exhaustion or dehydration.
3. Laxatives or cathartics are given the day before, then enemas until a clear return is obtained. If there is feces or a large amount of gas in the large intestine at the time of the examination the procedure may have to be repeated.
4. Barium studies interfere with many other studies. Check to make sure that this study does not interfere with other studies.

During the Procedure

1. The patient is in the lateral recumbent position with a catheter in the rectum. Administer the barium slowly by means of gravity, while the radiologist observes the filling of the colon on the fluoroscope. The patient is rotated into various positions so that all flexures and loops of the colon may be visualized.
2. When the fluoroscopic examination is completed, films are made of the filled colon.
3. Assist the patient to the bathroom to evacuate the barium sulfate solution.
4. A double contrast examination may follow the above procedure. After the evacuation of the barium sulfate, air is injected into the colon. The air is outlined on x-ray because the mucosa of the colon retains a coating of barium. This procedure is used to visualize polyps.

Postprocedure

1. Provide food and fluids after the test. Encourage fluids as the extensive preparation may have produced dehydration.
2. Allow the patient to rest. This examination is the most fatiguing of all the radiographic studies. The patient is weak, thirsty, and tired.
3. Cleansing enemas or cathartics may be prescribed because of the danger of impaction. Inform the patient to expect white stools.

4. If no enemas or cathartics are given, inform the patient to expect white stools for 24 to 72 hr after the test.
5. Observe and chart the passing of barium.

Signed Consent

Not required

BARIUM SWALLOW

The radiographic examination of the esophagus is usually done as a part of the procedure known as the upper gastrointestinal series. However, it may be done as a separate procedure if only the function and structure of the esophagus is to be evaluated. The barium swallow is used to visualize such conditions as hiatal hernia, esophageal strictures or spasms, diverticula, malignant growths, gastroesophageal reflux, and swallowed foreign bodies.

Normal Results

Normal function and structure of the esophagus

Nursing Implications

Preprocedure

1. Explain the procedure to the patient in terms appropriate to the patient. Answer any questions. The procedure is not uncomfortable.
2. Hold food and fluids from midnight until the exam is completed.
3. Barium studies interfere with results of many other studies. Check to make sure that the barium swallow is sequenced so it will not interfere with other studies.

During the Procedure

1. Take the patient to the radiology department. The patient is placed on a tilt table. The patient assumes an upright standing position behind a fluoroscopic screen.
2. Explain to the patient that he will be asked to swallow several mouthfuls of barium sulfate. Barium sulfate solution usually has a consistency of malted milk, and is flavored with either strawberry or chocolate.
3. The patient is rotated on the table to various degrees as films are taken. The patient will assume both supine and prone positions.
4. Special techniques
   • If a foreign body such as a pin or fishbone has lodged in the esophagus, the patient may be asked to swallow a cotton ball saturated with barium to help localize the obstruction.
   • When hiatal hernia or gastroesophageal reflux is suspected, the patient is asked to cough or bear down.
5. The procedure usually takes 20 to 45 min.

Postprocedure

1. Provide food and fluids after completion of the test.
2. Allow the patient to rest.

3. A cathartic may be given to eliminate the barium. Inform the patient to expect white or light-colored stools.
4. If no cathartic is given, inform the patient to expect white or light-colored stools 24 to 72 hr after the test.
5. Observe and chart the passing of the barium. Retained barium may cause bowel obstruction or an impaction in the rectum.

Signed Consent
Not required

CT SCAN (Computed Axial Tomography)
Tomography is a special x-ray technique that visualizes specific layers of tissue. It is much more sensitive than regular x-rays and creates a three-dimensional appearance. Tissues of different densities absorb the x-ray photons differently. Air will appear as black images, bone as white, and soft tissue as gray. By providing a three-dimensional view of tissue, layer by layer, abnormalities can be precisely located. When the CT scan is applied to the right upper quadrant of the abdomen, the viewer can visualize a distended gallbladder, dilated bile ducts, gallstones in the gallbladder or biliary tree, and cysts and tumors in the liver and pancreas.

Normal Results
Abdominal organ structure; absence of abnormal masses

Nursing Implications
Preprocedure
1. Inform the patient of the purpose of the test and the procedure. Reassure him that it is safe, noninvasive, and easily tolerated. The patient will receive no more radiation than he would with conventional x-rays. If possible, show the patient photographs or drawings of the equipment.
2. The procedure should be scheduled before any barium studies are done, as retained barium can obscure organs.

During the Procedure
1. The patient is transported to the radiology department.
2. The patient is placed in the supine position in the scanner. His head remains outside. Some patients express fears of claustrophobia. Reassure the patient that this is common.
3. Instruct the patient to lie as quietly as possible. Sedation may be necessary if the patient cannot remain immobile.
4. The patient feels no sensations as the scanner moves around his body.

Postprocedure
No specific nursing care measures are required.

Signed Consent
Not required

CHOLANGIOGRAPHY

This procedure is similar to the cholecystography except that the dye is injected intravenously rather than given orally. Cholangiography should not be performed if the patient has liver cell disease. The test is used primarily to visualize the cystic, hepatic, and common bile ducts for the detection of stones, strictures, and tumors. Cholangiography may be performed preoperatively, operatively, or postoperatively. Postoperatively the test is used to determine if the T-tube drain can be removed. The dye can be injected into the T-tube and films made immediately. If the ducts are patent, the T-tube is removed. The following nursing implications apply mainly to preoperative cholangiography.

Normal Results

Normal appearance of the cystic, hepatic, and common bile ducts

Nursing Implications

Preprocedure

1. Instruct the patient about the purpose of the test and procedure. Question the patient about allergies. The procedure is contraindicated for patients with sensitivity to iodine or seafood.
2. A cathartic may be given the afternoon prior to the procedure.
3. Hold food and fluids from midnight until after the completion of the test.
4. Since the procedure takes 2 to 4 hr, provide the patient with fat-free liquids to prevent dehydration.

During the Procedure

1. Take the patient to the radiology department. A preliminary film is taken.
2. A small amount of contrast material (Chlorografin) is given intravenously. If the patient has no hypersensitivity reaction, the remainder is given slowly.
3. A series of films are made starting 20 min after the injection and continuing at 20 min intervals until the biliary ducts and gallbladder visualize.

Postprocedure

1. Provide food and fluids.
2. Allow the patient to rest.
3. Observe the patient for any untoward reactions from the dye such as nausea, vomiting, elevated temperature. A persistent elevated temperature may be indicative of inflammation of the bile ducts.

Signed Consent

Required

PERCUTANEOUS TRANSHEPATIC CHOLANGIOGRAPHY

This procedure is used to differentiate obstructive jaundice from hepatocellular or nonobstructive jaundice. It detects liver dysfunction, the presence of gallstones, and injury to or obstruction of the bile ducts. Using fluoroscopy, a very thin caliber needle is introduced into the liver until bile comes out through the needle. A contrast dye is injected through the needle and any obstructed or distended bile ducts can be visualized with the fluoroscopy.

Normal Results

Normal functioning of the liver, gallbladder, and patent hepatic and bile ducts

Nursing Implications

Preprocedure

1. Explain the procedure to the patient. The patient is given a local anesthetic but may experience some transitory pain when the liver capsule is entered.
2. Evaluate the patient's clotting mechanisms prior to the procedure. Prothrombin time and platelet count should be normal.
3. Have the patient fast prior to the procedure.
4. Premedicate the patient to relieve anxiety if prescribed.

During the Procedure

1. The patient is taken to the radiology department and placed in the supine position on the x-ray table.
2. The skin over the area of the liver is cleansed, draped, and a local anesthetic is given.
3. Under fluoroscopy, a thin caliber needle is inserted into the liver at the right costal margin.
4. The needle is slowly withdrawn and suction is applied until a bile duct is entered and bile is aspirated. Then radiopaque dye is injected and the hepatic and biliary ducts can be observed on fluoroscopy.

Postprocedure

1. If the examination indicates the need for surgery, it is usually performed several hours after the procedure.
2. Observe the patient closely for signs of bile leakage or hemorrhage.
3. Take vital signs every 4 hr for 24 hr or more frequently if indicated. Observe for decreased blood pressure, increased pulse, pain, temperature elevation, chills, and abdominal distention.

Signed Consent

Required

CHOLECYSTOGRAPHY

A cholecystography examination is a series of x-ray films taken at intervals to evaluate the functioning of the gallbladder and to detect the presence of disease or gallstones. The patient is given an oral radiopaque dye (Telepaque, Oragrafin, or Priodax), which is then absorbed from the small bowel into the bloodstream. If the liver is functioning normally, it will remove the dye from the bloodstream, excrete it with the bile and concentrate it in the gallbladder.

Bile containing the dye is excreted through the common bile duct when the patient is fed a fatty meal. Gallstones are not usually radiopaque but may be seen as shadows when the gallbladder is filled with a radiopaque dye. If the gallbladder does not visualize, this usually indicates an obstruction in the ducts or a diseased gallbladder that cannot concentrate the dye. This study is effective only if the patient has a normally functioning liver and normal gastrointestinal absorption.

Normal Results

Normal appearance and functioning of the gallbladder

Nursing Implications

Preprocedure

1. Explain the purpose of the test and the procedure to the patient. Inform the patient that there should be no pain or discomfort.
2. Obtain an allergy history from the patient as the procedure is contraindicated in the patient who is sensitive to iodine. If the patient does not know if he is sensitive to iodine, ask him if he is sensitive to seafood. Seafood contains iodine.
3. Give the patient a fat-free supper the evening prior to the exam. Inform the patient that this is done so that the gallbladder will not be stimulated by any fats and can thus concentrate the dye.
4. Give the contrast medium tablets (usually Telepaque) after the evening meal. The tablet dose is calculated by patient's body weight and the tablets are given at 5 min intervals to minimize nausea. Most patients do not experience any side effects. If nausea, vomiting, diarrhea, or dysuria do occur, notify the physician.
5. Check to see if the patient is to have any other tests using iodine, such as protein-bound iodine tests or iodine uptake. These should be scheduled first or they may have to be delayed several months. Schedule any barium studies after the gallbladder series, as barium will interfere with visualization of the gallbladder.

During the Procedure

1. Take the patient to the radiology department. Films of the dye-filled gallbladder are made.
2. Give the patient a fatty meal to stimulate the gallbladder to empty. This usually takes 15 to 20 min. Films are taken at intervals as the gallbladder empties.
3. Inform patient that the total time for the series is approximately 1 hr.

Postprocedure

1. Provide food and fluids for the patient.
2. Allow the patient to rest.
3. If the gallbladder does not visualize on x-ray or is poorly visualized, the test is usually repeated the next day. Inform the patient that this is a usual occurrence if the gallbladder is diseased.

Signed Consent

Not required

ENDOSCOPY

An endoscopy is a study in which the inside of a body structure is visualized by means of a lighted tube. Today most endoscopies, particularly those of the upper gastrointestinal tract, are done by means of flexible fiberoptic scopes. Some endoscopies of the lower gastrointestinal tract are still done using the rigid, lighted metal tubes such as the proctoscope and the sigmoidoscope.

The fiberoptic scope can be inserted into areas of the body that are not easily accessible or not directly visualized by means other than surgery. The scope consists of bundles of thin, flexible, transparent fibers through which light is transmitted to different regions of the gastrointestinal tract. An illuminated image is reflected back to the viewer. Most endoscopes are equipped with channels for passing other instruments such as biopsy forceps, cytology brushes, cauteries, and irrigating cannulas.

In addition to being a diagnostic tool, endoscopies may be used for treatments such as the removal of polyps, retrieval of foreign objects (pins, fishbones, etc.), and the cauterization of sites of internal bleeding.

UPPER GASTROINTESTINAL ENDOSCOPY

The upper gastrointestinal endoscopy or esophagogastroduodenoscopy (EGD) is used to visualize the lining of the esophagus, stomach, and the first part of the duodenum. The EGD is used to detect and diagnose the presence of hiatal hernia, esophagitis, strictures, esophageal varices, upper gastrointestinal bleeding, gastric ulcers, and malignancies. An EGD may also be used to obtain cytology and biopsy specimens. The procedure may be done in a special endoscopy suite, the outpatient department, or at the patient's bedside.

Normal Results

Normal appearance of the esophagus, stomach, and duodenum

Nursing Implications

Preprocedures

1. Explain the procedure to the patient in terms appropriate to the patient. Tell the outpatient to bring someone with him to assist him in returning home. Explain to the patient that the procedure is exhausting and uncomfortable but not painful. The patient will not be able to speak during the procedure.
2. Hold food and fluids for at least 8 hr prior to the examination. This is done to prevent aspiration and enhance visualization.
3. Remove any dentures, eyeglasses, jewelry, or any constricting garments.
4. Have the patient void/defecate to prevent embarrassment or discomfort.
5. A sedative is usually given ½ to 1 hr prior to examination to lessen

apprehension. Sometimes atropine is given to decrease saliva and gastric secretions. Observe the patient for any untoward reactions to these medications.

During the Procedure
1. The physician will anesthesize the patient's throat either by having the patient gargle with a local anesthetic or by swabbing the throat. The anesthetic may cause the tongue and the throat to feel swollen.
2. As soon as the gag reflex disappears, place the patient in a dorsal recumbent position. For esophageal endoscopy, the head and shoulders should extend over the edge of the table. The nurse should support the patient's head. For gastroscopy, the patient is placed in the left lateral recumbent position. The patient must remain perfectly still. A general anesthetic may be given to children and to patients who cannot be cooperative.
3. The physician guides the endoscope as the patient swallows. Explain to the patient that a gagging sensation may occur.
4. The physician may introduce air through the scope. This distends the area being examined and provides for better visualization. The patient may experience a feeling of fullness or bloating. Some patients may have cramping.
5. If specimens are obtained, place them in specimen bottles, label, and send them to the lab. Photographs may be taken also.
6. Explain that the procedure takes from 15 min to 1 hr.

Postprocedure
1. Check the patient's vital signs and keep the siderails up until the sedative medication has worn off.
2. Observe for any signs of GI perforation such as bleeding, fever, dysphagia, and pain.
3. Do not give any food or fluids until the gag reflex returns (usually about 3 to 4 hr). Test the gag reflex by gently touching the back of the throat with a cotton swab or tongue blade. If the patient is an outpatient, have him remain in the endoscopy suite until sedation has worn off and the gag reflex has returned.
4. The patient may have a sore throat. Give throat lozenges or normal saline gargle as prescribed by the physician.

Signed Consent
Required

COLONOSCOPY (Fiberoptic Colonscopy)
Fiberoptic colonoscopy is a more valuable technique than proctosigmoidoscopy in that a larger portion of the intestine can be examined. The colon can be examined as far as the ileocecal valve. The colonoscopy is especially valuable in differentiating inflammatory disease from neoplastic disease. The colonoscopy allows the physician to examine and remove specimens, polyps, and foreign bodies. Photographs may also be taken during the examination.

Normal Results

Normal structures and appearance of the colon

Nursing Implications

Preprocedure

1. Explain the procedure to the patient in terms appropriate to the patient. Include sensations that the patient may experience.
2. Place the patient on a clear liquid diet 24 to 72 hr prior to the procedure. Some physicians require the patient to fast for 8 hr prior to the procedure.
3. Give cathartics or laxatives 1 to 3 dy prior to the procedure as prescribed by the physician.
4. Give enemas the night before as prescribed by the physician or hospital policy.
5. Premedicate the patient with a mild sedative as prescribed.
6. Advise outpatients to bring someone with them to assist them home.

During the Procedure

1. Place the patient in the left lateral recumbent position. The position may need to be changed as the physician inserts the scope into various segments of the colon.
2. Explain to the patient that a digital rectal exam usually precedes the procedure in order to dilate the rectum and to make sure there are no major obstructions. The patient may feel the urge to defecate when the digital exam is performed or as the scope is inserted.
3. The physician passes the colonoscope the entire length, then slowly withdraws it for better visualization. Specimens for biopsy and cytology may be taken. Polyps may be excised. Air is introduced as part of the procedure to distend the lumen of the bowel. The patient may experience cramping sensations.
4. The procedure may take 30 min to 3 hr to complete.

Postprocedure

1. Check the patient's vital signs. Allow the patient to rest. Outpatients should rest for 30 min to 1 hr before leaving the hospital. Outpatients should not leave unaccompanied.
2. Give the patient food and fluids.
3. Observe stools for gross bleeding. Report any complaints of abdominal pain to the physician. Instruct the outpatient to observe and report any changes in stool or presence of abdominal pain.

Signed Consent

Required

GASTRIC ANALYSIS

The analysis of gastric contents is done to determine whether the patient is able to secrete hydrochloric acid (HCL), the degree of acidity in the stomach, and the volume of HCL. Gastric analysis is an important aid in diagnosing the presence of conditions such as benign ulcers, carcinoma, Zollinger–Ellison syndrome, and pernicious anemia, as well as for the effectiveness of a vagotomy.

A nasogastric tube is inserted prior to the procedure. Gastric fluid specimens are aspirated for analysis. A baseline analysis or an analysis of the gastric secretions without histamine stimulation is usually done first. This is followed by an analysis of secretions, which have been stimulated by the introduction of histamine or Histolog (betazole hydrochloride).

For those patients who cannot tolerate insertion of a nasogastric tube, a tubeless analysis may be performed. The tubeless analysis uses a dye (Diagnex Blue), which is given orally. The dye is released when the gastric acidity has a pH of 3.5 or less. The dye is absorbed in the small intestine and excreted in the urine. The reliability of the tubeless analysis is often questioned, especially if the patient has pyloric obstruction, vomiting, diarrhea, liver damage, urinary tract obstruction, or has had gastric surgery.

Normal Results

Fasting Residual Volume	20 to 100 ml
pH	< 2.0
Basal acid output (BAO)	0 to 6 mEq/hr
Maximal acid output after histamine stimulation (MAO)	5 to 40 mEq/hr
BAO/MAO ratio	< 0.4

Nursing Implications

Preprocedure

1. Explain the procedure to the patient. Inform the patient that smoking will be prohibited on the morning of the test, as it stimulates gastric secretions. Try to control any other extraneous stimulation.
2. If histamine is to be used, perform a skin test to determine possible sensitivity. The histamine test will be contraindicated for patients with a positive skin test reaction or patients with a history of asthma, urticaria, and hypertension.
3. Withhold food and fluids for 12 to 14 hr prior to the test. Do not give prior to the test any drugs that affect gastric secretions such as cholinergics, anticholinergics, sedatives, or tranquilizers.

During the Procedure

1. Place the patient in bed in a high Fowler's position with the head slightly flexed for the insertion of the nasogastric tube. The tube is inserted and basal stomach contents are aspirated. The specimen is sent to the lab for analysis of acidity and pH.
2. Administer histamine or Histolog intravenously according to physician's orders. Often when histamine is used, an antihistamine will be administered 30 min after the basal specimen is collected and 1 hr

before the histamine is injected (augmented histamine test). This will decrease the severity of any side effects of the histamine.

3. Aspirate specimens of gastric contents every 15 to 20 min for 1 hr and send to the lab.
4. Take the patient's pulse and blood pressure immediately after administering the histamine. Inform the patient that he may feel warm and flushed and may develop a headache. Have epinephrine available to be used if the patient develops a severe reaction to the histamine.

Postprocedure
1. Provide food and fluids for the patient.
2. Continue to observe for any side effects of histamine.

Signed Consent
Required

TUBELESS GASTRIC ANALYSIS
Normal Results

If there is free hydrochloric acid in the stomach, the dye (Diagnex Blue) will be excreted by the kidneys within 2 hr.

Nursing Implications
Preprocedure
1. Explain the procedure to the patient.
2. Withhold food after the evening meal, but the patient may have water as desired.

During the Procedure
1. Have the patient void early on the morning of the procedure. This specimen is discarded.
2. The patient is given caffeine sodium benzoate (a stimulant for acid secretions) with a glass of water.
3. One hour later ask the patient to void. The specimen is saved as a control specimen.
4. A dye (Diagnex Blue) is then administered orally with water. If the gastric pH is 3.5 or less, the dye will be released, absorbed through the small intestine, and excreted in the urine. The urine will be a blue color.
5. Save all urine excreted within the next 2 hr and send to the laboratory.

Postprocedure
1. Give the patient food and fluids.
2. Inform the patient that urine may be blue or green for several days following the procedure.
3. If there is an absence of dye color in the urine, the direct gastric analysis using histamine or Histalog may be done.

Signed Consent

Check the hospital policy.

LIVER BIOPSY

A biopsy of the liver is useful in establishing the cause of liver disease. A specially designed needle is inserted through the chest or abdominal wall into the liver and a small piece of hepatic tissue is removed. This procedure is indicated for patients with abnormal liver function studies, unexplained hepatomegaly, hepatitis, cirrhosis, and suspected liver malignancy.

Normal Results

Normal hepatic cellular appearance and structure when examined microscopically.

Nursing Implications

Preprocedure

1. Explain the procedure to the patient. Assess the patient's ability to be cooperative. The patient must be able to hold his breath and remain very still when the needle is being introduced into the liver.
2. Check the patient's prothrombin time. If it is prolonged, the biopsy should not be done. Bleeding time and the platelet count should also be within normal limits.
3. Vitamin K may be administered for several days prior to the examination and after the biopsy is taken. Blood may be typed and cross-matched.
4. Take baseline vital signs.
5. Hold food and fluids for several hours prior to the test according to hospital policy.
6. Administer a sedative 30 min prior to the test if prescribed.
7. The procedure is usually done in the patient's room with the patient in his bed.

During the Procedure

1. Have the patient lie in the supine position with his right arm under his head.
2. The skin is cleansed and a local anesthetic is injected into the skin and the liver capsule by the physician.
3. The patient is instructed to take several breaths and hold on expiration while the biopsy needle is inserted and the specimen is withdrawn. The patient may then resume breathing normally.
4. A simple dressing is placed over the aspiration site.
5. The specimen should be sent immediately to the laboratory.
6. The procedure usually takes only about 10 min.

Postprocedure

1. Take vital signs every 30 min for 4 hr and then hourly for the next 8 hr. Observe for signs of hemorrhaging.

2. Have the patient lie on his right side with a small pillow or folded bath blanket under the right costal margin. This applies pressure and prevents bleeding. This position should be maintained for several hours.
3. Instruct the patient to stay on bedrest for 24 hr.
4. Administer vitamin K to prevent bleeding if prescribed.

Signed Consent

Required

LIVER SCAN (Radioisotope Scanning)

Radioisotope scanning is very helpful for evaluating the structure, position, and function of the liver and gallbladder. This scan is a noninvasive procedure that allows visualization of organs and regions within organs that cannot be seen on ordinary x-ray film. Chemical compounds (radionuclides) containing minute amounts of radioisotopes are injected intravenously and are taken up by different types of liver cells. The radioisotopes emit gamma rays, which are picked up by scanning devices similar to Geiger counters. The scanner converts radiation emissions into electrical impulses, which can be viewed on an oscilloscope screen and recorded as dots on x-ray film or paper. Scans may be done on an inpatient or outpatient basis.

Normal Results

Normal concentration of radioisotope showing normal size, shape, and position of the liver

Nursing Implications

Preprocedure

1. Explain the procedure to the patient. There is no discomfort during the scan. Many patients worry about radiation hazards, especially since the radioisotopes are injected into them. Inform the patient that the dose of radiation received in most scans is less than that received during a single chest x-ray. The scanning device does not emit radiation, it only receives it.
2. Assess the patient's ability to remain still during the scanning procedure.
3. Obtain the patient's history of allergies. Some patients may have allergic reactions to certain radionuclides such as ^{131}I rose bengal, an iodine-based compound.
4. Inform the patient that several scans will be done at various intervals to observe the isotope uptake in the liver and the filling of the gallbladder. A final scan is usually taken 24 hr later.

Postprocedure

1. The patient is taken to nuclear medicine department or to radiology department and given an intravenous injection of a radioisotope.
2. The patient is placed on a table and in 10 to 20 min the scan begins. The scanning device travels slowly back and forth over the area to be scanned as the patient lies quietly.

Signed Consent

Required

PROCTOSIGMOIDOSCOPY

The proctosigmoidoscopy is an inspection of the anus, rectum, and sigmoid colon using a rigid metal tube with a light source. This procedure is used mainly for the detection and diagnosis of malignancies. It can be used also for evaluating hemorrhoids and ulcerative colitis, obtaining biopsy specimens, and excising polyps. All patients over the age of 40 should have this examination included as part of their routine physical assessment.

Normal Results

Normal appearance of the colon, rectum, and anus

Nursing Implications

Preprocedure

1. Explain the procedure to the patient in terms appropriate to the patient. Include an explanation of the sensations the patient may expect to feel.
2. The patient does not need to fast. A light evening meal and light breakfast may be allowed.
3. Laxatives, enemas, or suppositories may be given the night before the exam. No preparation is given to the patient with suspected ulcerative colitis.
4. The examination is emotionally upsetting to many patients. Prepare the equipment prior to bringing the patient into the room to decrease the patient's apprehension.

During the Procedure

1. Place the patient in the knee–chest position. For some patients, such as the elderly, the left lateral recumbent position is used. Many treatment rooms and endoscopy suites have specialized tilt tables that help the patient to assume and maintain the knee–chest position.
2. The physician usually performs a digital rectal examination first to dilate the sphincter and make sure there are no major obstructions. The endoscope is then gradually inserted to its full length and slowly withdrawn. The patient may feel the urge to defecate when the digital exam is performed and as the endoscope is inserted.
3. Air is sometimes introduced into the colon to separate mucosal folds. Some patients experience gas pains during this procedure.
4. Biopsy specimens may be obtained. Polyps may be excised.
5. The procedure takes approximately 10 min. Observe the patient carefully, as dizziness and light-headedness often occur. The nurse may want to take the patient's pulse periodically.

Postprocedure

1. Have the patient rest in a horizontal position for a few minutes before standing. Have the outpatient rest for 30 min to 1 hr before leaving the hospital.

2. Notify physician if rectal bleeding or severe abdominal pain occur.

Signed Consent

Required

ULTRASONOGRAPHY (Echography)

Ultrasonography is another safe, noninvasive method of visualizing the abdominal organs. The test is especially valuable in demonstrating large distended, obstructed gallbladders and stones within the gallbladder. The test is also helpful for identifying cystic lesions and abscesses of the liver and pancreas, pseudocysts, pancreatitis, and carcinoma.

Ultrasonography uses high frequency inaudible sound waves to form images that can be viewed on an oscilloscope and recorded on photographic film. Sound waves are directed into the body by a transducer, a device that converts electrical energy into sound waves. The sound waves make contact with structures in the body and are reflected back to the transducer, which converts them electronically into a picture.

Normal Results

Normal pattern image indicating normal size and position of the organ or body structure studied

Nursing Implications

Preprocedure

1. Inform the patient of the procedure. Tell him of its safety and that only sound waves will be introduced into his body. Instruct the patient to lie still while the procedure is in progress. If possible, show the patient photographs or drawings of the equipment.
2. Sedation may be necessary if the patient is a child or a person who cannot remain still.
3. Fasting is sometimes required before gallbladder ultrasound in order to allow for the greatest dilation of the gallbladder.
4. The procedure should be done before any barium studies, as barium will alter ultrasound transmission.

During the Procedure

1. The patient is taken to the ultrasonography suite.
2. The patient is placed in a supine position. An oil or gel is spread on the patient's skin and on the transducer to facilitate the sound wave passage. Then the transducer is moved back and forth over the area to be studied at various angles and directions. Results are viewed on an oscilloscope and recorded in photographs.

Postprocedure

1. There are no specific nursing care measures other than helping the patient remove the gel or oil from the abdomen.

Signed Consent

Not required

UPPER GASTROINTESTINAL SERIES AND SMALL BOWEL EXAM

The upper gastrointestinal series is a radiographic visualization of the esophagus, stomach, and duodenum. The small bowel exam visualizes the small intestine and includes all of the small intestine up to and including the ileocecal junction. The small exam may be done as a separate procedure, although it usually follows the upper gastrointestinal series. These procedures are used to help diagnose such conditions as hiatal hernia, presence of foreign bodies, thickening of gastric wall, gastric ulcers, malignancies, congenital anomalies, pyloric stenosis, and obstructions.

Normal Results

Normal anatomical appearance of the esophagus, stomach, and small intestine

Nursing Implications

Preprocedure

1. Instruct the patient about the procedure. Inform the patient that there will be no discomfort but that the procedure may require several hours if the examination of the small bowel is included. Suggest that the patient take some reading material or other diversionary activity with him to the radiology department.
2. The patient is given a light supper such as soup, toast, Jello, tea, poached egg the night before and then instructed to fast until the examination is completed.
3. Barium studies interfere with many other studies. Check to make sure that these studies are sequenced so they will not interfere with other studies.

During the Procedure

1. The patient assumes an upright standing position behind a fluoroscopic screen and drinks a suspension of flavored barium sulfate. The table is then tilted in several different positions while films are made.
2. If a small bowel exam is to be done, tell the patient to drink additional barium and that x-ray films will be taken at 30 min intervals. The test is complete when barium enters the ileocecal junction.
3. The upper gastrointestinal series takes 20 to 45 min to complete. The small bowel examination may take 2 to 6 hr.

Postprocedure

1. Provide food and fluids after completion of the test.
2. Allow the patient to rest. The procedure may be exhausting for some patients.
3. A cathartic may be administered to eliminate the barium. Inform the patient to expect white stools.
4. If no cathartic is given the patient should expect white stools 24 to 72 hr after the test.

5. Observe and chart the passing of the barium. Retained barium may cause bowel obstruction or impaction in the rectum.
6. A follow-up film may be made 24 hr after the barium meal.

Signed Consent

Not required

BIBLIOGRAPHY

Beck ML: Guiding your patient . . . a step at a time . . . through a colonoscopy. Nursing 81, 11:28–31, 1981

Beck ML: Preparing your patient physically for an esophagogastroduodenoscopy. Nursing 81, 11:88–96, 1981

Beck ML: Preparing your patient psychologically for an esophagogastroduodenoscopy. Nursing 81, 11:28–30, 1981

Beck ML: Tests: what to do when they call for inserting gastrointestinal tubes. Nursing 81, 11:74–76, 1981

Beck ML: Three common gastrointestinal tests—and how to help your patient through each. Nursing 81, 11:44–47, 1981

Beck ML: Two intestinal tests: one oral, one anal. Nursing 81, 11:20–24, 1981

Brunner LS, Suddarth DS: Textbook of Medical-Surgical Nursing, 4th ed. Philadelphia, JB Lippincott, 1980

Fischbach FT: A Manual of Laboratory Diagnostic Tests. Philadelphia, JB Lippincott, 1980

French RM: Guide to Diagnostic Procedures, 4th ed. New York, McGraw-Hill, 1975

Garb S: Laboratory Tests in Common Use, 6th ed. New York, Springer, 1979.

Given BA, Simmons SJ: Gastroenterology in Clinical Nursing, 3rd ed. St Louis, CV Mosby 1979

Guyton AC: Textbook of Medical Physiology, 4th ed. Philadelphia, WB Saunders, 1971

Haughey CW: Understanding ultrasonography. Nursing 81 11: 100–104, 1981

Luckmann J, Sorenson KC: Medical-Surgical Nursing: A Psychophysiologic Approach. Philadelphia, WB Saunders, 1980

Phipps WJ, Long BC, Woods NP: Medical-Surgical Nursing. St Louis, CV Mosby, 1979

Price SA, Wilson LM: Pathophysiology, Clinical Concepts of Disease Processes. New York, McGraw-Hill, 1978

Skydell B, Crowder AS: Diagnostic Procedures. Boston, Little, Brown and Co, 1975

Thorpe CJ, Caprini JA: Gallbladder disease: Current trends and treatments. Am J Nurs 80:2181–2185, 1980

Tilkian SM, Conover MB, Tilkian AG: Clinical Implications of Laboratory Tests. St Louis, CV Mosby, 1979

Wallach J: Interpretation of Diagnostic Tests, 3rd ed. Boston, Little, Brown and Co, 1978

6

Tests Related to Metabolic Function

Harriett L. Riggs

OVERVIEW OF PHYSIOLOGY AND PATHOPHYSIOLOGY

Metabolism in the human body can be defined as chemical reactions within the cells that convert proteins, carbohydrates, and fats into energy. This energy is needed for physiologic processes, such as structural growth, muscle activity, and brain development.

NORMAL METABOLISM

Proteins

Proteins, when ingested, are broken into amino acids for absorption, whereby they can be synthesized into body proteins that are necessary for growth and repair of body tissues. Amino acids are the principal constituents of proteins. Normally, unused amino acids are further broken down in the liver into urea and fatty acids. Urea is excreted by the kidneys. Fatty acids are converted to glucose and stored as glycogen, primarily in the liver and muscles, or converted to body fat.

Fats

Ingested fats are converted to fatty acids and glycerol for absorption in the gastrointestinal tract. Subsequently, they are reconverted to neutral fats for storage in adipose tissue or broken down to form carbon dioxide and water. The liver plays an important function in the metabolism of fats, as well as of carbohydrates and proteins.

Carbohydrates

In the process of carbohydrate digestion, carbohydrates are reduced to monosaccharides such as glucose, galactose, and fructose in order to be absorbed by the body. Subsequently, the galactose and fructose are converted to glucose for use by body cells. Galactose must be converted by liver cells into glucose. Fructose is converted primarily to glucose during absorption through the epithelial cells. Most of the remaining fructose is then converted in the liver. When glucose is oxidized in body cells to water and carbon dioxide, energy is released to provide for growth, muscular contraction, and other cellular activities.

PATHOPHYSIOLOGY: GENETIC ORIGIN

An inborn error of metabolism is usually caused by defects in the structure or function of protein molecules within the body. Most metabolic disorders are of genetic origin and are inherited by transmission of an abnormal gene from parent to child.

Abnormal genes may be autosomal dominant, autosomal recessive, or sex linked. The gene conveys the instructions for development of one single characteristic such as color of the eye or color of the hair. There may be several thousand genes on each chromosome.

Chromosomes are a part of the nucleus of every body cell. The characteristic number of chromosomes in each cell of a human being is 46. Through the process of cell division, each mature spermatozoon and each mature ovum carry 23 single chromosomes that combine during fertilization to form the 46 chromosomes. The genes of each chromosome pair have the same function.

Twenty-two pairs of chromosomes are alike in both the male and female and are called autosomal chromosomes. The twenty-third pair is called the pair of sex chromosomes. These chromosomes are not matched as in the autosomal ones but are different in the male and female and are important in sex determination. In the female the sex chromosomes are paired similarly to the autosomal ones and are referred to as XX. In the male, one chromosome is an X, identical to the female X, and the other is a Y, resulting in a pair of XY chromosomes.

Although abnormal genes can be inherited from one or both parents in the same manner as normal genes are inherited, the abnormality can also result from mutations or changes in the structure of the gene.

Autosomal Recessive Disorders

A carrier of an autosomal recessive disorder has both a normal and an abnormal gene but has no evidence of the disease. In this case, the normal gene is the dominant gene and its characteristics are the ones expressed in the human organism.

Each child born to parents who are both carriers of, or who both possess an autosomal recessive gene for the same disorder, statistically has a 25% chance of having the disease, a 50% chance of being a carrier like the parents, and a 25% chance of being completely free of the defective gene. This is the pattern of inheritance usually seen in autosomal recessive disorders. Phenylketonuria (PKU) is an example of an autosomal recessive disorder.

Autosomal Dominant Disorders

The usual pattern of inheritance of autosomal dominant disorders is observed when one parent has the disorder and the other parent is free of the disease. The affected parent usually has one normal gene and one abnormal gene. The abnormal gene is the dominant gene, and its characteristics are the ones expressed in the human organism. The unaffected parent has both normal genes. Each child conceived by this union has a 50% chance of having the disease like the affected parent and a 50% chance of having only normal genes.

Sex-linked Genetic Disorders

Sex-linked genetic disorders usually are referred to as X-linked disorders because the defective gene is carried on the X chromosome. The pattern of inheritance of a recessive gene on the X chromosome is expressed by all males who carry the gene but rarely is seen in the female. This results because of the pairing of the recessive gene with a dominant gene on the X chromosomes.

If the female who carries the recessive gene marries a normal male, each daughter of their union will have a 50% possibility of having only normal genes and a 50% possibility of carrying the defective gene. The sons of the female carrying the recessive gene will have a 50% possibility of being normal and a 50% possibility of having the disorder. An affected male will transmit the recessive gene to all his daughters and to none of his sons, since the gene is only in the X chromosome.

The difference in X-linked recessive and the X-linked dominant disorders is that the dominant disorders are rare and occur twice as often in females as in males. The affected male transmits the gene to all of his daughters and to none of his sons, since the gene is found on the X chromosome. The pattern of transmission by affected females follows the same pattern as that of an autosomal dominant disorder. Autosomal dominant and sex-linked (X-linked) metabolic disorders will not be discussed in this text.

ENZYME DISORDERS

Most disorders described as inborn errors of metabolism are those disorders in which there is a decrease or absence of enzymatic activity within the cell. An enzyme is a body protein that controls metabolism by serving as a catalyst in chemical reactions within the cell. The basic defect in the enzymatic activity of inborn errors of metabolism is congenital, meaning that the infant is born with a genetic defect. However, the age at which the defect becomes clinically evident varies.

Many disorders can be diagnosed early in life, such as PKU and galactosemia. Other disorders, such as gout, are not fully manifested until adulthood. Other diseases are symptomlesss until the affected individual is exposed to certain stressors, such as drugs or foods. The hemolytic anemia of glucose-6-phosphate dehydrogenase deficiency (G-6 PD) is an example of this category of disorders.

Phenylketonuria and galactosemia are examples of genetic disorders caused by enzyme deficiencies. These disorders, if not treated in early infancy, produce severe developmental problems.

PKU

The apparent genetic defect in PKU is the absence of phenylalanine hydroxylase, a liver enzyme necessary for the conversion of phenylalanine into tyrosine in the pathway of protein metabolism. Phenylalanine is an essential amino acid needed for the production of protein in the human body. Tyrosine, another essential amino acid, is necessary for the formation of thyroxin (a thyroid hormone). Tyrosine is also necessary for the formation of dopamine and norepinephrine, which are substances that enhance the passage of nerve impulses from one neuron to another.

The neonate with PKU appears normal at birth, suggesting that the brain developed normally during intrauterine life. However, the infant with PKU is unable to continue normal brain growth. After birth, the critical period for brain development occurs as cells divide during the first 6 months of life. Later, growth of brain tissue results from an increase in protein, DNA, and lipid content of the already existing cells. This growth process continues until about the age of 5 or 6 years.

During this period of growth, myelination of the large nerve fibers takes place. The process is most active during the first 2 years of life. Myelination is the development of the myelin sheath around these fibers. The myelin sheath increases the rapidity of the nerve impulses as they progress along the nerve fibers. Any interference with the myelination process would decrease the potential for transmission of nerve impulses.

When the infant with PKU begins to ingest milk proteins, which contain phenylalanine, the deficiency of the enzyme becomes evident. As a result phenylalanine and its metabolites accumulate in excess amounts of blood, urine, and cerebrospinal fluid.

- Since the body is unable to metabolize the ingested phenylalanine, there is a rise in serum phenylalanine, which is accompanied by a low tyrosine level.

- After the serum level of phenylalanine reaches approximately 12 to 15 mg/100 ml, phenylalanine in the form of phenylpyruvic acid is spilled in the urine.

- This occurs in the newborn at about 3 weeks of age, since it is necessary for the newborn to have had enough protein intake to elevate the serum levels for urinary spillage to occur.

Metabolism of tyrosine is also necessary for the formation of melanin, the pigment which gives color to hair and skin.

- Because tyrosine production is inhibited, children with PKU usually begin to exhibit a decrease in pigmentation during the first year of life. As a result, most of the affected children are fair, blond, and blue-eyed.

- Other early apparent manifestations of the excess of phenylalanine and its derivatives are vomiting, irritability, an eczematoid skin rash, or a characteristic mousey, musty odor. The odor, usually noted in the first 2 to 3 months of life, is attributed to the presence of phenylacetic acid, a by-product of phenylpyruvic acid, in the urine and in sweat.

- The great majority of children who are not diagnosed and not begun on dietary treatment in early infancy experience permanent and profound mental retardation from exposure to the high serum levels of phenylalanine.

GALACTOSEMIA

Another inborn error of metabolism, galactosemia, is also an autosomal recessive disorder. Galactosemia is associated with failure to thrive in newborns, liver dysfunction, mental retardation, cataracts, and gastrointestinal disorders. These disorders appear to result from the decreased activity of the enzyme galactose-1-phosphate uridyl transferase. This enzyme is one of those needed to complete the metabolism of lactose to galactose and subsequently to glucose. When a deficiency of the enzyme is present, the galactose is not metabolized. Galactose accumulates in the blood, causing elevated blood levels. Galactose metabolites accumulate in body tissues, especially in the neurons and in the renal epithelium.

- When the newborn with galactosemia ingests milk, vomiting and diarrhea occur within the first week of life. This infant is often classified as a failure to thrive infant.

- Cataracts have also been observed as early as the first few days of life.

- Liver cell injury is caused by the galactose metabolites and may cause elevated bilirubin levels.

- Other complications of galactosemia include a fatty liver, ascites, edema, and infections.
- Galactosemia may cause elevated blood galactose levels, galactosuria, hyperchloremic acidosis, albuminuria, and aminoaciduria.

LACTOSE INTOLERANCE

An intolerance to the dietary disaccharide lactose, especially in the form of milk, is called lactose intolerance. This intolerance to dietary lactose results from a deficiency of the enzyme, lactase. The epithelial cells of the mucosa of the small intestine contain the disgestive enzymes. These enzymes act upon food products during the processes of digestion and absorption. One of these enzymes is lactase, which is necessary for splitting the disaccharide lactose into the monosaccharides, glucose, and galactose. Lactase is present in the brush border of the epithelial cells where it facilitates the hydrolysis of lactose.

Lactose intolerance is classified as primary, secondary, or congenital. Lactose intolerance is considered a primary disorder when there is no evidence of any present or previous underlying intestinal disease. Secondary lactose intolerance occurs in the presence of other gastrointestinal disorders. Primary and secondary lactose intolerance is relatively common.

Congenital Lactose Intolerance

Congenital lactose intolerance, which is evident at birth, is rare and believed to be inherited as an autosomal recessive disorder. Although there is no apparent change in the histology of the gastrointestinal mucosa, there is evidence of little or no lactase produced in the brush border of the epithelial cells. Lactase appears to be diminished or absent.

Although the normal newborn has an abundance of the enzyme lactase and is able to digest lactose, the amount of lactase in the human being diminishes with maturation. Adults are unable to tolerate equivalent amounts of lactose-containing food substances that they previously tolerated in infancy.

- In children who develop primary lactose intolerance, symptoms of intolerance to milk and milk products can begin as early as 3 or 4 years of age.
- Many adolescents or young adults who claim a dislike for milk, may have eliminated milk products from their diet because of symptoms of intolerance.
- North American blacks, Asians, and Mexican Americans appear to have a higher incidence of lactose intolerance.

Secondary Lactose Intolerance

Secondary lactose intolerance is observed more frequently because of its association with other intestinal diseases. If the surface cells of the intestine are injured, such as with celiac disease or gastroenteritis, lactase production is diminished. Milk and milk products are not tolerated. This intolerance is temporary. Intolerance to lactose may also occur after gastrointestinal surgery. After gastrectomy, lactose products are rapidly delivered to the intestine. The existing lactase in the intestine is insufficient to break down the large amount of lactose. After resection of the small bowel, the supply of lactase available for breakdown of lactose in the diet is reduced.

- When lactose cannot be broken down by the enzyme lactase, the lactose remains in the lumen of the intestine, fluids are retained by osmosis, and reabsorption of fluids and electrolytes is prevented.

- Bowel distention results and peristalsis is stimulated causing diarrhea. When the lactose reaches the large bowel, intestinal bacteria act on the lactose to release lactic acid hydrogen.

- The stool is watery, frothy, acid, sour smelling, and irritating to the perianal skin. Since the lactose is not digested and absorbed, its presence in the stool is evidenced by a positive reaction to reducing sugars.

OTHER DISORDERS

Pathophysiologic findings of other metabolic diseases vary according to the body tissue affected by the faulty product or by the absence of the production of an essential product. These obscure diseases are seen rarely and are beyond the scope of this text.

BLOOD TESTS
BLOOD AMINO ACIDS

The concentration and distribution of amino acids in the blood are partially dependent upon the type of protein ingested, the excretion of waste products of protein metabolism by the kidneys, and the synthesis of protein by body cells. The blood concentration of amino acids will rise slightly soon after a meal. Only a slight rise in blood concentration will occur, since the amino acids are rapidly absorbed by the body cells. The concentration of each type of amino acid remains relatively stable unless there is interference with the metabolism of the specific amino acid. This interference with metabolism will occur in PKU.

When overflow of specific amino acids is detected in the urine, or screening tests for some metabolic disorders are positive or questionable, quantitative measurement of blood levels of the amino acid are desirable.

GALACTOSEMIA SCREENING—BLOOD

The basic defect in galactosemia lies in the hereditary absence of the enzyme galactose-1-phosphate uridyl transferase. This enzyme is normally present in red blood cells. An effective screening method is used to detect the presence or absence of the enzyme in the red cells. Two different techniques are used. One is the methylene blue technique, and the other is a spot test using ultraviolet light. In both tests a color change or fluorescence is expected if the enzyme is present. The test is also useful in monitoring the effectiveness of therapy.

Laboratory Results
Normal

Color change or evidence of fluorescence

Positive for Galactosemia

No color change or fluorescence

Nursing Implications

Procedure for Collection/Storage of Specimen

1. A specimen of blood is obtained by venipuncture.
2. Micromethod is used for newborns and infants. Obtain the blood specimen using a heel stick. (For details, see page 218.) Capillary blood saturates a strip of prepared filter paper.

Possible Interfering Factors

1. Because the enzyme is relatively unstable, it is recommended that the test be done only if local laboratory facilities are available for processing.
2. Carriers of the disorder may show a normal finding.

Patient Care

1. Avoid repeated heel stick to prevent development of fibrotic tissue in the heel.
2. Check the puncture site for bleeding. Apply a pressure dressing if the bleeding persists.

Parent Education

1. Inform the primary caretaker of the need for obtaining a blood specimen.
2. Instruct the primary caretaker in observing puncture site for further bleeding.

Signed Consent

Not required

GALACTOSE TOLERANCE TEST

The galactose tolerance test was once used widely in the diagnosis of galactosemia. It is no longer recommended for infants in whom galactosemia is suspected because of the possibility of associated hypoglycemia and hypokalemia. Doses of galactose, which are determined by the patient's weight, are administered orally or intravenously to the fasting patient. Urine and blood specimens are collected periodically over a 5-hr period, as in the glucose tolerance test.

ORAL LACTOSE TOLERANCE TEST

The oral lactose tolerance test measures the amount of lactose absorbed. It does not measure the amount of lactose that remains in the lumen of the bowel and that produces the undesirable consequences of lactose intolerance. Therefore, the oral lactose tolerance test is not effective in the diagnosis of lactose intolerance.

The test may be a more valid test of infant intolerance to lactose. The standard test dose of lactose more closely correlates with the amount of lactose that is ingested during one feeding by an infant. The test dose of lactose may not correlate with the amount of lactose that is ingested at one time by an older child or adult.

Lactose is given by mouth to individuals suspected of having lactase deficiency or lactose intolerance. A 240-ml glass of milk contains about 12 g of lactose. This is considerably less lactose than the 2 g/kg of body weight test dose of lactose that is used for older persons. The person who is unable to tolerate the test dose of lactose may well be able to tolerate the usual dietary intake of lactose. The oral lactose tolerance test is useful as a screening procedure for lactose intolerance.

Laboratory Results
Normal Range

The blood glucose peaks between 15 and 60 min after ingestion of lactose. The rise in blood glucose levels is greater than 25 mg/dl over the fasting level.

Range with Lactose Intolerance

- Rise in blood glucose is less than 20 mg/dl over the fasting level.

Associated Findings with Lactose Intolerance

- The patient may develop abdominal cramps and watery diarrhea within 2 to 6 hr.
- Disaccharides may be present in the stool.
- The stool pH is strongly acidic.

Nursing Implications
Procedure for Collection/Storage of Specimen

1. See glucose tolerance test.
2. Weigh the patient prior to the procedure.
3. Keep the patient NPO for 8 hr prior to the test.
4. Obtain two blood glucose levels during the fasting period.
5. Give a 10% solution of lactose. The dosage is to be 2 to 2.5 g of lactose per kilogram of body weight. If there is a history of severe intolerance to lactose, reduce the dosage to 1 g lactose per kilogram of body weight.
6. The solution is ingested orally by the patient. Instruct the patient to ingest all of the solution.
7. Record the exact time of ingestion.
8. Obtain blood glucose samples from capillary sticks or from venipuncture at 15-, 30-, 90-, and 120-min intervals.
9. Collect all stools for 24 hr after the administration of the lactose.
10. Observe the hydration status of the patient. Excessive fluids and electrolytes can be lost from the bowel.

Possible Interfering Factors

1. For reasons unknown at this time, many persons who tolerate lactose in the diet develop diarrheal stools that contain reducing substances.
2. The results are influenced by the rate with which gastric contents are emptied.

3. The tests are sensitive only to the amount of lactose absorbed rather than to the amount that is not absorbed and remains in the bowel.

Patient Care

1. Record and report the reactions of the patient during the test.
2. Observe the patient closely for abdominal cramping and watery stools.
3. Notify the physician if gastrointestinal symptoms occur.
4. Notify the physician if diarrhea occurs in order that serum electrolytes may be drawn.
5. If diarrhea causes fluid and electrolyte imbalances, replace fluids and electrolytes as prescribed by the physician.

Patient Education

1. Instruct the patient or primary caretaker in the purpose of the test and possible side effects.
2. Caution the patient or primary caretaker to report the onset of diarrhea.

Signed Consent

Not required

GUTHRIE TEST FOR PKU

Most states require a screening test for PKU for all newborn infants. The Guthrie test is the most widely used test for this screening process. The test is usually done prior to the newborn's discharge from the hospital. The newborn must drink milk protein for a minimum of 3 days prior to the test in order for the phenylalanine levels in the blood to increase to a detectable level. The test should be repeated in a clinic or in the physician's office before the infant is 3 weeks old.

The Guthrie test is a bacterial inhibition procedure. Blood is introduced into a specially prepared culture medium that contains *Bacillus subtilis* spores. Bacterial growth takes place if the blood is abnormally high in phenylalanine.

Laboratory Results

Normal Results

Negative—no growth of bacteria

Abnormal Results

Positive—growth of bacteria indicates serum phenylalanine greater than 4 mg/dl

Nursing Implications

Procedure for Collection/Storage of Specimen

1. Cleanse the infant's heel with an antiseptic solution.
2. Keep the heel in a dependent position to encourage pooling of peripheral blood.
3. Apply a warm, moist cloth to the heel to encourage dilation of peripheral vessels.
4. Puncture the heel on the lateral aspect of the sole with a sharp, sterile lancet.

5. Collect the blood on circles of prepared filter paper. Each circle must be completely filled with blood. Press the infant's heel against the center of the filter paper until the circle is filled. Observe both sides of the circle to ascertain if blood has saturated the circle.
6. Cleanse the heel and place a sterile adhesive dressing over the puncture site.
7. Place the lancet in the disposal container for dirty needles.

Possible Interfering Factors

1. Increases in phenylalanine levels may occur in infants with low birthweight (less than 5 lb at birth), liver disease, and galactosemia.
2. Because most tests are done after the newborn has been on milk (protein) for only about 24 hr, it is possible to miss a significant number of children with PKU.

Patient Care

1. Avoid repeated heel sticks. This can cause a fibrotic area on the infant's heel.
2. Check the puncture site for bleeding. Apply a pressure dressing if the bleeding persists.

Parent Education

1. Explain to the parent or primary caretaker that the test is a screening test to detect genetic diseases. The test is done on all newborns.
2. Inform the parent that the test involves taking a small sample of blood from the infant's heel.
3. If the test is to be repeated, obtain an appointment for the infant to return to the clinic or the physician's office.
4. Explain to the parent the importance of repeating the test, when this is necessary.

Signed Consent

Not required

QUANTITATIVE PHENYLALANINE BLOOD LEVELS

When an abnormal phenylalanine level is obtained in a screening program, repeated measurements of phenylalanine level are done on the infant's blood. The blood levels are correlated with a ferric chloride urine test. A positive ferric chloride urine test and abnormally elevated blood phenylalanine levels establish the diagnosis of PKU.

Laboratory Results

Normal Range

Adults	1.9 to 2.2 mg/dl
Newborn Infants	1.6 to 2.6 mg/dl
Child with PKU	16 to 46 mg/dl
Maintenance level for child with PKU	3 to 10 mg/dl

Nursing Implications
Procedure for Collection/Storage of Specimen

Small amounts of venous blood are needed. Many laboratories use micro-techniques, which require even smaller amounts of blood.

Patient Care

The infant or child is appropriately prepared according to age as for any other venipuncture. Restrain the infant if necessary with a mummy or papoose-type restraint in order to keep the infant from moving during the venipuncture.

Patient Education

1. Instruct the parent or primary caretaker in the importance of following the dietary regime.
2. Instruct the parent or primary caretaker in the need for periodic evaluation of serum phenylalanine levels. As the child grows older, foods are added to the diet. Most authorities believe the diet can be discontinued by the age of 8 years.
3. The child's protein intake is determined by the phenylalanine levels, which are monitored at regular intervals.
4. Instruct female patients on the importance of having periodic monitoring of the serum phenylalanine levels throughout their reproductive years.
5. Explain to the patient who has become pregnant the importance of regular phenylalanine monitoring. Pregnant women with a history of PKU should have phenylalanine levels measured at the first prenatal visit. Increased maternal levels of phenylalanine may cause intrauterine growth retardation, mental retardation, or a variety of congenital deformities.
6. Refer both parents of a child with PKU for genetic counseling.

Signed Consent

Not required

URINE TESTS
AMINOACIDURIA

The normal level of urinary amino acid excretion is relatively higher in infants than in adults. This reflects the infant's pattern of feeding. Increased amounts of amino acid excretion may be demonstrated in infants until the age of 6 months.

A metabolic disturbance may be suspected if there is an abnormal level of amino acid in the urine. If there is an abnormal level of amino acids in the urine, there may also be an elevated blood level of the same amino acid. After evaluation of the total urinary amino acid excretion, the presence and the amount of the specific amino acids in the urine can also be determined.

Aminoaciduria is also seen in untreated galactosemia and in the disease of phenylketonuria.

GALACTOSURIA

Persons with galactosemia spill galactose into the urine. The urine is therefore tested for the presence of galactose. The urine must be analyzed also for the presence of other sugars, especially glucose.

Laboratory Results
Normal Results

> Protein   Negative, 2 to 8 ml/dl of total protein
>
> Sugars (reducing substances) Negative

Significant Results with Galactosemia

- Copper reduction reagent, positive for all reducing substances (sugars)
- Enzyme test, negative for reducing substances
- Thin-layer chromatography, positive for specific sugars, such as galactose

Nursing Implications
Procedure for Collection/Storage of Specimen

See collection of urine specimens and testing for presence of sugars.

Possible Interfering Factors

1. Many laboratories routinely use a test that detects only the presence of glucose. Negative results may be interpreted as galactose-free.
2. Biliary atresia or hepatitis in infants will give positive results.

Patient Care

No special care

Patient Education

1. There is no special instruction for collection of specimens.
2. Instruct the parents or primary caretaker in restrictions.
3. As the child grows and new foods are introduced to the diet, explain to the parent the need for periodic evaluation to ascertain the status of the dietary compliance.
4. Teach the child how to comply with dietary restrictions. There is no evidence that dietary restrictions can be relaxed at any age.

Signed Consent

Not required

URINE TEST FOR PHENYLPYRUVIC ACID

Phenylpyruvic acid is excreted in the urine of persons who have a deficiency of a liver enzyme. This enzyme is needed to convert the amino acid phenylalanine into tyrosine. When the serum phenylalanine levels reach 12 to 15 mg/dl, phenylpyruvic acid can be detected in the urine. Phenylpyruvic acid is in the urine in abnormal infants between 2 to 8 weeks after birth.

Laboratory Results
Normal Results

No phenylpyruvic acid present in the urine.

Positive Results

> *Reagent strip.* Color changes indicate presence of 15 mg/dl or more of
> phenylpyruvic acid.
>
> *Ferric chloride test.* Transient color change to gray green or blue green.

Nursing Implications
Procedure for Collection/Storage of Specimen

Two methods can be used for screening purposes, the ferric chloride test
and the dipstick or reagent strip test.

1. *Ferric chloride test.* At least 5 ml of freshly voided urine are sent promptly
   to the laboratory. The specimen is refrigerated immediately after the
   voiding if it cannot be sent immediately to the laboratory.
2. *Dipstick or reagent method*
   a. Dip the strip into a sample of freshly voided urine or press the strip
      against a wet diaper containing freshly voided urine.
   b. In exactly 30 sec compare the strip to the color chart that accom-
      panies the bottle of dipsticks. The color chart indicates the concen-
      tration of phenylpyruvic acid in the urine: 0, 15, 40, and 100 mg.
   c. Record the test results in the patient's chart.

Possible Interfering Factors

1. Ketones in the urine may produce a false positive result, especially
   when the ferric chloride test is used. The dipstick method uses a different reagent source of ferric ions and is not as subject to interference
   from other substances.
2. Urine that is dilute, or urine with low specific gravity, will give unreliable results.
3. Phenylpyruvic acid is unstable when left at room temperature but stable
   under refrigeration.
4. The test is negative during the first week of life, even in children with
   PKU.
5. A positive result with the ferric chloride test can occur from the transient excretion of tyrosine.
6. Drugs that interfere with the test are salicylates and metabolites of
   phenothiazine derivatives.
7. A high bilirubin concentration will alter the reaction.

Patient Care
1. Use an infant urine collection bag to collect a routine urine specimen.
2. Remove the bag as soon as the infant has voided, and send the specimen
   to the laboratory.

Patient Education
Instruct the parent or primary caretaker to notify the nurse as soon as the
infant voids.

Signed Consent

Not required

STOOL TESTS
REDUCING SUBSTANCES IN THE STOOL

The disaccharides, glucose, lactose, and galactose are absorbed in the small intestine. When diarrhea occurs or when there are deficiencies of the enzymes necessary for breakdown of the sugars, these reducing substances are present in the stool. This test determines the presence of reducing substances in the stool.

Laboratory Results
Normal Results

Absence of reducing substances

Positive Results

0.5% sugar in two consecutive stools

Nursing Implications
Procedure for Collection/Storage of Specimen

1. Obtain a fresh stool specimen or stool that has been refrigerated for no more than 4 hr.
2. Drop 5 drops of liquid fecal material into a test tube.
3. Add 10 drops of water to the feces in the test tube.
4. Add a reagent tablet.
5. Watch the reaction. Do not shake the test tube.
6. When boiling stops, compare the resulting solution with the color chart that reports results from the 5-drop method.

Possible Interfering Factors

If the stool has not been refrigerated or tested immediately, bacterial fermentation will cause a low sugar content to be identified.

Patient Care

See discussion of collection of stool specimens.

Patient Education

Instruct the parent or caretaker in the importance of adhering to dietary restrictions when reducing substances are detected in the stool. For infants who are recovering from diarrhea and who have a temporary lactose intolerance, maintain the infant on a nonlactose formula until the ability to handle lactose is restored.

Signed Consent

Not required

STOOL pH

The pH of the stool is determined by the fermentation of bacteria and putrefaction of organic substances in the fecal material that takes place in the bowel.

Laboratory Results

Normal Results

Neutral or slightly alkaline

Nursing Implications

Procedure for Collection/Storage of Specimen

1. See discussion of collection of stool specimens.
2. Obtain a swab from a fresh stool specimen.
3. Obtain a rectal swab when unable to collect a stool.

Possible Interfering Factors

1. When excessive amounts of carbohydrates are present in the large intestine, the bacteria present cause fermentation to change the stool contents to strongly acid.
2. The process of protein breakdown can change the pH to alkaline.
3. Other conditions, especially steatorrhea, can produce highly acidic stools.

Patient Care

1. See discussion of collection of stool specimens.
2. To obtain a rectal swab, restrain the infant securely in the frog position. Gently insert a swab through the anal sphincter.

Patient Education

The purpose of the procedure is explained to the client or the primary caretaker.

Signed Consent

Not required

DIAGNOSTIC TESTS
AMNIOCENTESIS FOR GALACTOSEMIA

Galactosemia is one of the genetic disorders that can be diagnosed prenatally by amniocentesis. Cultured amniotic fluid cells have a deficiency of the necessary enzyme for galactose metabolism, galactose-1-phosphate uridyl transferase.

Nursing Implications

See Chapter 8 for care of the patient having an amniocentesis. Refer the patient for genetic counseling if a positive result is obtained.

INTESTINAL BIOPSY

A biopsy of the mucosal cells of the jejunum or duodenum is done to diagnose carbohydrate malabsorption. Lactose intolerance or lactase deficiency falls into the category of malabsorption. A lighted endoscope is introduced into the gastrointestinal tract and a tissue specimen is obtained. An analysis of the enzymatic activity of the tissue cells is done.

Normal Results

- Mucosal cells have no evidence of lesions.
- Mucosal lactase activity correlates with the activity of other enzymes present.

Positive Results

- Histologic changes can be microscopically identified in the mucosal cells.
- Enzyme activity in the cells is decreased.
- A decrease in the assayed activity of the enzyme lactase as compared to the activity of sucrase or isomaltase is significant.

Nursing Implications
Preprocedure

1. Explain the procedure to the patient or the primary caretaker. Use age-appropriate therapeutic play to prepare children.
2. Remove dentures, retainers, contact lenses, and other prosthetic appliances. Check child for loose teeth.
3. Administer preoperative medications as prescribed.
4. Encourage the primary caretaker to remain with the child at least until the procedure is begun.
5. Keep the patient NPO for 8 hr prior to the procedure to prevent aspiration and permit visualization of the duodenum.

During the Procedure

1. The physician may apply topical anesthesia to reduce gagging and discomfort during the procedure.
2. The procedure may be done under anesthesia in children and selected adults.
3. The scope is passed by the physician.

Postprocedure

1. Monitor vital signs until the patient has fully recovered from anesthesia.
2. Send the specimen to the appropriate laboratory promptly. Record the disposition of the biopsy specimen in the chart.
3. Keep the patient NPO for 2 to 4 hr until gag reflex has returned and the patient is fully recovered from general anesthesia.
4. Test the gag reflex by tickling the back of the pharynx with a tongue depressor.
5. Offer clear liquids as tolerated.
6. Advance the patient's diet as tolerated.
7. Explain to the parent that there may be a sore throat and reduced gag and swallowing reflexes following the procedure. Offer warm saline gargles to relieve pharyngeal discomfort.
8. Observe for signs of gastrointestinal perforation: abdominal pain,

subcutaneous emphysema, dyspnea, cyanosis, back pain, or abdominal rigidity.

9. Assess and record presence or absence of bowel sounds.
10. Assess and record breath sounds. Report any questionable finding.
11. Instruct the patient to relieve the feeling of fullness by passing flatus or by belching.

Signed Consent

Required

UPPER GASTROINTESTINAL SERIES IN LACTASE DEFICIENCY

When lactase deficiency is suspected, x-ray studies may be done to determine gastrointestinal structure and function. An upper gastrointestinal series with a small bowel follow-through may be done. (See the chapter on Digestive function for Upper Gastrointestinal Series.)

Normal Results

Normal gastrointestinal structure and function

Abnormal Results

There is an area of rapid dilatation of the intestine and an increased outpouring of fluid into the lumen in the area of the splenic flexure.

Nursing Implications

Preprocedure

Explain the procedure to the patient. Clarify for the patient the differences between this test and a routine upper gastrointestinal series.

During the Procedure

Fifty grams of lactose are added to the usual barium suspension.

Postprocedure

1. Observe and record the patient's response during the procedure.
2. Report to the physician and record the onset of diarrhea, type of stool, odor, amount, and frequency.
3. Assess the hydration status of the patient. The physician may order serum electrolytes to be drawn.
4. If fluid and electrolyte imbalance occurs, administer replacement fluids and electrolytes as prescribed to replace losses caused by the diarrhea.

Signed Consent

Not required

BIBLIOGRAPHY

American Academy of Pediatrics, Committee on Nutrition: The practical significance of lactose intolerance in children. Pediatrics 62, No. 2:240–245, 1978

Bauer JD, Ackermann PG, Toro G: Clinical Laboratory Methods, 8th ed. St Louis, CV Mosby, 1974

Berry, HK: The diagnosis of phenylketonuria, a commentary. Am J Dis Child 135:211–213, 1981

Bond JH, Levitt M: Use of breath hydrogen (H2) in the study of carbohydrate absorption. Am J Dig Dis 22, No. 4:379–382, 1977

Brunner LS, Suddarth DS: The Lippincott Manual of Nursing Practice, 2nd ed. Philadelphia, JB Lippincott, 1978

Copeland L: Chronic diarrhea in infancy. Am J Nurs 77:461–463, 1977

Davidsonn I, Henry JB: Todd-Sanford Clinical Diagnosis by Laboratory Methods. Philadelphia, WB Saunders, 1974

Donnell GN, Bergren WB: Mellituria. In Rudolph AM (ed): Pediatrics, 16th ed. pp 712–716. New York, Appleton-Century-Crofts, 1977

Eastham EJ, Walker WA: Adverse effects of milk formula ingestion on the gastrointestinal tract, an update. Gastroenterology 76, No. 2:365–374, 1979

Fischbach FT: A Manual of Laboratory Diagnostic Tests. Philadelphia, JB Lippincott, 1980

Gans SL, Ament M, Christie DL et al: Pediatric endoscopy with flexible fiberscopes. J Pediatr Surg 10, No. 3:375–380, 1975

Gleason WA, Tedesco FJ, Keating JP et al: Fiberoptic gastrointestinal endoscopy in infants and children. J Pediatr 85, No. 6:810–813, 1974

Gray GM: Intestinal disaccharidase deficiencies and glucose-galactose malabsorption. In Stanbury JB, Wyngaarden JB, Fredrickson DS (eds): The Metabolic Basis of Inherited Disease, 4th ed. New York, McGraw-Hill, 1978

Gross PT, Berlow S, Schuett VE et al: EEG in phenylketonuria, attempt to establish clinical importance of EEG changes. Arch Neurol 38, No. 2:122–126, 1981

Guyton AC: Textbook of Medical Physiology, 5th ed. Philadelphia, WB Saunders, 1976

Harrison M, Walker-Smith JA: Reinvestigation of lactose intolerant children: Lack of correlation between lactose intolerance and small intestinal morphology, disaccharidase activity, and lactose tolerance tests. Gut 18:48–52, 1977

Holdaway MD: Management of gastroenteritis in early childhood. Drugs 14:383–389, 1977

Koch R, Friedman EG: Accuracy of newborn screening programs for phenylketonuria. J Pediatr 98, No. 2:267–268, 1981

MacCready RA, Levy HL: The problem of maternal phenylketonuria. Am J Obstet Gynecol 113:121–128, 1972

Nitowsky HM: Biomedical aspects of gene action. In Rudolph AM (ed): Pediatrics, 16th ed. New York, Appleton-Century-Crofts, 1977

Nyhan WL: Disorders of amino acid metabolism. In Rudolph AM (ed): Pediatrics, 16th ed. New York, Appleton-Century-Crofts, 1977

Pettersson R, Dahlqvist A, Hatevig G et al: Borderline galactosemia. Acta Paediatr Scand 69:735–739, 1980

Ravel R: Clinical Laboratory Medicine, Clinical Application of Laboratory Data, 3rd ed. Chicago, Year Book, 1978

Segal S: Disorders of galactose metabolism. In Stanbury JB, Wyngaarden JB, Fredrickson DS (eds): The Metabolic Basis of Inherited Disease, 4th ed. pp 160–181. New York, McGraw-Hill, 1978

Sinclair L: Metabolic Disease in Childhood. Oxford, Blackwell Scientific Publications, 1979

Sisson JA: Handbook of Clinical Pathology. Philadelphia, JB Lippincott, 1976

Stanbury JB, Wyngaarden JB, Fredrickson DS: Inherited variation and metabolic abnormality. In Stanbury JB, Wyngaarden JB, Fredrickson DS (eds): The Metabolic Basis of Inherited Disease, 4th ed. pp 2–32. New York, McGraw-Hill, 1978

Thompson JS, Thompson MW: Genetics in Medicine, 2nd ed. Philadelphia, WB Saunders, 1973

Tourian AY, Sidbury JB: Phenylketonuria. In Stanbury JB, Wyngaarden JB, Fredrickson DS (eds): The Metabolic Basis of Inherited Disease, 4th ed. pp 240–255. New York, McGraw-Hill, 1978

Vangsted P: Galactosemia with cataract and persistent hyaloid artery. Acta Ophthalmol (Copenh) 58:812–818, 1980

Vorhees CV, Butcher RE, Berry HK:: Progress in experimental phenylketonuria: A critical review. Neurosci Biobehav Rev 5:177–190, 1981

Watts RWE, Baraitser M, Chalmers RA et al: Organic acidurias and amino acidurias in the aetiology of long term mental handicap. J Ment Defic Res 24:257–270, 1980

Whaley LF, Wong DL: Nursing Care of Infants and Children. St Louis, CV Mosby, 1979

7

Tests Related to Endocrine Function

Virginia A. Rahr

OVERVIEW OF PHYSIOLOGY AND PATHOPHYSIOLOGY

The endocrine system is made up of glands that synthesize and secrete hormones that are vital to life. Most hormones are secreted directly into the bloodstream by the endocrine glands and transported to specific target tissues where the hormones exert their effects.

Endocrine diseases are caused by either an excess or deficit in the secretion of one or more of the hormones. The chemical structure of hormones are proteins, peptides, amino acids, or steroids. Hormones need to be continually replaced by the body as they become metabolically inactive or are lost by urinary excretion. The endocrine system and the nervous system are integrated. Stimulation or disturbances of the central nervous system frequently alter the functions of the endocrine system. This integration is usually useful to the person's successful adaptation, but, under certain circumstances, may also produce disease conditions.

FUNCTION AND STRUCTURE

The endocrine system is involved in maintaining and regulating five vital body functions. These are the following:

- response to stress and injury
- regulation of metabolism and use of energy
- fluid and electrolyte balance
- reproduction
- growth and development

The endocrine system is primarily composed of seven glands:

- the pituitary
- the thyroid gland
- the parathyroid glands
- the adrenal glands
- the gonads
- islets of Langerhans of the pancreas
- the hypothalamus

PITUITARY

The pituitary gland, also called the hypophysis, is located in the brain. It was once called the "master gland" because it stimulates or regulates hormones of the other endocrine glands. However, it is now known to be regulated by the hypothalamus. Thus, the hypothalamus is the true master gland. The pituitary gland is about 1 cm in size and is located in the pituitary fossa of the sella turcica.

Hypothalamus Influence

The pituitary gland and the hypothalamus are closely interrelated by both vascular and central nervous system connections. The pituitary is connected to the hypothalamus by a structure known as the hypophyseal stalk. This connection is very important because the hypothalamus allows for the movement of "releasing factors" and "inhibiting factors" from the hypothalamus to the pituitary gland. The production and secretion of releasing or inhibiting factors are activated by stimuli from the brain. These factors from the hypothalamus reach the pituitary gland by a special vascular network.

The following factors are secreted by the hypothalamus:

- growth hormone releasing factor (GRF)
- growth hormone inhibiting factor (GIF)
- thyrotropin releasing factor (TRF)
- corticotropin releasing factor (CRF)
- follicle-stimulating hormone releasing factor (FRF)
- luteinizing hormone releasing factor (LRF)
- prolactin releasing factor (PRF)
- prolactin inhibiting factor (PIF)

There is also a thyrotropin inhibitory factor (which may be the same as GIF and is now called somatostatin).

This chapter will not include further discussion of the hypothalamic factors which influence the gonads, such as (FRF), (LRF), (PRF), and (PIF), nor of the gonadal hormones, as this material is covered in the chapter on reproductive function.

Since the pituitary gland has multiple functions, disorders or surgical removal of this gland have many serious effects on the body. Removal of the pituitary may require replacement of the hormones which are deficient. Hypersecretion of hormones from the pituitary, such as in certain pituitary tumors, may cause an excess of hormones.

ANTERIOR PITUITARY

The pituitary gland is composed of an anterior and a posterior lobe. The anterior pituitary responds to the blood-borne releasing or inhibiting factors, which are produced by the hypothalamus, by secreting or retaining certain hormones. Most anterior pituitary tropic hormones function by stimulating particular target organs to produce and release hormones. The growth hormone has no target organ that produces a hormone; most tissues are its target organs. The tropic hormones secreted by the anterior pituitary are the following:

- thyrotropin or thyroid-stimulating hormone (TSH)
- adrenocorticotropic hormone (ACTH)
- somatotropin or growth hormone (GH)
- the gonadotropins, which are the follicle-stimulating hormone (FSH) and luteinizing hormone (LH)
- prolactin

TSH

Thyrotropin (TSH) is necessary for the growth and function of the thyroid gland. The secretion of TSH is regulated by the balance between the stimulating effects of TRF and the inhibiting effect of the thyroid hormone serum level.

- When the thyroid hormone in the serum is low, increased TSH is secreted to increase the thyroid hormone level.

- If the thyroid hormone level is above normal, decreased TSH is secreted. This physiologic control is called the negative feedback mechanism and is one of a number of normal control mechanisms in the endocrine system.

- Rarely, disorders in secretion of TSH may cause either hypersecretion or hyposecretion of thyroid hormone.

ACTH

The adrenocorticotropic hormone (ACTH) regulates the growth of the adrenal cortex and its secretion of cortisone.

- Various biological stresses, such as trauma, hypoglycemia, bacterial infections, and hypoxia, cause increased secretion of cortisone.

- Excessive secretion of ACTH resulting from a dysfunction of the anterior pituitary, also results in hypersecretion of cortisone from the adrenal cortex.

GH

Somatotropin or growth hormone (GH) promotes the growth of bones, muscles, and various visceral organs. Growth hormone promotes use of fats as an energy source and has a carbohydrate and protein sparing effect.

- Disorders in secretion of growth hormone may result in giantism, dwarfism, or acromegaly.

(The functions of the gonadotropins and prolactin are discussed in the chapter on reproductive function).

POSTERIOR PITUITARY

The posterior lobe of the pituitary secretes antidiuretic hormone (ADH) and oxytoxin. Antidiuretic hormone is produced in the hypothalamus and is stored in the posterior pituitary. The posterior pituitary is connected to the hypothalamus by the nervous system rather than by the vascular system. The axons of the nerves regulate the release of ADH and oxytocin and carry the ADH and oxytocin to the posterior pituitary.

ADH

Antidiuretic hormone promotes reabsorption of water from the renal tubules and thus decreased excretion of water in the urine. Secretion of ADH is regulated by the amount of salt and other solutes in the blood.

- A deficiency of ADH results in a condition known as diabetes insipidus. In *diabetes insipidus,* large volumes of dilute urine are excreted and the body is unable to establish an appropriate water balance.

• A syndrome known as *inappropriate ADH secretion* is characterized by increased or persistent ADH secretion, resulting in excessive water retention. A concentrated urine or small volume is excreted, in spite of decreased sodium blood levels. The osmotic concentration of the blood becomes abnormally low because of the increased excretion of sodium in the urine and the retention of water.

Oxytocin

Oxytocin is also produced in the hypothalamus and stored in the posterior pituitary. Secretion of oxytocin from the posterior pituitary stimulates contraction of the uterus near the end of gestation and influences release of milk from the breasts in response to sucking stimulation.

THYROID

The thyroid gland is composed of two lobes connected by a thin isthmus and is located below the cricoid cartilage in the neck.

Disorders of the thryoid are related to an excess or deficit in the hormones produced by this gland. Thyroid enlargement (goiters), with or without abnormal hormone secretion, may also occur.

• Thyroid hormones are necessary for the normal development of the central nervous system. If they are deficient, mental retardation and delayed neurological maturation are seen in infants and children.

• In adults, hyposecretion of thyroid has many effects, one of which is mental sluggishness.

Thyroxine (T_4) and Triiodothyronine (T_3)

The principle hormones secreted by the thyroid gland are *thyroxine (T_4)*, and *triiodothyronine (T_3)*. Both T_3 and T_4 stimulate the oxidative reactions of most of the cells of the body, thus influencing the basal metabolic rate. These hormones are necessary for normal physical growth and development.

• Excessive secretion of T_3 or T_4, or both, results in a condition known as *hyperthyroidism*. The signs and symptoms represent an exaggeration of the normal functions of the thyroid hormones.

• For example, thyroid hormones control the rate of metabolism; in hyperthyroidism the metabolic rate is excessively increased, causing symptoms such as weight loss and heat intolerance.

Iodine

Adequate amounts of iodine intake are needed for healthy functioning of the thyroid gland. Iokine is absorbed from the small intestine into the circulation and is concentrated in the thyroid. It is a necessary product for formation of T_3 and T_4.

Calcitonin

Calcitonin is also a hormone produced by the thyroid gland. Calcitonin is released in the presence of increased blood calcium levels. Calcitonin's function is to lower serum calcium levels.

PARATHYROID

The parathyroid glands, of which there usually are four, are located behind the lobes of the thyroid gland. Two parathyroids are located behind the right thyroid lobe and two behind the left lobe. The parathyroid glands secrete parathyroid hormone (PTH), which is responsible for calcium and phosphate homeostasis in the body.

Parathyroid Hormone and Calcium Homeostasis

Serum calcium is maintained within normal limits by the interaction of PTH, calcitonin, and vitamin D. Vitamin D stimulates the absorption of calcium from the duodenum and upper jejunum. Vitamin D can also stimulate calcium resorption (or release) from bones and thus increase serum calcium. Parathyroid hormone increases serum calcium by stimulating gastrointestinal calcium absorption, calcium resorption from bone, and reabsorption of calcium by the kidney. *Calcitonin,* secreted by the thyroid, decreases serum calcium by decreasing gastrointestinal calcium absorption, calcium resorption from bone, and calcium reabsorption by the kidney.

Normally calcium homeostasis is maintained in that calcium input is equal to its output. Calcium output is controlled by the kidney and the gastrointestinal tract. Calcium is excreted in the urine and in the stool.

- When blood calcium levels are decreased (hypocalcemia), PTH secretion is stimulated and calcitonin secretion is suppressed.
- In the presence of increased blood calcium levels (hypercalcemia), PTH is suppressed and calcitonin secretion is stimulated.
- These controls allow for normal serum calcium levels.

Hyperparathyroidism

Hyperparathyroidism is a disorder in which increased PTH secretion causes increased gastrointestinal calcium absorption, calcium resorption from bone and reabsorption by the renal tubules. As calcium input becomes greater than its excretion, *hypercalcemia* results. Excessive parathyroid hormone also decreases reabsorption of phosphate by the kidney, thus increasing phosphate loss (hypophosphatemia).

Disorders other than hyperparathyroidism may cause excessive blood calcium levels. One example is increased resorption of calcium from the bones in patients with malignant metastases involving the bones. Long term immobility is another cause of increased loss of calcium from the bones and can result in hypercalcemia.

Hypoparathyroidism

Hypoparathyroidism is caused most frequently by damage or removal of the parathyroid glands during thyroidectomy. The results of decreased PTH seen in hypoparathyroidism are *hypocalcemia* and *hyperphosphatemia*. Vitamin D deficiency may also bring about hypocalcemia. Deficiency of vitamin D decreases the response of the gastrointestinal tract to PTH and less calcium is absorbed. Gastrectomy, resection of the small bowel and steatorrhea, as well as lack of adequate intake, may be causes of vitamin D deficiency.

PANCREAS

The pancreas has both endocrine and exocrine functions. Only endocrine functions will be discussed here. (See the chapter on gastrointestinal function for exocrine functions.)

Insulin

The beta cells of the islets of Langerhans of the pancreas secrete insulin. Insulin is a hormone that lowers blood glucose and assists in the transport of glucose from the blood into the cells. Glucagon, secreted by the alpha cells of the islets of Langerhans, has the opposite function—that of increasing blood glucose levels. Glucagon stimulates the breakdown of glycogen and the release of glucose by the liver, thereby causing an increase in blood sugar.

Diabetes Mellitus

Diabetes mellitus, the most common endocrine disorder, is related to an absence or deficiency of insulin production or resistance to insulin. An abnormally high blood glucose level (*hyperglycemia)* results. Increased glucagon secretion may also play a part in the pathophysiology of diabetes by augmenting production of hyperglycemia and ketonemia.

Hormones from other endocrine glands that increase blood sugar levels are the following: (1) growth hormone secreted by the anterior pituitary, (2) epinephrine secreted from the adrenal medulla, and (3) glucocorticoids (steroids) secreted from the adrenal cortex.

The chief function of insulin is to transport glucose from the bloodstream into the cells.

- When there is a complete or relative absence of insulin, metabolism of carbohydrate, fat, and protein are adversely affected.

- In the absence of insulin, the cells cannot receive adequate glucose, even if blood glucose levels are very high.

- As a compensatory mechanism, the body breaks down fats and uses them for energy.

- The end products of fat metabolism result in an abnormally high level of fatty acids and *ketone* bodies in the blood.

- Excessive amounts of ketone bodies result in ketoacidosis, or metabolic acidosis.

Protein synthesis is adversely affected when insulin is lacking, because insulin is needed for amino acid uptake by many cells and for conversion of these amino acids to protein. This is one reason for decreased rate of wound healing found in many diabetics.

Diabetics have a significantly increased incidence of vascular complications. An accelerated atherosclerotic process thought to be related to increased blood fatty acids, is associated with diabetes and results in conditions such as coronary artery disease, stroke, renal insufficiency, peripheral vascular disease and retinal changes.

Hypoglycemia

An abnormal increase in the secretion of insulin from the pancreas is much less common, but might be seen in some neoplastic disorders of the pancreas. Increased insulin secretion leads to an abnormally low blood glucose level (hypoglycemia). Hypoglycemia is more frequently seen in the diabetic patient who has received too much insulin or has skipped meals or has had an increased amount of exercise.

ADRENAL GLANDS

The adrenal glands are located at the superior pole of each kidney. The adrenal gland has two parts, the cortex (the outer part) and the medulla (the center). The adrenal cortex synthesizes and secretes four types of adrenocortical hormones:

- glucocorticoids (cortisol or hydrocortisone)
- mineralocorticoids (aldosterone)
- androgens
- estrogens

Cortisol and Cushing's Syndrome

Excessive secretion of glucocorticoids results in the clinical condition known as Cushing's syndrome. Hypersecretion of cortisol may be caused by a pituitary disorder in which excessive ACTH is produced and the adrenal cortex is overstimulated. A tumor or other disorder of the cortex, independent of the pituitary, may also cause hypersecretion. Signs and symptoms of Cushing's syndrome may also be caused by prolonged drug therapy with large doses of synthetic corticosteroids.

Aldosterone and Aldosteronism

Excessive secretion of aldosterone, the mineralocorticoid produced by the adrenal cortex, causes the disorder of aldosteronism. Fluid and electrolyte imbalances, specifically depletion of potassium and retention of sodium, are some of the metabolic effects of aldosteronism. Hypertension is one of the clinical manifestations.

There are two types of aldosteronisms: (1) primary and (2) secondary. Primary aldosteronism is caused by a tumor or hyperplasia of the adrenal cortex, which autonomously produces excessive aldosterone secretion. Secondary aldosteronism may result when blood supply to the kidneys is inadequate, which leads to stimulation of the renin–angiotensin system. Angiotensin stimulates increased production of aldosterone in a normal adrenal cortex. Plasma renin levels and plasma and urine aldosterone levels are important in the diagnosis of secondary aldosteronism.

Addison's Disease

An insufficient production of the hormones of the adrenal cortex causes Addison's disease. In Addison's disease there is a deficiency of the glucocorticoids, mineralocorticoids (aldosterone), and androgens. The major clinical manifestations are due to a deficiency of the glucocorticoids and aldosterone.

- Lack of cortisol results in hypoglycemia, weakness, and inability to withstand stress. Lack of aldosterone results in the inability to conserve sodium and excrete potassium.

- The sodium depletion may cause hypotension and may be a life-threatening emergency. The cause may be decreased pituitary ACTH production (secondary adrenocortical insufficiency) or a disease of the adrenal cortex (primary adrenocortical insufficiency). In the case of secondary adrenal insufficiency, aldosterone secretion remains intact, since it is largely independent of ACTH (depends more on the renin–angiotensin system).

Catecholamines and Pheochromocytoma

The adrenal medulla contains chromaffin cells which synthesize and secrete hormones known as catecholamines. The most active components of the adrenal catecholamines are epinephrine (adrenalin) and norepinephrine. Metabolic changes eventually convert these hormones into vanillylmandelic acid (VMA), which is excreted in the urine.

Pheochromocytoma is an uncommon tumor that originates from chromaffin cells and results in hypersecretion of the catecholamines. Chromaffin tissues may be located in abdominal or pelvic areas, however most tissues of this type are located in the adrenal medulla. Most pheochromocytomas are benign.

- The major clinical manifestation of pheochromocytoma is paroxysmal hypertension.

- Other symptoms, such as increased heart rate, profuse perspiration, and pounding headaches, are also related to increased circulating catecholamines.

(Disorders of the gonads are discussed in the chapter on reproductive function).

BLOOD TESTS
CALCIUM (Ca^{++})

The parathyroid glands secrete parathyroid hormone, which maintains a normal balance between calcium and phosphorus blood levels.

Hyperparathyroidism, usually caused by an adenoma, is the endocrine dysfunction that causes abnormally increased serum calcium levels. Decreased phosphorus levels also result.

Hypoparathyroidism causes abnormally decreased serum calcium levels and increased phosphorus levels. Hypothyroidism may occur after surgery involving the thyroid and parathyroid glands. (For details related to this test, see page 92.)

DEXAMETHASONE SUPPRESSION TEST

Patients with Cushing's syndrome have abnormally increased levels of plasma cortisol. In normal persons, the drug dexamethasone (Decadron) suppresses ACTH secretion, which, in turn, causes decreased cortisol secretion. Patients with Cushing's syndrome do not respond to dexamethasone, since cortisol secretion in Cushing's syndrome is not dependent on ACTH.

Laboratory Results
Normal Values

In the absence of Cushing's syndrome, the cortisol level falls <5 μg/dl after the administration of dexamethasone.

In the presence of Cushing's syndrome, plasma cortisol levels remain >10 μg/dl.

Nursing Implications
Procedure for Collection/Storage of Specimen

1. Dexamethasone 1.0 to 2.0 mg is given orally between 10 P.M. and midnight.
2. A blood sample of 10 ml is drawn at 8 A.M. the following morning.

Possible Interfering Factors

Failure of cortisol suppression after dexamethasone in the absence of Cushing's syndrome may be seen in the following conditions:

- acutely ill patients
- patients receiving phenytoin (Dilantin) or estrogen-containing drugs.

Patient Care
Observe the patient for signs and symptoms of Cushing's syndrome.

Patient Education
1. Explain the test and its purpose to the patient.
2. A second test using a higher dose of dexamethasone may be ordered if there is nonsuppression using the low dose of dexamethasone.
3. If Cushing's syndrome is confirmed, reinforce the physician's plan for further studies or treatment.

Signed Consent
Not required

GLUCOSE OR FASTING BLOOD SUGAR (FBS)

The glucose level is a blood measurement for glucose levels. The test is most frequently done to diagnose and monitor the patient with diabetes mellitus. Since the test is done after the patient has fasted, the test is referred to as the fasting blood sugar (FBS).

Conditions other than diabetes mellitus that may increase the blood glucose level (hyperglycemia) include the following: stress, certain drugs, chronic liver or renal disease, and hypokalemia.

The following endocrine disorders can also increase blood glucose levels: Cushing's syndrome, pheochromocytoma, hyperthyroidism, and acromegaly.

The following conditions may decrease blood glucose levels (hypoglycemia): pancreatic islet cell tumor, anterior pituitary hypofunction, Addison's disease, extensive liver disease, and steatorrhea. Hypoglycemia may also occur under certain conditions in the diabetic who is on insulin therapy.

Laboratory Results
Normal Range

Adult	Fasting Serum	70 to 110 mg/dl
	Fasting Whole Blood	60 to 110 mg/dl
Pediatric	Fasting Serum	60 to 105 mg/dl
	Fasting Whole Blood	50 to 90 mg/dl

Fasting serum glucose levels of >150 mg/dl are considered diagnostic of diabetes mellitus. There is normally a slight elevation of glucose during pregnancy. A fasting or nonfasting glucose level of <60 mg/dl signifies hypoglycemia.

Nursing Implications
Procedure for Collection/Storage of Specimen

1. Collect a sample of venous blood while the patient is in a fasting state.
2. Send the blood sample to the laboratory as soon as possible after collection. It should be refrigerated at 4°C.

Possible Interfering Factors

1. A delay in processing the specimen may result in a falsely lowered value.
2. The following drugs may increase the blood glucose to above normal levels:

   - steroids
   - estrogens
   - diuretics
   - phenytoin (Dilantin)
   - nicotinic acid
   - phenothiazines

Patient Care

1. If diabetes mellitus is diagnosed, initiate a comprehensive teaching plan including diet, insulin, exercise, and prevention of complications.
2. Observe the patient for signs and symptoms of abnormally high or low blood glucose levels.
3. Use the same method of testing each time. Results may vary with different tests.

Patient Education

Explain the test to the patient. Be certain that the patient understands that no food or liquids other than water are allowed after midnight prior to the test.

Signed Consent

Not required

GROWTH HORMONE (Somatotropin)

Baseline growth hormone (GH) levels are unreliable in the evaluation of patients with growth hormone excess or deficit. Therefore, GH stimulation and suppression tests are used.

In patients with overproduction of growth hormone, such as in giantism or acromegaly, there is lack of GH suppression in response to administration of 100 g of oral glucose. Normally GH levels decrease after glucose administration.

The usual clinical situation for assessing GH is the child who fails to grow. GH deficiency may be caused by a pituitary tumor, trauma, infection, or the cause may be unknown. There are several methods to stimulate GH. One method is by oral administration of L-dopa, another is by intravenous injection of regular insulin. In both methods there is expected to be a rise in serum GH levels. If GH deficiency is present, the rise is absent or subnormal. Definite evidence of GH deficiency should be assessed by using both the L-dopa and insulin methods.

Laboratory Results
Normal Values

- Basal serum GH levels at 8:00 A.M. are 5 ng/ml or lower in adults and in children after infancy. In the newborn period basal levels are high (15 to 40 ng/ml). Normally GH levels decrease to 2 ng/ml 1 to 2 hr after glucose administration.

- After L-dopa or insulin administration, an increase of >7 ng/ml from the basal (baseline) value is considered a normal response.

Abnormal Values

- Patients with acromegaly have elevated baseline GH levels and fail to suppress GH in response to glucose.

- Patients with GH deficiency have absent or subnormal responses to L-dopa and insulin stimulation tests.

Nursing Implications
Procedure for Collection/Storage of Specimen
Testing for elevated GH levels

Blood (10 ml) for GH and glucose is obtained before, and 1 and 2 hours following, ingestion of 100 g of glucose.

Testing for deficiency of GH levels (L-dopa method)

1. With the patient fasting, L-dopa is administered orally (500 mg for adults and children weighing more than 35 kg, 250 mg for children between 20 and 35 kg, and 125 mg for children weighing less than 20 kg.
2. Blood (10 ml) is drawn at 0, 30, 60, 90, and 120 min after L-dopa administration.

Insulin method

1. With the patient fasting, regular insulin is injected in a dose of 0.05 to 0.1 u/kg.
2. Hypoglycemia (20 to 40 mg/dl 30 min after insulin administration) is documented. Intravenous glucose should be on hand in case severe hypoglycemia symptoms develop.
3. Blood samples are collected at 0, 30, 45, 60, 90, and 120 min after insulin administration.

Possible Interfering Factors

1. Many factors such as eating, exercise, stress, and sleep can increase baseline serum GH levels.
2. A decreased GH response to regular insulin may be seen in the following conditions:
   - obese individuals
   - persons on high carbohydrate diets
   - glucocorticoid therapy
   - hypothyroidism

Patient Care

1. Keep the patient in a resting, stress-free environment during the test.
2. When regular insulin is given as the GH stimulation test, observe the patient very carefully for symptoms of severe hypoglycemia. Have intravenous glucose available if needed.

Patient Education

1. Explain the test and its purpose to the patient. Children may be assisted in their coping abilities by using therapeutic play activities.
2. Relate further teaching to the problem that may be found. If abnormal results are not found, the patient and family may also need support.

Signed Consent

Not required

PHOSPHORUS

Hypoparathyroidism is an endocrine disorder that can lead to increased serum phosphate levels. Phosphate levels are inversely related to calcium levels. When blood calcium is abnormally decreased, blood phosphate is abnormally increased and *visa versa*. Depression of phosphate levels, or hypophosphatemia, is normally associated with hyperparathyroidism in patients with normal renal function. (For details related to this test, see page 95.)

PLASMA ADRENOCORTICOTROPIC HORMONE (ACTH)

ACTH, which is secreted from the anterior pituitary, regulates the secretion of hormones from the adrenal cortex. Plasma ACTH levels may be done to diagnose dysfunctions of the pituitary gland or the adrenal cortex. Plasma

ACTH levels are generally low in patients with an adrenal tumor, because the excessive production of cortisol causes the negative feedback cycle to decrease ACTH secretion. Plasma ACTH levels are increased when there is a primary adrenal deficiency, as the negative feedback cycle attempts to stimulate production of cortisol. Greatly elevated ACTH levels are found in ectopic ACTH-producing tumors or in pituitary adenomas that cause increased secretion of ACTH.

Laboratory Results
Normal Range

Plasma ACTH at 8 A.M. 20 to 100 pg/ml

Nursing Implications
Procedure for Collection/Storage of Specimen

1. At 8 A.M. 10 ml of blood is drawn.
2. The tube should contain heparin and 1.25 mg of N-ethylmaleimide, which prevents the degradation of ACTH for at least 72 hr at room temperature.

Possible Interfering Factors

None reported

Patient Care
Observe the patient particularly for any signs and symptoms of cortisol excess, such as in Cushing's syndrome.

Patient Education
Explain the test and its purpose to the patient.

Signed Consent
Not required

PLASMA CORTISOL
Cortisol is the most potent and abundant steroid hormone secreted by the adrenal cortex. Plasma cortisol may be used as a screening test for Cushing's syndrome or a suspected hormone-secreting tumor of the adrenal cortex. Normally there is a diurnal variation of plasma cortisol. Highest levels occur around 6 to 8 A.M. and lowest levels usually occur about midnight. Approximately one half of the early morning level is present at 4 to 5 P.M. This normal diurnal variation is not seen in Cushing's syndrome, and cortisol levels are increased. However, the test is not always valid because of the episodic nature of cortisol secretion. Blood samples may be obtained when the adrenal cortex is not abnormally active, even in the presence of Cushing's syndrome.

Laboratory Results
Normal Range

7 to 25 μg/dl at about 8:00 A.M.

<10 μg/dl at about 8:00 P.M.

Nursing Implications

Procedure for Collection/Storage of Specimen

1. A venous blood sample is obtained at 8:00 A.M. and probably again at 8:00 P.M.
2. The specimen should be sent to the laboratory immediately. Delay in processing the specimen may yield a falsely decreased value because of cortisol uptake by red blood cells.
3. Several blood samples may be drawn during the day to determine if diurnal variation is present.

Possible Interfering Factors

Elevated plasma cortisol levels may be seen in the following conditions:

- stress, which causes increased cortisol secretions
- chronic liver disease or chronic renal failure, which cause decreased cortisol metabolism
- women on estrogen-containing medications, which cause increased synthesis of corticosteroids

Patient Care

1. Observe the patient for signs and symptoms of Cushing's syndrome.
2. Decrease sources of stress for the patient during the testing period if possible.

Patient Education

1. Explain the test and its purpose to the patient. The patient may be especially concerned if several blood specimens are taken within a 24-hr period.
2. Encourage the patient to be as relaxed as possible during the testing period, as stress can increase cortisol secretion.

Signed Consent

Not required

PLASMA RENIN ACTIVITY

Renin is an enzyme produced by the kidney. The production of renin is influenced by the pressure of blood flowing through the afferent arteriole into the glomerulus of the kidney. Factors such as decreased arterial pressure and renal ischemia cause increased amounts of renin to be secreted. Renin activates angiotensin II, which stimulates the production of aldosterone by the adrenal cortex. This sequence of activities causes sodium reabsorption, blood volume expansion, and increased blood pressure. It is important to evaluate plasma renin activity in selected hypertensive patients. This test is useful in patients who have excessive aldosterone secretion, to differentiate between primary and secondary aldosteronism. Increased renin activity is normally seen in patients with hypokalemia or sodium and blood volume depletion. Upright posture also increases renin secretion. Renin cannot be measured directly, but an estimate of its production can be made by examining plasma renin activity.

Laboratory Results

Normal Range

Normal values vary widely depending on laboratory technique.

Normal Plasma Renin Activity (ng/ml per hr)

Condition	120 mEq Na*	10 mEq Na* (low Na intake)
8 A.M. recumbent	0.3–1.5	1.2–3.4
8 A.M. upright	0.6–2.3	2.9–5.9
Noon, upright	0.8–1.9	3.1–9.1
Noon, after oral administration of furosemide (Lasix) 80 mg at 8 A.M.	1.8–7.2	

*amount of Na intake for 3 days prior to the test

Normally plasma renin activity increases in response to low sodium intake and upright posture. In patients with primary aldosteronism renin activity does not increase under these conditions. Patients with secondary aldosteronism have abnormally elevated values and may have a greatly increased response to upright posture.

Nursing Implications

Procedure for Collection/Storage of Specimen

1. Ensure that the specified sodium diet has been followed, as prescribed by the physician.
2. Obtain a venous blood specimen.
3. Place the specimen on crushed ice and send it to the laboratory at once.

Alternate Procedure

1. After drawing blood at 8 A.M. the patient is given an oral dose of 80 mg of furosemide (Lasix).
2. The patient is asked to remain in an upright posture until noon, when a second blood sample is obtained.
3. This procedure may be indicated for outpatients when very specific salt intake is difficult to control.

Possible Interfering Factors

High values may be seen in the following conditions:

- patients receiving diuretics (volume and sodium depletion)
- patients receiving estrogen-containing medications
- patients receiving antihypertensive drugs (except for apresoline and methyldopa)
- hypokalemia
- upright posture

Patient Care

1. Carefully assess the patient's blood pressure readings, as plasma renin activity evaluation is usually associated with diagnosing certain types of hypertension. Most antihypertensive medications are withheld for 1 to 2 wk before the test.
2. If a diet with specified sodium intake has been prescribed by the physician, make sure the patient eats the prescribed foods and none other. Notify the physician or laboratory if the patient is unable to comply.

Patient Education

1. Explain the test and its purpose to the patient.
2. Explain dietary or drug changes ordered prior to the test.

Signed Consent

Not required

PROTEIN-BOUND IODINE (PBI), BUTANOL-EXTRACTABLE IODINE (BEI)

The PBI and BEI are tests that measure the amount of organic iodine bound to protein in the blood. The level of PBI and BEI reflects thyroid function. The PBI was once used widely. Its use now is limited, because any condition that increases or decreases the level of proteins that carry thyroxine also falsely increases or decreases the amount of PBI. Iodine-containing drugs also cause inaccurate results. The BEI is similar to the PBI but is more accurate and less likely to be influenced by drugs containing iodine.

Increased PBI and BEI levels are found in hyperthyroidism and in acute thyroiditis. Pregnancy may normally cause a mild increase in the PBI. Decreased PBI and BEI levels are found in hypothyroidism and myxedema, chronic thyroiditis, and in nephrosis.

Laboratory Results

Normal Range

PBI	4.0 to 8.0 µg/dl
BEI	3.5 to 6.5 µg/dl

Nursing Implications

Procedure for Collection/Storage of Specimen

1. Obtain a venous sample of at least 3 ml.
2. Schedule the test before any other diagnostic tests which use iodine. Common diagnostic tests using iodine in the contrast media are the IVP, gallbladder x-ray, myelogram, and CT scan.

Possible Interfering Factors

1. A diet high in iodine, such as seafood and iodized salt, may interfere with test results.
2. False elevations occur after the use of iodine-containing contrast media,

such as is used in the IVP, gallbladder x-rays, myelograms, CT scans, and bronchograms. These substances interfere for varying lengths of times.

3. Numerous drugs interfere with the PBI and BEI. Some of the more common drugs include the following:

- thyroid hormones
- estrogens
- steroids
- multipurpose vitamin supplements containing A & D
- thiazide diuretics
- sulfonamides
- salicylates (high doses)

Patient Care

Observe the patient for signs and symptoms of thryoid abnormalities, such as hyper- or hypothyroidism.

Patient Education

1. Explain the test and its purpose to the patient.
2. Instruct the patient to eat an iodine-free diet for 3 dy prior to the test. No iodized salt should be used. Consult the dietary department for more specific information.
3. Explain to the patient why the physician may discontinue some drugs for about 1 wk before the test.

Signed Consent

Not required

SERUM THYROXINE (T_4), SERUM TRIIODOTHYRONINE (T_3), AND THYROID-BINDING GLOBULIN (TBG) TEST

Thyroxine (T_4) and triiodothyronine (T_3) are hormones synthesized and released by the thyroid gland. The primary screening test for hyperthyroidism is the measurement of serum T_4 concentration in the blood. Measurement of serum T_3 is also necessary, as some patients with hyperthyroidism have normal T_4 levels, but elevated T_3 levels. Serum T_3 and T_4 levels normally regulate the thyroid-stimulating hormone (TSH) secreted by the anterior pituitary gland.

The thyroid hormones, particularly thyroxine, circulate in the blood bound to three types of plasma proteins. Thyroxine-binding globulin (TBG) is one of these plasma proteins that is measured. Thyroid-binding globulin abnormalities may affect the results of thyroxine measurements.

In hyperthyroidism, T_4, T_3, and TBG serum levels are increased. Pregnancy may temporarily increase T_4 levels. In hypothyroidism T_4, T_3, and TBG serum levels are decreased. Normal pregnancy, menstruation, and liver disease may decrease T_3 levels. Serum T_3 levels may be increased in infancy.

Diseases that may cause increased T_3 levels are liver disease, severe nephrosis, atrial arrhythmias and fibrillation, metastatic cancer, COPD, polycythemia vera, uremia, and threatened abortion.

Laboratory Results
Normal Range

T_4	3.8 to 11.4% or 5.0 to 13.7 µg/dl
T_3	25 to 35% or 80 to 220 ng/dl
TBG	0.9 to 1.1

Nursing Implications
Procedure for Collection/Storage of Specimen

A venous blood sample is obtained. No radioactive substances are given.

Possible Interfering Factors

Drugs or conditions that may increase T_4 levels include the following:

- pregnancy
- estrogen-containing drugs
- clofibrate
- residual radioactivity from other tests

  Drugs that may decrease T_4 levels include the following:

- aminosalicylic acid
- corticosteroids
- lithium
- methylthiouracil
- reserpine
- sulfonamides
- chlorpromazine
- testosterone
- heparin
- tolbutamide
- diphenylhydantoin

  Drugs that may increase T_3 levels include the following:

- ACTH
- anabolic agents
- androgens
- anticoagulants (dicumarol and heparin)
- corticosteroids
- thyroid preparations
- diphenylhydantoin and diphenylhydantoxin

- phenylbutazone
- salicylates (high doses)
- heroin withdrawal
- methadone
- penicillin (large doses)
  Drugs that may decrease T_3 levels include the following:
- ACTH
- antithyroid drugs
- chlordiazepoxide
- corticosteroids
- estrogens, including oral contraceptives
- ipodate
- perphenazine
- thiazide diuretics
- sulfonylureas
  Drugs that may increase TBG levels include the following:
- chlormadinone
- oral contraceptives
  Drugs that may decrease TBG levels include the following:
- anabolic agents
- androgens

Patient Care

1. Observe the patient for signs and symptoms of thyroid dysfunction, especially hyperthyroidism or hypothyroidism.
2. Review the drugs the patient is taking. Inform the physician of any drugs that may interfere with the test results.

Patient Instruction

1. Explain the tests and their purpose to the patient.
2. If thyroid dysfunction is diagnosed, begin appropriate teaching of the patient.

Signed Consent

Not required

THORN ACTH TEST

The Thorn ACTH test is useful in the diagnosis of Addison's disease or to determine adrenal corticol function. The test can also be used to distinguish between hypofunction of the pituitary gland and disease of the adrenal cortex. When ACTH is administered intramuscularly it produces a decrease in the eosinophil count in persons whose adrenal cortex is functioning normally.

Laboratory Results

Normal

A 50% or greater decrease in the eosinophil count 4 hr after ACTH has been administered.

Adrenal Insufficiency

20 percent decrease in eosinophil count.

Nursing Implications

Procedure for Collection/Storage of Specimen

1. Withhold food after 8 P.M. prior to the morning of the test. Water is allowed.
2. A venous blood sample is drawn and an eosinophil count is done.
3. Administer ACTH as prescribed and note the exact time it was given.
4. A second venous blood sample is drawn 4 hr later and the eosinophil count is repeated.

Possible Interfering Factors

None reported

Patient Care

Observe the patient for signs and symptoms of adrenal cortical hypofunction.

Patient Education

1. Explain the test and its purpose to the patient.
2. If adrenal corticol insufficiency is diagnosed, teach the patient about management of the insufficiency. Cortisone therapy is likely to be prescribed.

Signed Consent

Not required

THYROID-STIMULATING HORMONE (TSH) OR SERUM THYROTROPIN

The TSH test is used to differentiate primary from secondary hypothyroidism and to indicate the level of thyroid gland activity. Primary hypothyroidism occurs when there is an intrinsic disease of the thyroid gland. Secondary hypothyroidism occurs when there is inadequate stimulation of the thyroid gland by TSH from the pituitary.

In the TSH test the ability of the thyroid gland to respond to an intramuscular injection of TSH is determined. In primary hypothyroidism, TSH values are high because the thyroid gland cannot produce enough thyroxine to inhibit TSH by way of the normal negative feedback cycle. In secondary hypothyroidism, after TSH administration, TSH values are low or normal because the pituitary is secreting inadequate amounts of thyrotropin. In cases of diminished thyroid reserve, such as in subtotal thyroidectomy or postradiation therapy to the thyroid, there is no response to TSH stimulation.

This test can be used even if the patient is receiving thyroid replacement therapy.

Laboratory Results
Normal Value

TSH < 5 μu/ml

Normally T_4 and radioactive iodine uptake is increased within 8 to 10 hr after TSH is administered.

Nursing Implications
Procedure for Collection/Storage of Specimen

After the prescribed amount of TSH is administered intramuscularly, collect blood samples at the intervals indicated by your laboratory.

Possible Interfering Factors

Iodine intake may antagonize TSH stimulation and cause decreased TSH values.

Patient Care
1. Observe the patient for signs and symptoms of hypothyroidism.
2. Restrict iodine intake if ordered. Consult the dietary department if necessary.
3. Take a nursing history to determine if the patient has a large intake of iodine such as in seafood, multivitamins, expectorants containing iodine, or salt.

Patient Education
1. Explain the test to the patient.
2. Relate further teaching to management of the problem identified by the test.

Signed Consent
Not required

TWO-HOUR POSTPRANDIAL BLOOD SUGAR (2-hr PPBS)
The 2-hour postprandial blood sugar test measures blood glucose two hours after the patient has eaten a high carbohydrate meal. This test is a more definitive screening test for diabetes than the FBS. In a nondiabetic, the blood glucose returns to normal two hours after eating. The blood glucose remains abnormally increased two hours postprandially in the untreated diabetic. Abnormally increased or decreased glucose levels would likely be found in the same conditions listed under the FBS.

Laboratory Results
Normal Range

After two hours	145 mg/dl for adults under 50 years old
	160 mg/dl for persons in their sixties
	180 mg/dl for persons older than seventy

Nursing Implications

Procedure for Collection/Storage of Specimen

1. Keep the patient fasting at least 8 hr prior to the test. Water is permitted.
2. Obtain a venous blood sample 2 hr after the patient finishes eating a high carbohydrate meal, usually breakfast.
3. Note the time the meal is completed and notify the laboratory.
4. The patient should not smoke during this period of time.

Possible Interfering Factors

Smoking may raise the blood glucose level.

Patient Care

Encourage the patient to eat all of the pretest meal.

Patient Education

1. Explain the procedure to the patient. Be sure the patient understands the reasons for eating all of the meal prior to the test.
2. If diabetes is diagnosed, begin teaching the patient about the disease and its management.

Signed Consent

Not required

GLUCOSE TOLERANCE TEST (GTT)

The GTT may be done when the FBS or the 2-hr postprandial blood glucose levels are abnormally elevated but not conclusive for diabetes. The GTT may also be ordered to assist in the diagnosis of hypoglycemia, malabsorption syndrome, Cushing's syndrome, and acromegaly. Glucose intolerance is most frequently related to diabetes mellitus, but many other conditions can cause increased blood glucose levels. The GTT is indicated when there is suspected diabetes, and when one or more of the following conditions exist:

- obesity
- recurrent infections
- family history of diabetes, especially adult-onset
- women who have given birth to large infants or who have had stillbirths, abortions, or premature labor
- transient hyperglycemia or glycosuria during stressors such as pregnancy, surgery, or infections
- episodes of hypoglycemia of unknown cause

Laboratory Results

Normal Range

FBS	70–120 mg/100ml
30 min	155 mg/100ml
1 hr	165 to 180 mg/100 ml

2 hr	140 mg/100 ml (160 mg 100 ml for the elderly, *i.e.,* age 70)
3 hr	80 to 120 mg/100 ml

All urines should be negative for glucose.

Hypoglycemia—blood glucose is below normal (<60 mg/100 ml) after 2 hr and up to 4 or 5 hr. High insulin levels, or hyperinsulinism, cause the hypoglycemia.

Nursing Implications

Procedure for Collection/Storage of Specimen

1. Have the patient eat a diet containing at least 300 g of carbohydrate for 3 dy prior to the test.
2. Obtain a venous blood sample of 7 ml after the patient has fasted overnight.
3. Have the patient drink a concentrated liquid glucose preparation. The liquid should contain 1.75 g of glucose per/g of body weight. All of the solution must be taken. The patient is encouraged to drink the solution quickly.
4. Obtain blood and urine samples at intervals of 30 min, 1, 2 and sometimes 3 or 4 hours after ingestion of the glucose.
5. Allow the patient to drink water, but no other liquids during the test.

Possible Interfering Factors

1. The following drugs may influence the test and should be discontinued before the test.
   - hormones, including oral contraceptives
   - hypoglycemic agents
   - diuretics, especially the thiazides
   - salicylates
   - nicotinic acid
   - ferrous ascorbinate
   - lithium
   - phenothiazines
   - metapyrine
2. Insulin or oral hypoglycemics should not be given until after the test is completed.
3. Inability of the patient to drink or retain all of the glucose solution may cause inaccurate results.
4. Smoking may cause increased glucose levels.
5. A weight-reduction diet prior to the test can decrease carbohydrate tolerance and yield increased blood glucose levels.
6. Bedrest over a lengthy period of time may influence glucose tolerance. The patient should be ambulatory preceding the test.
7. Surgery, febrile illnesses, and other stressors may cause increased glucose levels.

8. Many disease conditions other than diabetes can cause abnormal blood glucose levels. (For more information related to blood glucose levels, see page 238.)

Patient Care

1. Observe the patient for any reactions during the test. Sweating, weakness and faintness may occur between the second and third hours. This response is normal and transient unless hyperinsulinism is present. Protect the patient who feels faint from injury.
2. Collect urine and blood samples at the specified time. Record the time on the specimens.

Patient Education

1. Explain the procedure and its purpose to the patient. Outpatients especially benefit from written instructions.
   a. Remind the patient to eat a normal, high carbohydrate diet for at least 3 dy before the test.
   b. The patient must fast for 8 to 12 hr before the test.
2. Allow no food or liquids other than water during the test.
3. Encourage the patient to drink water during the test to facilitate obtaining urine samples needed for testing. The patient should empty the bladder with each voiding.
4. Instruct the patient not to smoke during the testing period.

Signed Consent

Not required

URINE TESTS
ALDOSTERONE (Plasma and 24-Hour Urine)

Aldosterone, a hormone produced by the adrenal cortex, may be measured in hypertensive patients. A small percentage of hypertensive patients have increased blood pressure related to elevated aldosterone levels. Elevated aldosterone levels may result from an adenoma of or hyperfunction of the aldosterone producing cells of the adrenals. This condition is known as primary aldosteronism. Conditions which increase renin production, such as renal ischemia, can also cause increased aldosterone production. This condition is called secondary aldosteronism. (For details related to this test, see page 91.)

Laboratory Results
Normal Range

Plasma aldosterone	5 to 25 ng/dl
24-hr urine aldosterone	5 to 20 μg/24 hr

Nursing Implications
Procedure for Collection/Storage of Specimen

1. Plasma

   A venous blood sample is obtained, preferably with the patient having

been in a recumbent position for 4 hr. The upright position increases aldosterone production.
2. 24-hr urine
   a. Use the usual procedure for collection of a 24-hr urine specimen.
   b. Be especially aware of diet and activity orders during the specimen collection time.

Possible Interfering Factors
Aldosterone secretion

- Increases in response to sodium depletion and blood volume depletion, which can be caused by diuretic therapy and low-sodium diets
- Increases when the patient is in an upright position. Bedrest may, therefore, decrease aldosterone levels
- Decreases in the presence of increased sodium intake and increased blood volume
- Is suppressed in the presence of hypokalemia

Patient Care
1. Monitor the patient's blood pressure at regular intervals. Aldosterone levels are most frequently indicated in a comprehensive work-up for hypertensive patients.
2. Follow the physician's instructions regarding sodium and potassium intakes. Record the patient's dietary intake.
3. Note special instructions regarding the patient's activity during the testing period.
4. Note whether the patient is currently taking any diuretic therapy or whether the patient is on a sodium-restricted diet.

Patient Education
1. Explain the tests and their purpose to the patient.
2. Explain the reasons for any dietary or activity changes that the physician may order during the testing period. Increased dietary sodium may be ordered temporarily to determine if this suppresses secretion of aldosterone.
3. Explain why diuretic drugs, which the patient may have been taking for hypertension, may be withheld during the testing period.

Signed Consent
Not required

FOLLICLE-STIMULATING HORMONE (FSH) AND LUTEINIZING HORMONE (LH)-24-HR URINE

FSH and LH are gonadotropic hormones secreted by the anterior pituitary gland. The level of these hormones excreted in the urine in 24 hours can indicate whether there may be an insufficiency of these hormones. Insufficiency of FSH and LH may produce dysfunction of the reproductive system. FSH and LH are necessary for ovulation in the female. In the male, FSH is necessary for sperm formation, and LH stimulates the secretion of androges.

Ovarian tumors producing increased estrogen can inhibit the FSH hormone by the negative feedback cycle and cause decreased urinary excretion of FSH. Increased FSH levels are seen often in Turner's syndrome.

Laboratory Results
Normal Range

> 10 to 50 M uu/ 24 hrs (mouse uterine units)

> The effect of these hormones in the uterus of an immature mouse or rat is measured.

Nursing Implications
Procedure for Collection/Storage of Specimen

1. Follow the usual instructions for a 24-hr urine collection.
2. Obtain a 24-hr container. Either a preservative is used or the specimen is refrigerated.
3. Note the exact starting and ending time of the specimen.

Possible Interfering Factors

None reported

Patient Care

In the nursing interview include assessment of the patient's reproductive function, such as amenorrhea in the female.

Patient Education

1. Explain the test and its purpose to the patient.
2. Be certain the patient understands the procedure for collection of the 24-hr specimen and the importance of saving all urine.

Signed Consent

> Not required

GLUCOSE

Glucose is not normally present in the urine. Presence of glucose in the urine is called glycosuria. Glycosuria is usually associated with diabetes mellitus. In hyperglycemia, when the glucose can no longer be reabsorbed by the renal tubules, glucose spills into urine. The point at which glucose can no longer be reabsorbed by the renal tubules is called the renal threshold. In most individuals the renal threshold is about 180 mg/dl. Renal disease affecting tubular glucose reabsorption may cause glycosuria, even when the blood glucose level is normal.

Laboratory Results
Normal

Negative, no glucose in the urine

Nursing Implications

1. To ensure accuracy of results, a double-voided specimen should be used. Have the patient empty the bladder and drink a glass of water. Collect a urine specimen 30 min to 1 hr later for testing.
2. The urine can be tested using the glucose oxidase reaction or by the tablet method. The strips are easier to use and faster than the Clinitest tablet method.
3. Use the color chart that accompanies the various methods to interpret the test results.

Possible Interfering Factors

1. Many drugs may cause a false-positive reaction when the Clinitest tablets are used. These drugs include the following:
   - ascorbic acid } in large amounts
   - aspirin
   - antibiotics (cephalothin, chloramphenicol, streptomycin, tetracycline, ampicillin)
   - sulfonamides
   - nitrofurantoin (Furadantin)
   - methenamine mandelate (Mandelamine)
   - L-dopa, methyldopa
   - aminosalicylic acid (PAS) and isoniazid (INH)
   - penicillin
   - probenecid (Benemid)
   - any type of reducing sugar (lactase, galactose)
2. False-positive reactions are extremely rare using the Tes-Tape, Clinistix, or Diastix method, but false-negative reactions can occur. The following drugs may cause a false-negative reaction:
   - ascorbic acid in greater than 500 mg doses
   - aspirin in large doses
   - L-dopa in large doses
   - α-methyldopa in large doses
3. A urine specimen that is not double-voided may yield inaccurate results.

Patient Care

1. Review drugs that the patient is taking to determine if any may cause false-positive or false-negative results.
2. Notify the physician if the patient's urine test shows moderate or large amounts of glucose.
3. Keep an accurate record of all urine glucose test results.
4. If the patient is 5 or more mo pregnant use the Keto-Diastix test. All other tests will give inaccurate results owing to lactose secretion by the mother.

Patient Education

1. Teach the patient the importance of testing a double-voided specimen.
2. Instruct the patient to perform the urine test precisely according to the instructions included with the test materials.
3. After consultation with the physician, assist the patient to choose the test that best fits the patient's abilities and life style.
4. Teach the patient how to keep a record of test results and what the results mean.
5. Emphasize the need for the diabetic patient to test the urine 4 times a day during periods of illness and increased stress. Moderate or large amounts of glucose in the urine should be reported to a health professional.

Signed Consent

Not required

KETONES

Keto acids accumulate in the blood and spill into the urine of patients with ketoacidosis. Ketoacidosis is seen commonly in the diabetic but may also occur in starvation or alcohol intake. The keto acids are hydroxybuteric acid, acetoacetic acid, and acetone. Acetest tablets, Ketostix, or Keto-Diastix can detect only acetoacetic acid, one of the keto acids that is spilled into the urine during ketoacidosis.

Laboratory Results

Normal

No color change of the tablet or strip

Nursing Implications

Procedure for Collection/Storage of Specimen

1. To ensure accuracy of results, a double-voided specimen should be used. Have the patient empty the bladder, drink a glass of water, and then collect a urine specimen 30 min to 1 hr later for testing.
2. The test is done by placing a drop of urine on the acetest tablet or by dipping the Ketostix into the urine.
3. Use the color chart which accompanies the various methods to interpret the test results. The tablet or strip turns a purple color when acetone is present in the urine. A positive reaction results when there is a concentration ≥ 5 mg/dl of acetone in the urine.

Possible Interfering Factors

1. The following drugs may cause increased acetone or false-positive results:
   - BSP dye
   - PSP dye
   - isoniazid toxicity
   - L-dopa

- paraldehyde
- phenazopyridine (Pyridium)

2. High protein diets or starvation may cause an acidic urine.

Patient Care

1. Notify the physician if the patient's urine contains moderate or large amounts of acetone. In the diabetic, this may indicate the need for increased insulin.
2. Keep an accurate record of all urine acetone test results.
3. Observe the patient for signs and symptoms of ketoacidosis.
4. Use the same method each time to test the urine, as results vary with each type of test.

Patient Education

1. Teach the patient the importance of testing a double-voided specimen to ensure accuracy of test results.
2. Instruct the patient in how to use the Ketostix strips or the Acetest tablets.
3. Teach the patient how to keep a record of test results and what the results mean.
4. Emphasize the need for the diabetic patient to test the urine for acetone 4 times a day during periods of illness and increased stress. Moderate or large amounts of acetone may indicate impending ketoacidosis and should be promptly reported to a health professional.

Signed Consent

Not required

17-KETOSTEROIDS (17-KS), 17-KETOGENIC STEROIDS (17-KGS), 17-HYDROXYCORTICOSTEROIDS (17-OHCS)

Steroids excreted in the urine can be divided into these categories: 17-ketosteroids (17-KS), 17-ketogenic steroids (17-KGS), and 17-hydroxycorticosteroids (17-OHCS). Measurement of these steroids in a 24-hr urine specimen is indicated in the evaluation of disturbances of the adrenal gland and testes.

17-ketosteroids are composed of adrenal hormones and metabolites of androgens from the testes. In males approximately one third of 17-ketosteroids are produced by the testes and two thirds from the adrenals. In women all of these steroids are produced by the adrenals.

17-ketogenic steroids are derivatives of glucocorticoids, produced by the adrenal cortex, and pregnanediol, which is also a substance reflecting adrenocorticol activity.

17-hydroxycorticosteroids are additional substances that reflect adrenocorticol activity. Decreased 17-KGS and 17-KS urinary excretion is generally seen in Addison's disease or hypofunction of the pituitary gland.

Increased levels of 17-KGS, 17-OHCS, and 17-KS may indicate hyperplasia of the adrenal cortex, such as in malignancy or Cushing's syndrome.

Increased amounts of these three types of steroids, especially the 17-KS, may be seen in virilizing syndromes, in children with precocious puberty or the adrenogenital syndrome.

Eclampsia of pregnancy, acute pancreatitis, and ACTH therapy may also cause increased levels of urinary steroids.

In addition, severe stress can cause increased levels of 17-KS and 17-KGS. KS levels may be increased in the third trimester of a normal pregnancy.

Laboratory Results
Normal Values (24-Hour Urine)

17-ketosteroids (17-KS)

Male:	8 to 18 mg per 24 hr
Female:	5 to 15 mg per 24 hr
Children:	<12 yr: <5 mg per 24 hr 12 to 15 yrs: 5 to 12 mg per 24 hr

After 25 USP units ACTH, IM: 50% to 100% increase

17-hydroxycorticosteroids (17-OHCS)

Male:	5.5 to 14.4 mg per 24 hr
Female:	4.9 to 12.9 mg per 24 hr

Lower in children. After 24 USP units ACTH, IM: A two- to four-fold increase can be expected.

Nursing Implications
Procedure for Collection/Storage of Specimen
1. Follow the usual instructions for a 24-hr urine collection. (For details related to this test, see p. 103.)
2. Obtain a 24-hr container containing a preservative.
3. Note the exact starting and ending time of the specimen.
4. The specimen is refrigerated after being sent to the laboratory.

Possible Interfering Factors

Drugs that may increase 17-KS levels include the following:

- chloramphenicol
- chlorpromazine
- cloxacillin
- dexamethasone
- erythromycin
- ethinamate
- meprobamate
- nalidixic acid
- oleandomycin
- penicillin
- phenaglycodol
- phenazopyridine
- phenothiazine
- quinidine
- secobarbital
- spironolactone

Drugs that may decrease 17-KS levels include the following:

- chlordiazepoxide
- estrogen
- meprobamate
- probenecid
- promazine
- reserpine

Drugs which may increase 17-OHCS levels include:

- acetazolamide
- ascorbic acid
- chloral hydrate
- chloramphenicol
- chlordiazepoxide
- chlormerodrin
- chlorpromazine
- chlorthalidone
- colchicine
- cloxacillin
- erythromycin
- digitoxin and digoxin
- cortisone
- ethinamate
- etryptamine
- glutethimide
- meprobamate
- hydralazine
- oleandomycin
- paraldehyde
- quinine
- quinidine
- spironolactone

Drugs which may decrease 17-OHCS levels include the following:

- aminoglutethimide
- estrogen
- calcium gluconate
- oral contraceptives
- corticosteroids
- diphenylhydantoin
- dexamethasone
- phenothiazine
- metotane
- reserpine

Patient Care

1. Observe the patient for signs and symptoms of excessive or deficient cortisone levels, such as in Cushing's syndrome or Addison's disease.
2. Review the drugs the patient is taking. Notify the physician of any drugs that may interfere with test results.

Patient Education

1. Explain the test and its purpose to the patient. Written instructions are helpful.
2. Explain why the physician may have temporarily stopped some of the drugs the patient has been taking.
3. Be certain the patient understands the importance of collecting all urine during the 24-hr period.
4. Encourage food and fluid intake during the testing period.

Signed Consent

Not required

VANILLYLMANDELIC ACID (VMA)

The VMA is a 24-hour urine test that measures the principal substances formed by the adrenal medulla and excreted in the urine. These substances include vanillylmandelic acid, epinephrine, norepinephrine, metanephrine, and normetanephrine. These substances are commonly referred to as catecholamines because they contain a catechol nucleus and an amine group. The primary metabolite of the catecholamine group is VMA. The VMA test is usually done when a person with hypertension is suspected of having a tumor of the chromaffin cells of the adrenal medulla. This type of tumor, usually benign, is called a pheochromocytoma. Pheochromocytomas secrete excessive amounts of catecholamines, causing abnormally increased urine VMA levels.

Slight to moderate increases in VMA and catecholamines may be found also in patients with neuroblastomas, ganglioneuromas, and ganglioblastomas. Progressive muscular dystrophy and myasthenia gravis may cause slight to moderate increases in catecholamines.

Laboratory Results
Normal Range

VMA

| Adults | up to 9 mg per 24 hr |

Children

Age in years	*mg per 24 hr*
Under 1	less than 1
1 to 5	1 to 3
6 to 15	1.5 to 4
Over 15	over 2.5

Catecholamines

Adults

Epinephrine	100 to 230 µg/24 hr
Norepinephrine	100 to 230 µg/24 hr
Metanephrine	24 to 96 µg/24 hr
Normethanephrine	12 to 288 mg per 24 hr

Children

Age in years	*Norepinephrine*	*Epinephrine*
Under 1	10.6 ± 3.4 µg/24 hr	1.3 ± 1.2 µg/24 hr
1 to 5	18.8 ± 17	3.2 ± 2.7
6 to 15	37.4 ± 16.6	4.8 ± 2.4
Over 15	50.7 ± 15.7	7.1 ± 3.3

Nursing Implications
Procedure for Collection/Storage of Specimen

1. Follow the usual instruction for a 24-hr urine collection.
2. Obtain a 24-hr container containing a preservative.
3. All medications, especially antihypertensives should be discontinued before the test.
4. Note the exact starting and ending time of the specimen.
5. The specimen is refrigerated after being sent to the laboratory.

Possible Interfering Factors

VMA (possible increases)

1. For VMA determinations, a vanilla-free diet is given for 5 dy prior to the test. Laboratories vary in restrictions required, but coffee, tea, chocolate, ice cream, and other vanilla-containing foods are definitely not permitted. Other foods that may increase VMA levels include the following:

   - fruit, especially bananas
   - fruit juice
   - cheese
   - cider vinegar
   - gelatin foods
   - salad dressing
   - carbonated drinks, except gingerale
   - jelly and jam
   - candy and mints
   - cough drops
   - chewing gum
   - foods containing artificial flavoring or coloring
   - licorice

2. Severe decrease in food intake can increase VMA levels. Therefore the patient should not be NPO during the test.

3. Drugs that may increase VMA levels include the following:

   - aspirin
   - bromsulphalein
   - glycerol guaiacolate
   - mephenesin
   - chlorpromazine
   - para-aminosalicylic acid (PAS)
   - methocarbamol
   - methylene blue
   - nalidixic acid
   - oxytetracycline
   - penicillin
   - phenazopyridine
   - phenosulfonphthalein (PSP)
   - sulfa drug
   - isoproterenol
   - levodopa
   - lithium
   - nitroglycerin

VMA (possible decreases)

1. Drugs that may decrease VMA levels include the following:
   - clofibrate
   - cloridine
   - guanethidine drugs
   - imipramine
   - methyldopa
   - monoamine (MAO) inhibitors
   - reserpine
2. False decreased levels may be caused by alkaline urine or renal insufficiency, which causes impaired excretion of VMA.
3. Radiographic iodine contrast agents, such as IVP dye, may decrease VMA levels, and especially metanephrine levels.

Catecholamines

1. Increased levels may be caused by vigorous exercise.
2. Drugs that may interfere with catecholamine levels include the following:
   - ampicillin
   - ascorbic acid
   - chloral hydrate
   - epinephrine
   - erythromycin
   - hydralazine
   - methenamine
   - methyldopa
   - nicotinic acid
   - quinine
   - quinidine
   - tetracycline
   - vitamin B complex

Patient Care

Carefully assess for increased blood pressure readings and other symptoms of sympathetic stimulation in the patient with a possible pheochromocytoma. Blood pressure increases may be paroxysmal.

Patient Education

1. Explain the test and its purpose to the patient. Written instructions are needed especially for the outpatient, since many foods must be avoided for at least 2 dy prior to the test.
2. Explain why the physician may have temporarily stopped some of the drugs the patient has been taking.
3. Encourage the patient to rest, drink, and eat adequate amounts of food and avoid stress during the test.

4. Be certain the patient understands the importance of collecting all urine during the 24-hr period.

Signed Consent

Not required

DIAGNOSTIC TESTS
THYROID ECHOGRAM (Ultrasound)

The thyroid echogram, or ultrasound study, can be used to determine the size of the thyroid to demonstrate the depth of abnormalities such as nodules and to differentiate cysts from solid masses. Ultrasound involves passing sound waves into internal body structures. Images of these structures are displayed in picture form. Some limitations of the thyroid echogram are that very small nodules may not be detected by the echogram. Also, cysts near the thyroid gland may be mistaken as originating from thyroid tissue. This study is done in conjunction with the radioactive iodine uptake test. The echogram may be done alone in some instances, such as with pregnant patients when the radioactive iodine uptake test is contraindicated.

Normal Results

Pattern image showing normal size and shape of the thyroid gland. Echos are uniformly reflected throughout the gland.

Nursing Implications
Preprocedure

Explain the test and its purpose to the patient. There is no preparation prior to the test. The test takes approximately 30 min. There is no pain or discomfort involved.

During the Procedure

1. The ultrasound technician places the patient supine on the examining table with the neck hyperextended. A pillow can be placed under the patient's shoulders for comfort.
2. Oil is applied to the patient's neck to serve as a conductor of sound waves.

Postprocedure

1. Encourage the patient to resume normal activities.
2. If thyroid abnormalities are found, reinforce the physician's plan for further study or treatment.

Signed Consent

Not required

RADIOACTIVE IODINE (RAI)
UPTAKE TEST AND THYROID SCAN

The radioactive iodine uptake test and the thyroid scan are used in the evaluation of the size, position, and function of the thyroid gland. It is especially useful in the evaluation of patients with hyperthyroidism and thyroid masses or nodules. Benign and malignant masses characteristically have varying patterns of ^{131}I uptake. Areas of increased uptake, called "hot spots" most often signify benign adenomas. Areas of abnormally decreased uptake or "cold spots" more often signify malignancy.

A dose of 3 to 5 μ Ci of radioactive iodine (^{131}I) is administered orally. After a specified time the amount of ^{131}I absorbed or taken up by the thyroid gland is measured by use of a scanner. The test measures the ability of the thyroid gland to concentrate iodide. Abnormally increased ^{131}I uptake is seen in conditions such as hyperthyroidism and benign adenomas. Cirrhosis of the liver and renal failure may cause elevated uptake, but this does not signify hyperthyroidism. Decreased uptake may be seen in hypothyroidism or Hashimoto's thyroiditis.

Normal Results

Normal ^{131}I uptake by the thyroid gland, as follows:

1 to 13% absorbed after 2 hr

2 to 25% absorbed after 6 hr

15 to 45% absorbed after 24 hr

Normal size and position of thyroid. Evenly concentrated ^{131}I in thyroid gland.

Nursing Implications

Preprocedure

1. Explain the procedure and its purpose to the patient.
2. Have the patient in a fasting state prior to the test. Water, tea, or coffee without sugar or cream are allowed.
3. Explain to the patient and family that the radioactive material that is given is very small and will not be harmful. The patient will not emit "radioactivity."
4. Assure the patient that the procedure is painless, but mention that it is time consuming.
5. Ask the female patient if she may be pregnant. The ^{131}I uptake test is contraindicated during pregnancy and in lactating women.
6. Assess the patient for drugs or foods that may cause a lowered ^{131}I uptake, which includes the following:

   - Iodine-containing drugs, such as Lugol's solution and SSKI.
   - Radiographic contrast media received from 1 wk to a year previously (Consult the Nuclear Medicare Department for specific policies).
   - Thyroid medications taken 1 to 2 wk prior to the test.
   - Antithyroid drugs, such as propylthiouracil, taken 2 to 10 dy prior to the test.
   - Miscellaneous drugs, such as thiocyanate, perchlorate, nitrates, sulfonamides, tolbutamide (Orinase), corticosteroids, PAS, isoniazid, phenylbutazone (Butazolidin), thiopental (Pentothal), antihistamines, ACTH, aminosalicylic acid, and coumarin anticoagulants.
   - Cabbage and enriched breakfast cereals

7. Assess the patient for drugs that may cause an increased ^{131}I uptake including the following:
   - TSH
   - estrogens
   - barbiturates
   - lithium carbonate
   - phenothiazines taken 1 week prior to the test.

8. Explain to the patient that no iodine-containing products should be taken for at least 1 week prior to the test. A written list of foods containing iodine should be given to the patient. Consult the Nuclear Medicine Department if iodine products were taken more than 1 wk prior to the test.

9. Explain to the patient that several scans at varying intervals, such as 2 hr, 6 hr, and 24 hr after ^{131}I intake, are required. It is crucial that the patient return to the laboratory at these exact times. Therefore do not schedule other activities at these times.

During the Procedure

1. The Nuclear Medicine Staff administers the [131]I. The patient should not eat for 1 hr after taking the [131]I. Normal diet can be resumed after 1 hr.

2. Be aware that diarrhea, vomiting, or diuresis after the administration of the ^{131}I can decrease absorption and interfere with test results.

3. Remind the patient to remain very still during the scanning procedure.

Postprocedure

1. If a thyroid abnormality is found, provide the patient with support and appropriate teaching. The hyperthyroid patient may be irritable and hypersensitive.

Signed Consent

Required

WATER DEPRIVATION TEST

The water deprivation test is a test used when diabetes insipidus is suspected. The patient who has diabetes insipidus has inadequate ADH, which is produced by the hypothalamus and excreted from the posterior pituitary. Inadequate ADH results in the excretion of very large volumes of dilute urine. Other conditions such as psychogenic polydipsea may also cause polyuria. In persons with normal ADH secretion, after several hours of controlled water deprivation the urine becomes more concentrated. In diabetes insipidus the patient will continue to have polyuria and will not be able to concentrate the urine. The serum osmolality is relatively higher than that of the urine specific gravity. Dehydration occurs easily when water intake is controlled in the patient with diabetes insipidus.

Normal Range

Serum osmolality	280 to 295 mOsm/Kg
Urine osmolality	300 to 600 mOsm/Kg

In diabetes insipidus:
Before water deprivation

Serum osmolality	285 to 320 mOsmol/Kg (Normal to ↑)
Urine osmolality	<200 mOsmol/Kg (↓)

No fluids for 6 hr

Serum osmolality	Greater than before dehydration
Urine osmolality	Less than maximal concentration

After Pitressin (ADH) administration:

Serum osmolality	decrease
Urine osmolality	increase

Nursing Implications
Preprocedure

1. Explain the test to the patient. The patient may feel extremely thirsty during the test.
2. Remove all sources of fluids from the patient's immediate environment.
3. Obtain baseline urine and serum osmolality measurements as ordered.
4. Weigh the patient and obtain baseline vital signs.

During the Procedure

1. Make certain that the patient does not drink water or other fluids.
2. Observe the patient carefully for dehydration. Record urinary output and note significant changes in vital signs. The test may need to be discontinued if more than 3 to 5% of body weight is lost before the fluid deprivation time is completed.
3. Obtain urine and blood samples to be tested for osmolality at the time specified.
4. Administer vasopressin (Pitressin) (ADH) as prescribed.
5. Obtain urine and blood samples, at the time specified after ADH has been administered.
6. Offer support to the patient, as the test may be difficult and the patient may crave fluids.

Postprocedure

1. If diabetes insipidus is diagnosed, teach the patient how to administer the vasopressin (Pitressin) or other similar medication prescribed by the physician.
2. Continue to observe the patient's intake and output until the patient is well stabilized on the medication. Additional urine and blood samples may also need to be sent to the laboratory for analysis of osmolality.

Signed Consent

Not required

BIBLIOGRAPHY

Camunas C: Transphenoidal hypophysectomy. Am J Nurs 80, No. 10: 1820–1823, 1980

Fischbach F: A Manual of Laboratory Diagnostic Tests. Philadelphia, JB Lippincott, 1979

Hamburger JI: Thyroid testing: cost-benefit considerations. J Nucl Med 22, No. 7: 655–1981

Jubiz W: Endocrinology: A Logical Approach for Clinicians. New York, McGraw–Hill, 1979

Kindenlehrer DA: Thyroid function tests. American Family Physician 21, No. 5: 116–20, 1980

McHenry LE, Loebel JE, Saxe P: The case for routine screening of thyroid functions. J Fla Med Assoc 67, No. 2:1, 1980

Mestman JH: Outcome of diabetes screening in pregnancy and perinatal morbidity in infants of mothers with mild impairment in glucose tolerance. Diabetes Care 3, No. 3: 447–452, 1980

Moss JM: Pitfalls to avoid in diagnosing diabetes in elderly patients. Geriatrics 31, No. 10:52–55, 1976

Phipps W, Long BC, Woods NF: Medical-Surgical Nursing: Concepts and Clinical Practice. St Louis, CV Mosby, 1979

Price BA, Wilson LM: Pathophysiology: Clinical Concepts of Disease. New York, McGraw–Hill, 1978

Skydell B, Crowder AS: Diagnostic Procedures: A Reference for Health Practitioners and A Guide for Patient Counseling. Boston, Little, Brown and Co, 1975

Surks MI: Assessment of thyroid function. Ophthalmology 88, No. 6. 476–478, 1981

Tilkian SM, Conover MB, Tilkian AG: Clinical Implications of Laboratory Tests. St. Louis, CV Mosby, 1979

Vasyukova EA, Zefinova GS, Smirnova OI: Age disturbance of glucose tolerance and diabetes mellitus. Human Physiol 5, No. 2: 131–134, 1979

8

Tests Related to Reproductive Function

Ruth Tucker

OVERVIEW OF PHYSIOLOGY AND PATHOPHYSIOLOGY

The reproductive system plays an important role in the sexual and emotional responses of the male and female. In addition to procreation, the reproductive system produces hormones that cause the development of the primary and secondary sex characteristics. Primary female sex characteristics include enlargement of the fallopian tubes, uterus, vagina, and external genitalia. In the male, primary sex characteristics include enlargement of the penis, scrotum, and testes. Secondary sex characteristics for both the male and female influence distribution of body hair, voice pitch, skin texture, and metabolism.

Clinical signs and symptoms may occur as a result of primary disorders of the reproductive system. Other disorders of the body that may affect the reproductive system include endocrine and metabolic disorders, such as thyroid gland disorders, adrenal disease, pituitary disorders, and diabetes mellitus.

Factors that can produce dysfunction in the reproductive system include the following:

- functional or structural abnormalities
- abnormal hormonal balance
- infectious or inflammatory processes
- abnormal tissue growth

FUNCTIONAL/STRUCTURAL ABNORMALITIES
FEMALE: NORMAL ANATOMY

The principle internal organs of the female reproductive tract include the ovaries, fallopian tubes, uterus, and vagina. These organs are primarily responsible for the sexual and reproductive functions of the female.

Ovaries

The ovaries are the primary sex organs (gonads) of the female, acting as endocrine glands as well as reproductive organs. The ovaries produce ova and secrete the hormones, estrogen, and progesterone. Appropriate amounts of the pituitary gonadotropins, follicle-stimulating hormone and luteinizing hormone, estrogen, progesterone, and androgens must be present for the ova to mature and be released.

Fallopian Tubes

The fallopian tubes are muscular canals that extend from the uterus to the ovaries. Fertilization of the ovum by the sperm takes place in the fallopian tube. Peristaltic movements within the tubes transport the ovum from the ovary to the uterus.

Uterus

The uterus serves the primary function of child-bearing. The upper portion of the uterus, or body of the uterus, changes with the hormonal cycle.

Endometrial tissue normally lines the uterine wall. During the monthly cycle, this lining of endometrial tissue grows in preparation for implantation of a fertilized ovum. If fertilization does not occur, this lining is sloughed off during menstruation and the rebuilding of the lining begins. If implantation does occur, the uterus provides a place for the fetus to grow until the time for delivery. At that time, the muscular uterine walls begin to contract and expel the fetus.

Cervix

The cervix forms the lower end of the uterus. It provides a channel for the menstrual flow from the uterus to the vagina, secretes mucus to facilitate the movement of the sperm, and dilates during labor to allow passage of the fetus from the uterus.

Vagina

The vagina provides an outlet for the menstrual flow, receives the penis during intercourse, and allows for passage of the fetus during childbirth. Lubrication for the vagina is furnished primarily by secretions from the cervix and Bartholin's glands. Vaginal secretions are normally acidic.

External Female Genitalia

The external female genitalia has several functions. The clitoris serves as the "nerve center" during sexual excitement. Protection of the clitoris and the urethra is provided for by the labia majora and labia minor. Lubrication of the external genitalia prior to intercourse is provided by secretions from Skene's glands and Bartholin's glands.

ENDOMETRIOSIS

Endometriosis is a disorder resulting from the presence of endometrial tissue that is functioning outside the uterus. Endometriosis is usually confined to the pelvis, but may involve structures outside of the reproductive organs such as the bowel and bladder and abdominal wall.

- Symptoms caused by the proliferative growth and function of the endometrial tissue may include bleeding, pelvic pain during the menstrual cycle, a feeling of fullness in the lower abdomen, painful sexual intercourse, and painful defecation.
- Infertility may result from a decrease in the peristaltic movements of the fallopian tubes or blockage of the fallopian tubes as a result of scarring.

MALE: NORMAL ANATOMY

The male reproductive system is composed of the seminiferous tubules and epididymis of the testes, the vas deferens, the prostate gland, the seminal vesicles, the ejaculatory duct, and the internal urethra (the bulbourethral glands, urethra, and the penis). The functions of the male reproductive system include secretion of the male sex hormones, production of sperm, and performance of the male sexual act.

Testes

The testes are the primary sex organs or gonads of the male. Sperm production takes place in the seminiferous tubules of the testes as a result of stimulation by the gonadotropic hormones. The sperm empty into the epididymus, which lead into the vas deferens. The vas deferens enters the prostate gland. The seminal vesicles, which are located on each side of the prostate, pass into the ejaculatory duct to empty into the internal urethra. While in the tubules, the sperm are incapable of fertilizing an ovum and lack the ability to move. The maturation process that occurs in the epididymis gives the sperm the capabilities of motility and fertilization. Mature sperm are stored primarily in the vas deferens.

Scrotum

The scrotum acts as a protective organ for the testes. The seminiferous tubules, epididymis, and a portion of the vas deferens are located in the scrotal sack. High temperatures increase the rate of metabolism in the sperm and cause the life of the sperm to be greatly shortened. Very high temperatures can prevent sperm production and may cause sterility. The contractile tissue of the scrotum relaxes when body or environmental temperatures rise. This allows the testes to hang from the body, which keeps the temperature of the testicles lower than body temperature. When exposed to cooler temperatures, the scrotum contracts, pulling the testes close to the body for warmth.

Seminal Vesicles

The seminal vesicles are secretory glands. The mucoid secretion produced by the seminal vesicles contains nutrients and other substances of value to the sperm.

Prostate Gland

The prostate gland is located just below the bladder and surrounds the urethra. The prostate gland secretes an alkaline fluid that combines with secretions from the vas deferens during ejaculation. Semen, which is the combined secretions from the vas deferens, seminal vesicles, prostate gland, and the bulbourethral glands (Cowper's glands), has an average pH of approximately 7.5. Sperm become actively motile in an environment with a pH above 6.0 to 6.5. This alkaline liquid enhances the motility and fertility of the sperm.

Penis

The penis is primarily composed of erectile tissue. Erectile tissue is composed of large cavernous venous sinusoids that fill with blood as a result of parasympathetic stimulation. Physical or psychological sexual stimulation may cause the penis to become erect. The urethra passes through the penis. The urethra serves as a passageway for urine from the bladder and for the passage of semen. Semen is ejaculated from the penis and deposited in the female vagina during intercourse. The tip of the penis or the glans penis serves as the "nerve center" during sexual excitement. The Cowper's gland and other glands secrete mucus that aid in lubrication during intercourse.

ABNORMALITIES OF THE TESTES

Failure of the testes to descend from the abdomen into the scrotum is a structural abnormality. Normally, the testes descend through the inguinal canals into the scrotum during the latter part of fetal development. Testosterone, secreted by the fetal testes, appears to stimulate the testes to move into the scrotum.

- Malformed testes are often responsible for an insufficient amount of testosterone production causing failure of the testes to descend.

- Testes that remain in the abdomen are exposed to high temperatures, which may prevent sperm production. This causes destruction of the cells that produce sperm and infertility may result.

ABNORMAL HORMONAL BALANCE
FEMALE SEX HORMONES

Hormones that influence the female reproductive system originate in three major sites: the hypothalamus, the anterior pituitary gland, and the ovaries. The hypothalamus produces the hypothalamic-releasing factors, follicle-stimulating hormone releasing factor (FRF) and luteinizing hormone releasing factor (LRF). These hormone-releasing factors from the hypothalamus stimulate the anterior lobe of the pituitary gland to produce the gonadotropic hormones, follicle-stimulating hormone (FSH) and luteinizing hormone (LH). FSH and LH stimulate the ovaries to produce estrogen and progesterone.

Estrogen

The ovaries are the primary producers of estrogen. Estrogen is also produced by the adrenal cortex in minute amounts. Large quantities of estrogen are produced by the placenta during pregnancy. Three natural estrogens are present in significant quantities in the blood of females: β-estradiol, estrone, and estriol.

Estrogen is responsible for the development of primary and secondary sex characteristics of the mature female. It promotes tissue growth of the internal reproductive organs (fallopian tubes, uterus, vagina), enlargement of the external genitalia, and pelvic broadening. Estrogens promote growth of the breasts and the milk-producing structure. Estrogen affects the rate of skeletal growth, metabolism, skin texture, hair distribution, and electrolyte balance.

The estrogens are oxidized to estriol principally in the liver. Excretion of the by-products is primarily through urine and bile.

Progesterone

Almost all the progesterone is secreted by the corpus luteum. Small amounts of progesterone are produced by the adrenal glands. Large quantities of progesterone are produced by the placenta during pregnancy.

Progesterone's major functions are to prepare the endometrium for implantation of the fertilized ova, to maintain pregnancy, and to prepare the breasts for lactation. Progesterone is broken down principally in the liver. Pregnanediol, the major end product of progesterone metabolism, is excreted partially through the urine.

Androgens

Androgens, the male hormones produced by the adrenal glands in small quantities, seem to have an insignificant effect on the female under normal circumstances.

Menstrual Cycle

The FSH, LH, estrogen, and progesterone are responsible for the cyclic changes seen in the female menstrual cycle. With increases in FSH and LH, the ovary begins to demonstrate follicular changes. The levels of estrogen then increase, which inhibits the pituitary output of FSH. Production of LH increases during this part of the cycle. A surge of LH and possibly FSH is noted just prior to ovulation. Following ovulation, production of progesterone increases dramatically with accompanying drops seen in the production of FSH, LH, and estrogen.

Proliferation of the endometrial tissue is noted during the period when estrogen levels are high. Progesterone, working with estrogen, brings about secretory changes in the endometrium. The uterine lining becomes lush with nutritive secretions and becomes very vascular. This environment is conducive to implantation and growth of a fertilized ovum. If implantation does not occur, there is a sudden reduction in both estrogen and progesterone. Endometrial tissue growth ceases and the superficial layers of endometrium begin to slough off. Menstruation takes place.

If fertilization and implantation occurs, the trophoblastic cells of the fertilized ovum secrete human chorionic gonadotropin hormone (HCG). The HCG level continues to rise until approximately seven weeks after ovulation and drops to a low level by the sixteenth week after ovulation. The purpose of HCG is to stimulate the corpus luteum to continue to produce large amounts of estrogen and progesterone. Under the influence of these two hormones, the endometrium continues to grow and produce the nutrients necessary for successful implantation and early development of the placenta and other fetal tissues. After the sixteenth week of pregnancy, the placenta takes over the role of estrogen and progesterone production and the HCG level drops.

HORMONAL IMBALANCES IN FEMALES

Inadequate levels of estrogen may result in abnormalities in female sexual development.

- Abnormalities in secretion of FSH and/or LH may cause infertility, since the ovaries are not stimulated to ovulate.
- Deficiencies in progesterone may result in an inability to maintain a pregnancy.

- The interrelationships of estrogen, progesterone, FSH, and LH are responsible for the menstrual cycle. Abnormal secretion of any of these hormones interrupts the cyclic changes that occur normally. Irregular periods, ammenorrhea, or increases or decreases in the amount of menstrual flow are commonly noted changes.

- Major imbalances in the production of the primary female hormones, estrogen and progesterone, and the male hormones, androgens, may cause hirsutism and virilization in the female.

MALE SEX HORMONES

The male sex hormones orginate in three major sites: the hypothalamus, the anterior pituitary gland, and the testes. Hormone-releasing factors from the hypothalamus stimulate the anterior lobe of the pituitary gland. The pituitary responds by secreting the gonadotropic hormones, FSH, and LH.

FSH seems to stimulate the conversion of primary spermatocytes to secondary spermatocytes in the seminiferous tubules. Testosterone is needed to complete this maturation phase of the sperm. *LH* stimulates the Leydig cells of the testes to produce testosterone. *Testosterone* is the most abundant and potent of the androgens. The adrenal glands also produce androgens but to a lesser amount than the testes.

Testosterone

The primary function of testosterone is development of the primary and secondary sexual characteristics of the mature male. It promotes tissue growth of the penis, scrotum, and testes, and also affects distribution of body hair, pitch of the voice, thickness and texture of the skin, rate of metabolism, fluid and electrolyte balance, and bone growth. Testosterone is broken down by the liver and excreted into the urine and bile.

Estrogen

Small amounts of estrogen are produced by the testes or as a by-product of the breakdown of testosterone. Small amounts of estrogen can normally be found in the male's urine. The function of estrogen in the male is not known.

HORMONAL IMBALANCE IN MALES

- Inadequate levels of the androgens, primarily testosterone, may result in abnormalities in male sexual development. Growth of the penis, scrotum, and testes, which normally occur during puberty, may be absent. Major imbalances in the production of androgens and estrogen may cause feminization of the male.

- Imbalances in the secretion of LH, FSH, and testosterone may reduce or eliminate sperm production. Sperm may be produced, but a lack of testosterone may retard the maturation process. Immature sperm lack the ability to move and are incapable of fertilizing an ova, resulting in infertility.

- Interstitial tumors of the testes can produce abnormally high quantities of testosterone. This causes excessive development of the sexual organs and of the secondary sexual characteristics.

INFECTIOUS OR INFLAMMATORY PROCESSES

In the female, the thick vaginal epithelium and the acid secretions of the vagina provide natural barriers to infection. Decreased estrogen levels, alterations in vaginal pH, and thin vaginal mucosa may be factors that predispose women to develop vaginal infections. These factors may also increase the danger of trauma to the vaginal mucosa from intercourse.

Estrogen levels during the reproductive years appear to play an important role in the thickness of the vaginal epithelium. Lower estrogen levels, which occur prior to puberty and along with menopause, produce thinning of the vaginal epithelium.

VAGINAL pH CHANGES

Estrogen, Döderlein's bacilli, and lactic acid production maintain the acidity of the vaginal secretions. Alkaline changes in vaginal pH secretions occur naturally during the menstrual cycle and pregnancy.

- Medications, such as antibiotics that eliminate the naturally occurring organism Döderlein's bacilli, can alter vaginal pH.
- Disease processes such as diabetes mellitus and certain pathogenic organisms can cause the vaginal pH to change to a neutral or alkaline pH.
- Acute illnesses, malnutrition, and emotional disturbances can also increase susceptibility to vaginal infections.

INFECTIONS

The most frequent causative organisms for infections of the reproductive system include *Candida albicans, Trichomonas vaginalis, Treponema pallidum, Neisseria gonorrhoeae, Herpes simplex* virus type II, *Escherichia coli, Pseudomonas, streptococci*, and *staphylococci*.

Pathogenic organisms may be introduced during intercourse, childbirth, or the postpartum period, or during operative procedures such as dilatation and curettage (D and C) or abortion. Poor personal hygiene practices may also introduce pathogens to the reproductive system.

Infection and inflammation are two processes that may occur simultaneously. In the male, infections spread from the urinary tract to the reproductive organs. These processes may also originate in one portion of the reproductive system and then spread until that entire system is involved.

Gonorrhea

Infection and inflammation in the reproductive system may cause scarring of tubal tissue with resultant sterility. The venereal disease caused by *Neisseria gonorrhoeae* is a good example of this type of process. This organism is introduced during intercourse and spreads by way of the vagina to the uterus to the fallopian tubes and eventually to the entire pelvis. *N. gonorrhoeae* is one of the most frequent causes of pelvic inflammatory disease (PID).

Syphilis

Infections such as syphilis may begin in the reproductive system and eventually become systemic infections causing problems such as fever, malaise, sore throat, and damage to major organs such as the liver, heart, and central nervous system.

Herpes

Herpes virus can also cause infections. The virus may be dormant or may become acute. During the acute stage, lesions develop on the external genitalia, which become ulcerations. The infection is usually self limiting and no serious problems develop for the adult. However, an infant who is delivered vaginally to a woman who has herpes virus present in the vagina may develop the disease. Death results in a large percentage of these infants. Serious eye and central nervous system damage has been identified among infants who survive.

Prostatitis

In the male, prostatitis, or inflammation of the prostate, is a very common affliction. It may be caused by infection originating in the reproductive system or elsewhere in the body. The natural antibacterial factor found in prostatic fluid offers protection against many of the bacteria that may cause prostatic and urinary tract infections in men.

Sterility

High temperatures from systemic infections originating outside the reproductive tract, such as mumps, may cause sterility in males. This condition may be temporary if only the sperm are destroyed. However, sterility may be permanent if there is degeneration of all the cells of the seminiferous tubules.

Other Causes

In addition to infection, other causes of inflammation include parasites, chemical irritants, systemic disease, drug sensitivities and allergies, and injuries.

- Pediculosis pubis (lice) and scabies (itch mite) are parasites that may be present on the external genitalia.
- Common chemical irritants include soaps, douches, deodorants, and bubble bath.
- Some systemic diseases, such as diabetes and uremia, may cause inflammation or provide an environment conducive to infection in the reproductive system.
- Aspirin, chlortetracycline, antihistamines, iodides, and phenacetin are examples of drugs that may produce symptoms of sensitivity and allergies in the reproductive system.
- Vulvar itching (pruritis), erythema, urticaria, swelling, and ulceration of the skin may result from inflammation caused by chemical irritants and medications.

- Injuries may result from accidents, sexual intercourse, childbirth, or radiation treatments.

BREAST INFECTION

Infections of the breast are seen most frequently during lactation. Pathogenic organisms enter through cracked or infected nipples. Infection may also result from engorged tissue, which creates a blockage of the milk ducts.

ABNORMAL TISSUE GROWTH

Abnormal tissue growth may be benign or malignant. Benign neoplasms include condyloma accuminata (venereal warts), fibroid tumors, polyps, and cysts. Condyloma accuminata are most commonly noted on the external genitalia. However, venereal warts may also occur in the vagina and on the cervix.

In women, the cervix, uterus, ovaries, and breasts are common sites for both benign and malignant tissue growth. Fibroid tumors are most often located within the uterine muscle. Polyps occur primarily on the cervix or within the uterus. The ovaries are common sites for cyst formation.

Benign conditions of the breast may include fibrocystic disease, fibroadenomas, lipomas, and intraductal papillomas. Though seen more frequently in women, neoplasms involving breast tissue occur infrequently in men.

The most common site for abnormal tissue growth in the male is the prostate gland. Excessive tissue growth (hyperplasia) and malignant diseases are the most frequent causes of prostate gland disorder. Hyperplasia is usually a benign disorder.

BLOOD AND URINE TESTS
HORMONES INFLUENCING THE REPRODUCTIVE SYSTEM

Hormone level determinations are used to evaluate the functioning of various organs. The products of hormone metabolism are excreted in the urine. These metabolic products are the compounds upon which chemical analysis is based. Hormones that can be evaluated by urine analysis include the following:

- estrogen (estradiol, estrone, estriol)
- progesterone (pregnanediol)
- follicle-stimulating hormone
- luteinizing hormone, testosterone
- 17-ketosteroids, 17 hydroxycorticosteroids
- human chorionic gonadotropin

Most of these hormones and their metabolic by-products can also be identified by serum analysis using radioimmunoassay techniques.

FOLLICLE-STIMULATING HORMONE (FSH), LUTEINIZING HORMONE (LH)

Hormone-releasing factors from the hypothalamus stimulate the anterior lobe of the pituitary gland to secrete FSH and LH. In the female, FSH and

LH stimulate the ovaries, bringing about the cyclic changes of the menstrual cycle. In the male, FSH and LH seem to stimulate the production of testosterone and the production and maturation of sperm.

Decreased amounts of FSH and LH may cause abnormal menstrual cycles and infertility and may indirectly cause failure of the development of sexual characteristics.

Increased levels of FSH and LH may occur in the following:

- primary ovarian inadequacy
- midcycle of menstrual cycle
- menopause
- castration
- Turner's syndrome
- hypogonadism

Decreased levels of FSH and LH may occur in the following:

- pituitary insufficiency
- hypothalamic disorders
- pituitary tumors
- follicular and luteal phases of menstrual cycle
- central nervous system disorders
- ovarian tumors
- usage of depressant drugs

Laboratory Values

FSH

Serum	0.10–0.46 u/ml	
24-hr urine	Follicular phase	5 to 20 IU
	Midcycle	15 to 60 IU
	Luteal phase	5 to 15 IU
	Menopause	50 to 100 IU
	Males	5 to 25 IU

LH

Serum	Preovulatory or postovulatory	5 to 22 u/ml
24-hr urine	Not tested	

PROGESTERONE

Progesterone is produced primarily in the ovaries and is responsible for preparation of the endometrium for implantation of the fertilized ova, maintenance of pregnancy, and preparation of the breasts for lactation.

Increased levels of progesterone are noted in the following:

- pregnancy

- the luteal phase of the menstrual cycle
- benign ovarian tumors
- ovarian carcinoma
- adrenal hyperplasia
- ACTH administration
- hyperadrenocorticism

Progesterone deficiencies are rare and usually occur along with estrogen deficiency. They may occur in the following:

- threatened abortion
- toxemia of pregnancy
- adverse change in fetal or placental status
- amenorrhea

Laboratory Results

Pregnanediol

Serum	Premenopausal	0.45 to 0.50 ng/ml
	Postmenopausal	0.15 to 0.20 ng/ml
24-hr urine		
Children	Negative	
Males	0 to 1 mg	
Females		
Preovulatory	0 to 1 mg	
Postovulatory	3 to 8 mg	
Pregnancy	60 to 100 mg	

ESTROGEN

The ovaries are the primary producers of estrogen. Estrogen is responsible for the development of the female sex characteristics. Increased levels of estrogen and progesterone in the male may cause feminization.

Increased levels of estrogen occur in the following:

- ovarian tumors
- adrenocortical tumors
- adrenocortical hyperplasia
- estrogen-producing tumors of the testes
- cirrhosis
- the menstrual cycle during ovulation
- pregnancy

Decreased levels of estrogen may occur in the following:

- lack of or inadequate ovarian development
- ovarian tumors such as arrhenoblastoma, lutein-cell tumor

- Simmon's disease
- usage of oral diethylstilbestrol or progesterone agents

Laboratory Results

Total estrogens

Serum	Male: 5 to 18 μg
	Female:
	Ovulation: 28 to 100 μg
	Luteal peak: 22 to 105 μg
	At menses: 4 to 25 μg
	Pregnancy: up to 45,000 μg
	Postmenopausal: 14 to 20 μg
24-hr urine	4 to 100 μg
	Rises with pregnancy with the largest increase after the 30th week of gestation

Estrone (E1)

Serum	Nonpregnant, midcycle: 2 to 25 μg
24-hr urine	2 to 25 μg

Estradiol (E2)

Serum	0 to 10 μg
24-hr urine	0 to 10 μg

Estriol (E3)

Serum	2 to 30 μg
24-hr urine	1 to 2 mg at 8 to 12 wk gestation
	12 to 25 mg at term

Possible Interfering Factors

Some drugs that may either increase or decrease estrogen levels include the following:

- phenothiazine
- tetracycline
- vitamins

TESTOSTERONE

Cells within the testes are the primary producers of testosterone. In the male, testosterone is responsible for the development of male sex characteristics and for the maturation of sperm. Excessive amounts of testosterone in the female can cause virilization.

Increased amounts of testosterone may occur in the following:

- tumors of the testes

- ovarian pathology such as polycystic ovary, arrhenoblastoma, hilar cell tumor

  Decreased production of testosterone may occur in the following:
- hypofunction of the testes
- lack of development of the testes
- decrease in testicular activity in normal aging

Laboratory Results

Testosterone

Serum	Female: 30 to 120 ng/dl
	Male: 400 to 1200 ng/dl
24-hr urine	Adult male,
	less than 60-years-old: 9 to 22 mg/ml

Nursing Implications

Procedure for Collection/Storage of Specimen

Serum
1. Fresh whole blood is collected by venipuncture.
2. The specimen may be collected at any time.

24-hr urine specimen
1. Use a bottle large enough for the entire specimen. Usually a 2000 ml size is ample.
2. Use preservatives as instructed by the laboratory. Preservatives should be added to the bottle prior to collection of the urine. If only the estrogen level is being tested, no preservative should be used.
3. If preservatives are not to be used, refrigerate the specimen during the collection period to inhibit bacterial growth.
4. Label the specimen container with date and start time as well as with date and end time, such as 12/15/80 at 0800 until 12/16/80 at 0800.
5. Send the specimen to the laboratory as soon as the specimen collection is completed.

Possible Interfering Factors
- incomplete specimen collection
- contamination of urine with feces or vaginal secretions
- certain medications (See each individual test for specific medications)

Patient Care

1. Observe for any obvious signs or symptoms of hormone production excesses or deficits.
2. Assess the patient; check current medications for any that may affect the test results.
3. Assess the patient's understanding of the procedure. Stress the importance that *all* urine must be collected.

4. Give emotional support as needed since this may be a trying time for the patient. The 24-hr urine collection will probably be just one of many tests being done.

Patient Education

1. Instruct the patient to void and discard the specimen at the start time. Then *all* urine must be collected for the next 24-hr period. End the collection period by having the patient void.
2. Caution the patient to collect urine prior to bowel movements.

Signed Consent

Not required

HUMAN CHORIONIC GONADOTROPIN

Human chorionic gonadotropin (HCG) is one of the earliest hormones secreted by trophoblastic tissue. Measurable amounts of HCG are secreted one week after the first missed menstrual period. During normal pregnancy, the HCG level rises and reaches a peak about 10 to 14 weeks of gestation. The HCG concentration begins to drop and reaches a lower level of about one-third of the peak, by the 100 to 130 days of gestation. It again begins to rise slightly. Higher than expected levels of HCG may be noted throughout this cycle with multiple gestations. Within one to six days after delivery, the hormone disappears from the maternal system. Persistent positive tests for HCG may indicate retention of placental tissue or the presence of a chorionic tumor.

In patients with a history of *spontaneous abortions*, serial determinations of the HCG level during the first trimester may be done. If the HCG level remains high in the presence of vaginal spotting, the pregnancy will probably continue. The HCG level will drop rapidly when abortion takes place.

About two-thirds of women with *ectopic pregnancies* will have increasing levels of HCG. However, there is less HCG being produced and the serum titers will be lower.

Premalignant and malignant tumors that secrete HCG include hydatidiform mole (molar pregnancy), choriocarcinoma, ovarian and testicular teratomas. A sustained elevation of HCG during pregnancy is suggestive of the presence of a molar pregnancy. The HCG level is indicative of the amount of viable tumor present. Quantitative measurement of the HCG level is crucial in the diagnosis, evaluation of success of therapy, and follow-up confirmation of remission.

Increased levels of HCG are noted in the following:

- early pregnancy
- multiple gestation (twins, triplets, etc.)
- retention of placental tissue
- hydatidiform mole (molar pregnancy)
- choriocarcinoma
- ovarian and testicular teratoma

Decreased levels of HCG are noted in the following:

- abortion
- ectopic pregnancy
- fetal death

Laboratory Results

HCG

Serum	Nonpregnant	none
	0 to 14 weeks gestation	rising
	10 to 14 weeks gestation	peak at approximately 100 U/ml
	15 weeks to term	decreasing to approximately 20 U/ml
*Urine	Nonpregnant	none
	Pregnant	present

Nursing Implications

Procedure for Collection/Storage of Specimen

Serum

1. Fresh whole blood is collected by venipuncture.
2. Specimen may be collected at any time.

Urine

1. Collect the urine in a clean, dry specimen bottle.
2. Collect at least 2 ounces of the first voided specimen in the morning.
3. Send the specimen immediately to the laboratory. HCG is stable for 4 mo in the freezer but only for 72 hr at room temperature or in the refrigerator.
4. Follow the instructions precisely when measuring the reagents and during the mixing, timing, and reading of the test results.

Possible Interfering Factors

False-positive readings may occur in the presence of the following:

- excessive secretion of pituitary gonadotropin (LH)
- proteinuria in excess of 1 g per 24 hr
- hematuria
- certain drugs: phenothiazine derivatives, chlorpromazine derivatives, thioridazine

False-negative readings may occur in the following:

- when testing with dilute urine specimen (low specific gravity)
- if the specimen is obtained too early in pregnancy

---

*Not accurate for quantitative measurement

Patient Care

1. Check with the physician concerning urine tests for pregnancy for women of childbearing age prior to surgery or radiologic testing or treatment.
2. Ask the patient for the date of her last menstrual period. Testing is usually not satisfactory until 1 to 2 weeks after the first missed period. Reliable results can be expected within 3 wk of the first missed menstrual period.
3. Instruct the patient to avoid *all* fluid intake after the evening meal.
4. Instruct the patient to collect the first voided specimen in the morning using specimen container provided.
5. Repeat the test if results are negative and the patient is suspected of being pregnant.
6. If pathology is diagnosed, provide emotional support for the patient and family. Observe for emotional patterns that indicate the need for professional consultation.

Patient Education

1. Instruct the patient in how to perform the test, if home pregnancy testing is desired.
2. Instruct the patient to have follow-up care by qualified medical personnel if a positive result is obtained from a pregnancy test.
3. Instruct the patient to consult with her physician if pregnancy tests are still negative after the second missed menstrual period.
4. Instruct the patient as to symptoms to report to the physician during pregnancy. Danger signs in pregnancy that may suggest molar pregnancy include:
   - symptoms of toxemia, which manifest in the first or second trimester of pregnancy, such as headache, visual disturbances, generalized edema, excessive weight gain
   - excessive nausea and vomiting or nausea and vomiting that lasts past the first trimester of pregnancy
   - vaginal bleeding that may be painless, irregular in occurrence, and ranging in color from dark brown to bright red
   - failure to feel fetal movement after 12 to 14 wk of pregnancy
5. Instruct the patient to continue regular appointments with the physician following molar pregnancy and during and following treatment for choriocarcinoma, ovarian teratomas, and testicular teratomas. Follow-up monitoring is important even though the patient may feel well. Weekly follow-up serum HCG levels is essential until normal levels are noted for three consecutive weeks; then monthly for at least six consecutive months after the first normal titer.
6. Explain to the patient that birth control measures should be used until remission is assured. Normal elevations of HCG during pregnancy would make evaluation of therapy difficult if not impossible. The patient may decide to become pregnant if the HCG titer has been negative

for 12 to 18 months. Normal pregnancies should be anticipated in the future although an increased incidence of spontaneous abortion may be noted.

Signed Consent

Not required

VDRL

The VDRL is one of the most common screening procedures for syphilis. The test is based on an antibody–antigen reaction. The antibody (reagin) that causes the reaction in the VDRL is believed to be an antibody against tissue lipids. Reagin formation may be induced by the release of lipids that occur from the normal wear and tear of the body. This reaction results in a precipitation, or flocculation. Positive reactions will occur within 2 to 6 weeks following the first infection. Biologic false-positive readings may occur normally, or may also indicate the presence of serious diseases other than syphilis.

Some instances in which biologic false-positive readings may occur include the following:

- narcotic addiction
- aging
- terminal malignancy
- smallpox vaccination
- viral diseases such as chickenpox, measles, infectious mononucleosis, pneumonia, etc
- malaria
- hepatitis
- leprosy
- pregnancy

The quantitative VDRL is used in diagnosis of syphilis and also in evaluation of the effectiveness of treatment. Blood titers are obtained.

Laboratory Results

Screening	
Normal	nonreactive
Abnormal (require further testing)	reactive, weakly reactive, borderline

Following successful treatment, readings should revert to negative; within 6 to 8 mo if treated in the primary stage or within 1 to 2 yr if treated after secondary manifestations. If treatment is given 2 or more years after the primary infection, the readings may never revert to nonreactive.

Quantitative

Adult

Titer 1:32 or less	most often indicative of primary syphilis
Titer 1:32 or above	most often indicative of secondary or late syphilis

Titer drops following treatment. Usually reverts to negative during primary and secondary stages following treatment. Seldom reverts to negative in late syphilis.

Newborn (cord blood samples initially)

If titer is higher than mother's titer, probably active infection exists in the infant.

Serial titers are done if the mother was treated during pregnancy.

Progressive fall in titer is indicative of successful treatment.

If titer remains the same or rises, it is indicative of unsuccessful treatment and active infection in the infant.

Nursing Implications

Procedure for Collection/Storage of Specimen

1. Information important for the laboratory to have: suspected diagnosis, vaccinations and dates, therapy, previous infections.
2. Fresh whole blood is collected by venipuncture.
3. Sample should be drawn before a meal if possible since excess chyle interferes with the reaction.
4. Sample should be sent to the laboratory before hemolysis occurs.

Possible Interfering Factors

- alcoholic beverage intake in past 24 hr
- food intake
- co-existing disease
- skin testing

Patient Care

1. Ask the patient if recent skin testing has been performed. Testing should not be done following skin testing.
2. If syphilis is confirmed, administer medication as prescribed by the physician.
3. Provide support to the patient as the time of diagnosis, treatment, and informing sexual partners may be a difficult period.

Patient Education

1. Explain to the patient to abstain from alcohol for 24 hr prior to testing.
2. Explain to the patient that if a positive reaction occurs, it is imperative to follow-up with more specific tests.

3. Stress the importance of treatment and follow-up testing to evaluate effectiveness of treatment.

4. Explain to the patient that it is crucial for *all* sexual contacts to be tested, so that they may receive treatment if necessary.

Signed Consent

Not required

DIAGNOSTIC TESTS
AMNIOCENTESIS

During pregnancy the fetus is surrounded by amnionic fluid. This fluid contains chemical components and cells shed by the fetus. During amniocentesis, a sample of amnionic fluid is removed from the amnionic sac for the purpose of analysis for genetic abnormalities and for evaluation of fetal status in high risk situations. Factors that may be identified include the following:

- Rh isoimmunization
- Fetal maturity
- Respiratory distress syndrome dangers
- Inborn errors of metabolism
- Fetal genetic abnormalities
- Fetal sex
- ABO blood grouping

Amniocentesis may also be used to remove fluid to reduce the discomforts caused by the excessive production of amnionic fluid in hydramnios.

Amniocentesis also provides a way for substances to be injected into the amnionic sac. Situations in which substances may be injected include: intra-uterine fetal blood transfusions, amniography, and second trimester abortion using hypertonic saline solution.

Trauma to the fetus, placenta, umbilical cord, or maternal structures, infection and abortion or premature labor are the major risks involved with amniocentesis. Hemorrhage from trauma may result in significant transfer of fetal blood to the mother.

Normal Results

Bilirubin

Present	less than 35 to 36 wk gestation
Absent	36 wk or more gestation
Increasing levels as pregnancy progresses	fetal hemolytic disease

Creatinine

Mature fetus	2 mg/dl

Fetal fat cells

Less than 35 to 36 wk gestation or less than 2500 g fetus	less than 10% to 20% total cells
Mature fetus	20% or more total cells

Lecithin/sphingomyelin ratio

Immature fetal lungs	less than 2:1
Mature fetal lungs	2:1 or greater

Enzymes

Inborn errors of metabolism	enzyme activity deficiency

Chromosomal analysis

Genetic abnormalities	abnormal number or types
Male fetus	XY
Female fetus	XX

The presence of meconium or blood in the amnionic fluid may interfere with the interpretation of results.

Nursing Implications
Preprocedure

1. The expectant couple should fully understand the purpose of the procedure and the risks involved prior to signing the consent forms.
2. Strive to reduce patient anxiety by explaining the procedure simply and speaking to common concerns.
   a. Discomfort is minimal and usually limited to the injection of the local anesthetic (burning) and needle insertion to withdraw the amnionic fluid (feeling of pressure deep in the pelvis).
   b. The fetus is free floating and usually moves should the needle come near.
   c. Amnionic fluid production is a continual process. Any fluid removed will promptly be replenished.
3. Record baseline maternal blood pressure and fetal heart rate.
4. The patient may wear a hospital gown to avoid the risk of Betadine staining of her clothing.
5. Anti-Rhoglobulin (RhoGAM) may be administered to the nonsensitized Rh negative woman.

During the Procedure

1. Place patient in a supine position with the right side elevated slightly to avoid supine hypotensive syndrome. Raise the head slightly to facilitate the relaxation of the abdominal muscles.
2. The procedure is a sterile procedure. The site for insertion of the needle is usually chosen following placental location by ultrasonography. Shave the area and prep with a Betadine solution.

3. After injection of a local anesthetic agent, a needle is inserted through the uterine wall into the amnionic sac.
4. Between 10 to 30 ml of amnionic fluid is withdrawn and placed into sterile, labeled tubes. The number of tubes may vary depending on the number and type of tests to be performed.
5. Wrap the tubes to avoid exposure to light. Aluminum foil may be used. This is crucial if bilirubin determinations have been requested.
6. Place the specimen in ice and deliver to the laboratory.

Postprocedure
1. a. Wash the Betadine from the abdomen with warm sterile water to avoid skin burns and cover the puncture site with a Bandaid.
   b. Monitor for 30 min to 1 hr (continuously) the fetal heart tones and uterus for contractions.
   c. Inform the patient of the time that results should be available.
2. Lower abdominal cramping may occur for a few hours following the procedure. Report uterine contractions to the physician.
3. Report vaginal spotting or leakage of amnionic fluid from the vagina to the physician.
4. Explain to the patient that she may resume normal activities without any restrictions.

Signed Consent
Required

CULDOSCOPY

Culdoscopy is a technique in which the pelvis, pelvic viscera, and adjacent organs and structures are visualized. The culdoscope is introduced into the peritoneal cavity through the cul-de-sac in the vagina. Most frequent indications for culdoscopy include the following:

- suspected ectopic pregnancy
- endocrine problems
- unexplained acute or chronic pelvic pain
- infertility
- pelvic masses of unknown nature

Normal Results
Normal anatomical structures

Nursing Implications
Preprocedure
1. Explain the procedure to the patient.
2. The patient should be kept NPO after midnight prior to the procedure.
3. Shave the perineal area or give an enema if prescribed by the physician.
4. Ask the patient to empty the bladder.

5. Check to be sure that the operative permit is signed and that requested laboratory test results are on the chart.
6. Give the preoperative medication as prescribed.

During the Procedure

1. Provide emotional support during the administration of the anesthesia.
2. Assist the patient to assume a knee–chest position. Steep Trendelenberg in lithotomy position may also be used, especially if the patient is under general anesthesia.

Postprocedure

1. While the cannula, the tube through which the culdoscope is passed, is still in place, assist the patient to lie flat on her abdomen. This pressure against the abdomen assists in the expulsion of any air introduced during the procedure.
2. Explain to the patient that some patients experience a "bloated" or full feeling in the abdomen, or slight shoulder pain resulting from residual air in the abdomen.
3. Postsurgical care should include the following activities:
   - monitoring vital signs frequently
   - assessing respiratory status
   - encouraging deep breathing and coughing
   - evaluating amount and character of vaginal discharge
   - assessing level of consciousness, orientation, and return of sensations
   - providing for the patient's safety by keeping the side rails up, having suction equipment available
4. Instruct the patient to abstain from intercourse for about 2 wk following procedure.

Signed Consent

Written consents for the surgical procedure and for the anesthesia are required.

CERVICAL BIOPSY
PUNCH BIOPSY (Schiller Test)

Punch biopsies may be done if an abnormal Pap smear is obtained. The punch biopsy may also be performed as part of the routine pelvic examination. In addition to abnormal Pap smears, indications for biopsies include the following:

- cervical erosions
- eversions
- leukoplakia
- ulcerations
- polyps

Cervical biopsies should not be performed, if acute or subacute pelvic inflammatory disease or acute purulent cervicitis is present. Following resolution of these diseases, a biopsy may be done.

The Schiller test is used to identify the area to be biopsied. The cervical tissue is saturated with Schiller's iodine solution. Normal cervical and vaginal epithelium will be stained by the iodine. Light-colored or unstained areas represent abnormal tissue and give a positive Schiller's test. Biopsies are obtained from all abnormally stained and nonstained areas.

Normal Results

Normal tissue samples

Nursing Implications

Preprocedure

1. Explain to the patient not to douche for at least 24 hr prior to the anticipated biopsy.
2. Instruct the patient about how the procedure will be done.

During the Procedure

1. The specimen is collected during a pelvic examination.
2. The cervix is dried and then stained with Schiller's solution.
3. Samples are taken from abnormally stained or nonstained areas. Each sample should include a portion of the adjacent stained area for comparison of normal and abnormal tissue. At the time the sample is taken, the patient may feel a pinch.
4. Prompt fixation of the specimen is essential. Bouin's solution is often used, or the specimen may be immersed in 10% formalin solution.
5. Tag each specimen with a description of the area from which the specimen was obtained. This is crucial when multiple biopsies are taken.
6. Cauterization should *never* be performed at the time of the biopsy. This could distort results if further biopsies are needed. Light cautery may be used to control bleeding. Bleeding is usually minimal.

Postprocedure

1. A tampon is inserted in the vagina to provide pressure to the site. The tampon may be removed in several hours.
2. The patient should observe for excessive bleeding. If more than vaginal spotting occurs, she should notify the physician.
3. Instruct the patient to abstain from intercourse or douches for 2 wk, or as instructed by the physician.
4. If the tissue sample is benign, the patient will be scheduled for an additional office visit. During this office visit, the abnormal area will usually be cauterized. If the tissue sample is malignant, further evaluation and treatment (radiation or surgery) will be necessary.

Signed Consent

Not required

CONE BIOPSY

Cone biopsy is indicated in the patient with abnormal cytologic smears or cervical biopsies, which are suggestive of premalignant or malignant lesions.

Cone biopsy may be used to diagnose or rule out the presence of invasive carcinoma. Cone biopsy may also be used to assess the degree of malignant invasion of the tissue, which is necessary for the physician to determine the appropriate treatment. Conization requires hospitalization and anesthesia.

Normal Results

Negative for cancer cells

Abnormal Results

Staging of cervical cancer

Stage 0	Carcinoma *in situ*, intraepithelial carcinoma
Stage 1	The carcinoma is strictly confined to the cervix (extension to the corpus should be disregarded)
Stage 2	Microinvasive carcinoma (early stromal invasion)

Nursing Implications

Preprocedure

1. The patient will be hospitalized.
2. General anesthesia is usually given. This procedure is usually followed by a dilitation and curettage.
3. Instruct the patient to abstain from intercourse or douching for 24 hr prior to the procedure. Intercourse or douching may traumatize the cervical epithelium and distort examination results.
4. Keep the patient NPO after midnight prior to the procedure.
5. Explain the procedure for the cone biopsy to the patient.
6. Give a perineal shave and enema if ordered by the physician.
7. Instruct the patient to empty the bladder. A foley catheter may be inserted.

During the Procedure

1. A cone-shaped segment of the cervix, including all of the endocervix, is removed in a single piece using a scalpel.
2. A silk suture or similar marker may be placed at 12 o'clock on the anterior lip of the cone to serve to orient the pathologist. Note the location of the suture on the laboratory slip.
3. Fix the specimen in the same manner as for punch biopsy.

Postprocedure

1. Leave vaginal packing in place for about 24 hr.
2. Instruct the patient that delayed bleeding occasionally occurs in 7 to 10 dy and should be reported to the physician.
3. The patient should abstain from intercourse or douches for 4 to 6 wk

following the procedure, or as directed by the physician. This is to allow time for healing.

Signed Consent

Written consents for the surgical procedure and anesthesia are required.

PAPANICOLAOU SMEAR (Pap Smear)

The pap smear is used as a screening test for cervical cancer. Cell samples are obtained from the cervix, endocervical canal, the posterior fornix and the vagina, and are examined for abnormal cells. Pap smears obtained from vaginal scrapings may also be used to evaluate estrogen levels. Estrogen levels are useful in evaluating hormonal levels in postmenopausal women, following surgical removal of the ovaries, and in hormonal therapy. Evaluation of breast tissue may also be done using the Pap smear method. Fluids or tissue from the mammary tissue are obtained by needle aspirations.

Normal Results

Cancer screening

A five-point scale is used in reporting results of Pap smears.

Class I	Negative, absence of atypical or abnormal cells
Class II	Atypical cytology, dysplasia, borderline but not neoplastic
Class III	Suspicious, cytology suggestive of but not conclusive of malignancy
Class IV	Probably positive, strongly suggestive of malignancy
Cancer V	Positive, conclusive for malignancy, cancer cells present

Hormonal evaluation

By determining the percentages of various types of normal vaginal cells, a qualitative estimate of estrogen levels may be obtained. The Maturation Index (MI) describes the relative percentage of parabasal, intermediate, and superficial cells found in the smear.

Preprocedure

1. Instruct the patient that the best time to have a Pap smear is 5 to 6 dy after the end of the menstrual period. Pap smears taken during menstrual flow may make interpretation difficult and may obscure atypical cells.
2. Explain to the patient not to douche or have sexual intercourse for at least 24 hr prior to the anticipated examination.
3. Ask the patient if she is taking any medications. Drugs such as tetracycline and digitalis may effect squamous epithelium. Birth control pills and other hormone-containing medications may influence hormonal evaluation results.

During the Procedure

1. Use water only to lubricate the speculum. Lubricant gels should be avoided.
2. Specimens may be collected by a combination of scraping and aspiration:
   a. A cotton-tipped applicator is introduced into the external cervical os and rotated. The specimen should be gently rolled onto the slide to avoid breaking or streaking the cells.
   b. A wooden or plastic spatula is rotated with gentle pressure after being inserted into the external os. The "scraping" should be deposited on a slide by slowly and firmly smearing the spatula against the glass surface.
   c. Aspirate the cervical canal.
3. If the purpose of the test is to evaluate endocrine status, scrapings should be taken from the lateral wall of the midportion of the vagina. This area is most sensitive to hormonal changes.
4. Immerse the slide into the fixative immediately. Fixation is complete within 30 min. The slide may stay in the fixative indefinitely without harm to the specimen. Remove the slide from the fixative and allow the slide to air dry. Spray fixatives may also be used. Follow the directions carefully.
5. Package the dried smears in wooden or cardboard holders.
6. In addition to the usual patient identification information, the following information should accompany the specimen to the laboratory:

   - date of onset of last menstrual period
   - presence of pregnancy
   - use of oral contraceptives and intrauterine devices
   - history of hormonal imbalance or dysfunction
   - current diagnosis
   - previous surgeries, particularly any gynecologic surgery
   - history of previous cancer
   - area from which the specimen was obtained

Postprocedure

1. Remind the patient that Pap smears should be done at least annually in conjunction with a complete physical examination. Women 20 years of age or older should have the Pap smear included in the annual physical exam. The peak incidence for carcinoma *in situ* of the cervix is between 30 to 40 yr of age. The peak incidence for invasive carcinoma is between 40 to 50 yr of age. High-risk groups for cervical cancer include women

   - starting intercourse in their teens
   - having multiple sexual partners
   - having many children
   - from low socioeconomic groups

2. Instruct the patient that any abnormal report will be discussed with her and will need follow-up by a physician.
3. "Do-it-yourself" techniques are still under study with varied results. Explain to the patient that these kits should not replace the annual physical examination.

Signed Consent
Not required

DILATATION AND CURETTAGE (D & C)

Dilatation and curettage (D & C) involves gradual dilatation of the cervix and scraping of the endometrium with a curette. Endometrial tissue may also be obtained using aspiration or suction methods. Indications for a D & C may include the following:

- elective abortion
- incomplete abortion
- dysfunctional vaginal bleeding
- removal of endometrial or endocervical polyps
- suspected endometrial or endocervical carcinoma
- retained placental fragments

Normal Results
Normal tissue samples

Nursing Implications
Preprocedure
1. The patient is usually hospitalized. The procedure may be done on an outpatient basis.
2. Keep the patient NPO after midnight prior to the procedure.
3. Explain the procedure to the patient.
4. Give a perineal shave and an enema as prescribed.
5. Instruct the patient to empty the bladder. A foley catheter may also be inserted.
6. Check to be sure that the operative permit is signed and that requested laboratory test results are on the chart.
7. Administer preoperative medication as prescribed.

During the Procedure
1. Support the patient during anesthesia administration.
2. If general anesthesia is used, keep stimuli (lights, noise, movement) to a minimum during the induction period.
3. Position the patient in a lithotomy position. The feet and ankles should be well padded. Arrange the stirrups to avoid pressure against the thighs and knees.
4. Vaginal and perineal scrubs may be ordered.
5. Label all specimens and immerse them in a preservative.

Postprocedure

1. Postsurgical care should include the following activities:
   a. monitoring vital signs frequently
   b. assessing respiratory status
   c. encouraging deep breathing and coughing
   d. evaluating amount and character of vaginal discharge
   e. assessing level of consciousness, orientation, and return of sensations
   f. providing for the patient's safety by keeping the side rails up, having suction equipment available
2. Prior to dismissal, explain to the patient that
   a. minimal bleeding and abdominal cramping may be expected
   b. no douches or chemical applications should be administered for 1 to 2 wk unless ordered specifically by the physician
   c. abstain from intercourse for approximately 2 wk or as directed by physician

Signed Consent

Written consents for surgical procedure and for the anesthesia are required.

HYSTEROSALPINGOGRAPHY

The hysterosalpingography is an x-ray and fluoroscopic procedure used to study uterine and fallopian tubes anatomy. This study can identify malformations or defects of uterine or tubal structures, patency of the tubes, or locations of tubal blockage. The study involves the instillation of a radiopaque substance into the uterus and the fallopian tubes. This procedure is usually done to determine a possible cause of sterility. It may also be done after tubal ligation to confirm that the tubes are adequately ligated to prevent pregnancy. The Rubin test usually precedes the hysterosalpingography.

Hysterosalpingography is contraindicated in the following:

- pelvic infection
- purulent vaginal discharge
- fever from any cause
- during menstruation or any abnormal uterine bleeding in a week preceding or following menstruation
- immediately following curettage
- suspected pregnancy
- serious cardiac or any other serious systemic disease

Normal Results

X-ray evidence of passage of the dye through the uterus and the fallopian tubes into the peritoneal cavity. Normal uterus and fallopian tubes.

Nursing Implications

Preprocedure

1. Assist the patient to schedule the test so that it is not performed 1 wk prior to or after menses.

2. Explain the purpose of the procedure to the patient and answer any questions the patient may have. Inform the patient that the procedure may cause discomfort.
3. Before the procedure, assess the patient's understanding of the study.
4. Instruct the patient to complete bowel preparation 1 to 2 hr prior to the scheduled procedure. A Fleets enema may be prescribed.
5. Instruct the patient in relaxation techniques that can be used during the procedure.
6. Instruct the patient to void prior to the procedure.
7. Give a sedative if prescribed by the physician.

During the Procedure

1. Assist the patient into a lithotomy position and drape the patient appropriately.
2. Keep the patient informed of activities as they occur during the procedure.
   a. A bimanual pelvic examination will precede the procedure.
   b. A speculum will be inserted into the vagina.
   c. The cervix will be prepped with an antiseptic solution.
   d. The cervix will be grasped with a tenaculum. This may hurt for a few seconds.
   e. A uterine sound will be passed through the cervix to dilate the endocervix and the internal os. This may also cause slight discomfort.
   f. A cannula will be passed into the uterus and 1 to 2 ml of dye will be instilled. The first x-ray will be taken and examined prior to continuation of the procedure.
   g. If the uterine cavity is normal in structure, an additional 2 to 8 ml of dye will be instilled. This action may cause uterine cramping. Additional x-rays will be taken to evaluate the structure of the fallopian tubes.
   h. If the dye fails to fill the tubes, spasm of the tubes may occur. Amyl nitrite may be used to eliminate the tubal spasm.
3. Encourage the patient to use relaxation techniques, particularly during times of discomfort.
4. Remain with the patient throughout the procedure.
5. Observe the patient's response to the procedure.

Postprocedure

1. Instruct the patient that a vaginal discharge may occur for 1 to 2 dy after the procedure. Provide a perineal pad for the patient to wear. The discharge may be bloody or contain the dye that was used during the procedure.
2. Give emotional support if the test results are not as anticipated by the patient.
3. Explain to the patient that transient dizziness and cramping may occur.
4. Assist the patient to schedule further tests as ordered by the physician.

Signed Consent

Not required

MAMMOGRAPHY

Mammography is a soft-tissue radiography used to detect breast cancer that may not be detectible by any other means. Mammography uses a low-energy x-ray beam to provide a contrast between soft tissue structures of the breast. Mammography is useful in the following situations:

- diagnostic screening for women who are at a high risk of developing breast cancer

- women with diffuse tissue irregularities owing to fibrocystic disease

- evaluation of the second breast when a lesion is identified in one breast

- recurring breast symptoms with not palpable abnormalities or with indefinite physical examination findings

Disadvantages of mammography include the following:

- malignancy is not identified in 5 to 15% of the cases of breast cancers

- inaccuracy in interpretation of results in the young woman because of the density of breast tissue

- a possible hazard of radiation-induced breast cancer exists

Normal Results

Normal structure of the breast

Benign breast masses

Shape	Round, oval, or lobulated
Border	Well-circumscribed, regular, smooth
Density	Homogeneous
Surrounding tissue	Displaced, not invaded
Calcifications	Few, coarse, widely scattered
*Secondary signs	None

Malignant breast masses

Shape	Variable, ragged, tentacled
Border	Irregular, poorly circumscribed
Density	Nonhomogeneous
Surrounding tissue	Infiltrated, retracted
Calcification	Numerous, uncountable, confined to area of lesion
*Secondary Signs	Frequently present

---

*Secondary signs might include retraction or distortion of the nipple, areola, or skin, increased size of veins of the breast, enlarged axillary lymph nodes.

Nursing Implications
Preprocedure

1. Explain the procedure to the patient. The procedure takes approximately one half hour and is not painful.
2. Clean the breast tissue and axillary area of any material or substance that might interfere with the passage of the rays through the tissue. Remove adhesive tape, bandages, gowns, and medications including deodorants and powders.
3. Instruct the patient to wear clothing that allows the top to be removed.

During the Procedure

1. A chest film is taken at the beginning of the procedure.
2. The patient is asked to identify any abnormalities of the breast tissue, such as lumps.
3. The breast is positioned against the film plate so that there are no skin folds, wrinkles, or air pockets.
4. The patient is placed in several positions and two or three x-rays are taken of the breast.
5. The radiologist may palpate the breasts following the x-rays.

Postprocedure

1. Explain to the patient that a repeat mammography may be ordered but this does not necessarily indicate that an abnormality was found. Improper positioning or x-ray techniques may result in x-rays that cannot be evaluated.
2. Teach or reinforce the technique for self-breast examination. Ask the patient to report any changes noted.

Signed Consent
Not required

PELVIC EXAMINATION

The pelvic examination is used to evaluate structures in the lower abdomen (bladder, rectum) and the reproductive system (ovaries, fallopian tubes, uterus, cervix, vagina, external genitalia). The examiner may use palpation (internal and external), inspection, and percussion to aid in the evaluation. Tests that may be done at the same time as the pelvic examination include the following:

- vaginal smear
- Pap smear
- postcoital test
- cervical biopsy
- culdoscopy

Normal Results
Normal female anatomical structures

Nursing Implications

Preprocedure

1. Explain to the patient that she should not douche for at least 24 hr prior to the anticipated vaginal examination. If diagnostic smears are to be obtained, douches dilute and wet the cells making satisfactory staining of the cells difficult.
2. Explain the examination procedure to the patient. Include in your explanation, a description of some of the sensations that might be experienced by the patient.
3. Instruct the patient in relaxation techniques.
4. Explain to the patient that an enema may be prescribed since a full rectum makes pelvic examination difficult and inconclusive.
5. Assist the patient to assume a lithotomy position. Raising her head slightly will facilitate the relaxation of the abdominal muscles. The buttocks of the patient should extend just beyond the edge of the examining table. Be sure that her legs are adequately supported. The patient should be as comfortable as possible.

During the Procedure

1. The examination begins with an inspection of the lower abdomen and external genitalia. If vaginal smears are to be obtained, this is done prior to the vaginal examination.
2. Bimanual abdominal–vaginal examination follows.
3. Instruct the patient to remain relaxed by breathing slowly and deeply.
4. Explain to the patient that feelings of pressure are to be expected as the speculum and the examiner's fingers are introduced into the vagina. The relaxed patient should feel minimum discomfort if no abnormalities or pathology are present.
5. Instruct the patient that she may be asked to strain down as if voiding or having a bowel movement, or to cough during the examination.
6. Speculum examination of the cervix and vagina follows the bimanual abdominal–vaginal examination. Do not apply lubricating jels to the speculum if cervical or endocervical smears are to be done. Lubricants spoil the staining characteristics of the cells obtained. Use warm water as a lubricant.
7. Rectal and bimanual abdominal–rectal examinations are done after the speculum examination is completed. Bimanual abdominal–vaginal–rectal examinations may also be done.

Postprocedure

1. Provide the patient with tissues for wiping the lubricant from the external genitalia.
2. Reinforce the physician's instructions regarding further testing or treatment.
3. Provide additional information when necessary.

Signed Consent

Not required

POSTCOITAL TEST

The postcoital test is part of the physical examination of infertile couples. Male and female factors are evaluated in relationship to fertility. The postcoital test provides information about the following factors:

- quality, quantity, and physical properties of cervical mucus
- degree and quality of sperm penetration
- intercourse technique (indirectly)
- indirect measurement of ovarian function

Normal Results

No normal value has been assigned to this test, although the following findings seem more conducive for pregnancy to occur:

- 5 to 20 actively motile sperm per high power field
- abundant cervical secretion that is crystal clear and free of leukocytes and epithelial cells
- consistency of cervical secretions such that it will form long threads (spinnbarkeit)
- fern pattern formed by cervical secretions dried on the slide

   Pregnancy is less likely to occur in the presence of the following findings:

- less than 5 actively motile sperm per high power field
- scanty, cloudy, viscid, and cellular cervical secretions
- failure of cervical secretions to form fern pattern on the slide

Nursing Implications

Preprocedure

1. Explain to the patient how to identify ovulation time. The ideal time for collection of the specimen is at ovulation time. The female may use the basal body temperature (BBT) chart. The time of ovulation is within 24 to 48 hr of the day in which there is a rise in basal body temperature. The test may be planned 15 to 16 dy prior to the expected onset of menses.
2. A series of tests may be performed (days 10, 12, 14 of the menstrual cycle).
3. Explain the importance of the optimal time interval for collection of the specimen. The optimal time interval is 2 to 6 hr between intercourse and the examination. The preferred time interval is within 4 to 6 hr after intercourse. The patient should not use precoital lubricants or postcoital douches.
4. The patient should use no douches, intra-vaginal medication, or lubricants during the 48 hr preceding the test.
5. Note the duration of abstinence prior to intercourse for the test.
6. Record the time interval between intercourse and examination.

During the Procedure

1. Use a dry speculum, no lubricant.
2. Specimen samples will be collected from the vagina. Samples are aspirated from various areas. Sperm motility and survival are expected to be greatest in specimens obtained from high in the endocervical canal.
3. Portions of the samples are allowed to air dry for evaluation of fern pattern formation. Other samples are evaluated immediately under the microscope for spermatozoa and cellular content.

Postprocedure

1. Abnormal readings should be verified two to three times before they are considered conclusive.
2. Attempt to identify causes for abnormal readings by
   - evaluating the basal body temperature chart
   - examining the cervix for evidence of cervicitis
   - identify intercourse technique used

Signed Consent

Not required

RUBIN TEST

The Rubin test is a nonsurgical test for evaluating the patency of the fallopian tubes. This test is indicated as part of the studies done for infertility.

A gas, usually carbon dioxide, is passed under pressure into the uterus by way of the vagina. The gas will pass from the uterus into the fallopian tubes and the peritoneal cavity if the tubes are patent. Presence of the gas in the peritoneal cavity can be determined by x-ray, auscultation, and reports by the patient of pain in the shoulder after assuming an upright position. If both tubes are blocked, no gas will be detected in the peritoneal cavity.

The Rubin test is often therapeutic in cases where some blockage of the tubes is present. The pressure from the gas may open the tubes and correct the existing problem.

The Rubin test is contraindicated in the following:

- pelvic infection
- purulent vaginal discharge
- fever from any cause
- during menstruation or any uterine or cervical bleeding
- immediately following curettage
- suspected pregnancy
- serious cardiac or any serious systemic disease

Normal Results

Abrupt drop in gas pressure readings from 80 to 120 mm Hg (torr) or more to 20 to 40 mm Hg (torr). Presence of gas in peritoneal cavity confirmed by x-ray, shoulder pain, or by gas sounds heard upon auscultation of the abdomen.

Abnormal Results

None of the above occurs

Nursing Implications

Preprocedure

1. Assist the patient to schedule the test prior to ovulation and at least 3 to 4 dy after the last day of her menses. The procedure is usually done in the doctor's office.
2. Explain the purpose of the procedure to the patient and answer any questions the patient may have. Inform the patient that the procedure may cause some discomfort.
3. Assess patient's understanding of the test.
4. Instruct the patient how to perform relaxation techniques that can be used during the procedure.
5. Instruct the patient to void prior to the procedure.

During the Procedure

1. Assist the patient to assume a lithotomy position and drape the patient appropriately.
2. Inform the patient of activities as they occur during the procedure.
   a. A bimanual pelvic examination will be performed initially.
   b. A speculum will be inserted into the vagina.
   c. The cervix will be prepped with an antiseptic solution.
   d. The cervix will be grasped with a tenaculum. This will hurt for a few seconds.
   e. A uterine sound will be passed through the cervix to dilate the endocervix and internal os. This will also cause slight discomfort.
   f. A cannula will be passed into the uterus and the gas will be introduced.
   g. If the test is normal, the patient may experience shoulder pain when she assumes an upright position. The pain may be sharp initially.
3. Encourage the patient to use relaxation techniques particularly during times of discomfort.
4. Use a stethoscope to auscultate either side of the abdomen while the gas is being introduced. Intermittent bubbling sounds will be heard if gas is passing into the peritoneal cavity.
5. Remain with the patient throughout the procedure.
6. Observe the patient's response to the procedure.

Postprocedure

1. Insert a tampon into the vagina to stop any cervical bleeding caused by the tenaculum. Instruct the patient to remove the tampon when she arrives home.
2. If shoulder pain persists, instruct the patient to lie with her hips ele-

vated. This discomfort is not cause for concern and should gradually subside and disappear.

3. Give emotional support if the test results are abnormal.
4. Explain possible reasons for abnormal results. Some common causes are tubal spasms, improper timing of the test during the menstrual cycle, and mechanical obstruction of the cannula.
5. Assist the patient in scheduling another Rubin test or other tests as ordered by the physician.

Signed Consent

Not required

SEMEN ANALYSIS

Semen analysis is a test that is used to evaluate male infertility. Evaluation of the semen should include the following:

- volume of fluid
- sperm count
- motility of sperm
- morphology of sperm
- viscosity of fluid
- pH of fluid

Laboratory Results

Volume

Normal	3 to 5 ml
Abnormal	Small amounts (1 to 2 ml)
	Large amounts (6 to 10 ml)

Sperm count

Normal	60 to 120 million/ml
Abnormal	Less than 20 million/ml associated with infertility

Motility of sperm

Normal	Active, forward movement	
Normal	*Percentage of active sperm*	*Hours after collection*
	70% to 90%	0 to 1 hr
	60% to 70%	2 to 4 hr
	50% to 60%	4 to 7 hr
	35% to 50%	7 to 10 hr
	25% to 35%	10 to 15 hr
Abnormal	Inactive, sluggish movement, higher percent of inactive	

Morphology of sperm

Normal — 60% to 90% normal form

Abnormal — Higher percentage of bizarre sperm forms are associated with infertility

Viscosity of fluid

Normal — Initial presence of coagulum which liquifies in 10 to 30 min

Abnormal — Failure of coagulum to liquify

p*H of fluid*

Normal — 7.2 to 7.6

Abnormal — Less than 7.2

Nursing Implications

Procedure for Collection/Storage of Specimen

1. Collect the specimen in the doctor's office. The specimen should be examined within 1 to 4 hr after collection.
2. Note the date and the exact time when the specimen was collected.
3. Note the method that was used to obtain the specimen.
   a. Masturbation is the best method.
   b. The use of the comdom during intercourse may damage spermatic morphology and motility. Powder or lubricants may act as spermicides. If a condom is used, the condom must be washed with soap and water and thoroughly dried.
   c. Coitus interruptus is not recommended since an incomplete specimen collection with the loss of the first portion of the ejaculate may result.
4. Avoid exposure of the specimen to heat or cold. Keep the specimen at room temperature.

Possible Interfering Factors

Inaccurate results may be obtained if

- A specimen contained that is not clean and dry is used.
- All the ejaculate is not included in the specimen collection.
- The specimen is exposed to temperature extremes.
- Ejaculation has occurred within 3 to 6 days of specimen collection.

Patient Care

1. Assess the patient for a history of factors that may influence sperm production. Some factors are infections or undescended testes. Environmental factors may also interfere with sperm transport such as blockage of the tubules from infection such as gonorrhea or from abnormal tissue growth.
2. Give emotional support to the couple as this is a difficult time for both.

Patient Education

1. Instruct the patient to abstain from ejaculation if possible for 3 to 6 dy prior to the test. Prolonged abstinence will decrease sperm quality and motility.
2. Instruct the patient to save *all* ejaculate in order to obtain an accurate analysis.
3. Give the patient a clean, dry glass container to collect the specimen. Do not use a condom or plastic jar.
4. Assure the patient that one abnormal reading is not diagnostic. A minimum of 3 specimens obtained at intervals of 2 to 4 wk should be evaluated if an abnormal reading is obtained.

Signed Consent

Not required

ULTRASONOGRAPHY

Ultrasonography is a diagnostic technique that uses high-frequency sound to form pictures of the internal structures of the body. Information gained through this test includes measurement of size, determination of shape and location, and actual movement of certain structures.

A definite diagnosis of pathology is not able to be obtained by ultrasonography. It is suitable for use as a screening device and as an adjunct to other tests for many normal and abnormal conditions of the reproductive system.

It is safe, quick, highly accurate, noninvasive, and relatively inexpensive. There is no exposure to radiation, which makes its use particularly valuable during pregnancy.

A scanner is passed over the abdomen to evaluate structures located within the abdomen. For evaluation of the prostate, the transrectal approach is used. A probe containing the transducer and scanner is inserted into the rectum.

Ultrasonography is useful in evaluating the following:

- uterine masses such as fibroids and myomas
- ovarian cysts and neoplasms
- endometriosis
- pregnancy including monitoring fetal growth and formation, fetal age, placental location, molar pregnancy
- presence and position of intrauterine contraceptive devices
- pelvic inflammatory disease
- breast tissue such as cysts, cancer
- prostate abnormalities
- effectiveness of treatment for gynecologic and prostatic cancer, and
- nongynecologic pelvic masses, such as pelvic, kidney, rectal or colon carcinoma.

Normal Results

Normal pattern image of the structure being evaluated.

Nursing Implications

Preprocedure

1. Explain the procedure and the purpose to the patient. Assure the patient that the procedure is painless.
2. Administer cathartics or enemas if ordered for bowel cleansing.
3. Instruct the patient to drink 3 to 4 glasses of liquid prior to the examination.
4. Instruct the patient not to void until after the test is completed.

During the Procedure

1. Assist the patient into a supine position. A pillow may be placed under the head for comfort. Slight elevation of the right side may be necessary to prevent supine hypotensive syndrome if the patient is pregnant.
2. Coat the abdomen liberally with a coupling agent such as mineral oil. Explain that this will allow the transducer to glide easily across the abdominal surface.
3. Remain with the patient.
4. Identify structures to the patient when appropriate.

Postprocedure

1. Assist the patient to remove the oil used as the coupling agent.
2. Provide emotional support if the test results indicate an abnormality.
3. Assist the patient in scheduling additional tests as necessary.

Signed Consent

Not required

Transrectal Approach

Preprocedure

1. Explain the procedure and its purpose to the patient. Assure the patient that only minor discomfort should be expected when the probe is inserted into the rectum.
2. Administer cathartics or enemas if ordered for bowel cleansing.
3. Instruct the patient to drink 3 or 4 glasses of liquid prior to the examination.
4. Instruct the patient not to void until after the test is completed.
5. Explain that the entire procedure requires only a few minutes.
6. Teach relaxation techniques to use during moments of discomfort.

During the Procedure

1. Assist the patient into position in the special chair that will be used. The rectum and scrotum should be situated over the opening in the chair seat.
2. Remain with the patient.

3. Inform the patient prior to insertion of the probe into the rectum.
4. Encourage the use of relaxation techniques.
5. Observe the patient's response to the procedure. Be particularly alert for signs of pain and faintness.

Postprocedure

1. Give emotional support if the test results indicate an abnormality.
2. Assist the patient in scheduling additional tests as necessary.

Signed Consent

Not required

BIBLIOGRAPHY

Baber HRK, Fields DH, Kaufman SA: Quick Reference to OB-GYN Procedures, 2nd ed. Philadelphia, JB Lippincott, 1979

Bacchus H: Essentials of Gynecologic and Obstetric Endocrinology. Baltimore, University Park Press, 1975

Bauer JD, Ackermann PG, Toro G: Clinical Laboratory Methods, 8th ed. St Louis, CV Mosby, 1974

Bibbo M: Screening of individuals exposed to diethyestilbestrol. Clinical Obstet Gynecol 22, No. E: 689–699, 1979

Chen C, Jones WR: Application of a sperm micro-immobilization test to cervical mucus in the investigation of immunological infertility. Fertil Steril 35, No. 5: 542–545, 1981

Cohen J, Hendry WF, Rosner D: Ultrasonography in diagnosis of breast disease. J Surg Oncol 14, No. 1: 39–96, 1980

Cole-Beuglet C, Goldberg BB, Kurtz AB, Rubin CS, Patchefsky AS, Shaber, GS: Ultrasound mammography: a comparison with radiographic mammography. Radiology 139 No. 3: 693–698, 1981

Davidsohn I, Henry JB (eds): Todd-Sanford Clinical Diagnosis by Laboratory Methods, 15th ed. Philadelphia, WB Saunders, 1974

Davis LE, Sperry S: The CSF-FTA text and the significance of blood comtamination. Ann Neurol 6, No. 1:68–69, 1979

Dmowski WP, Rezai P, Auletta FJ, Scommegna A: Abnormal FSH and LH patterns contrasting with normal estradiol and progesterone secretion in women with long-standing unexplained infertility. J Clin Endocrinol Metab 52, No. 6:1218–1224, 1981

Dyckman JD, Wende RD: Comparisons of serum and plasma specimens for syphilis serology using the reagin screen text. J Clin Microbiol 11, No. 1:16–18, 1980

Edinger DD, Watring WC, Anderson B: Hysterography as a diagnostic technique in endometrial carcinoma. Clin Obstet Gynecol 22, No. 3:29–35, 1979

Egan RL: Technologist Guide to Mammography, 2nd ed. Baltimore, Williams & Wilkins, 1977

Ellice RM, Morse AR, Anderson MC: Aspiration cytology versus histology in the assessment of the endometrium of women in a menopause clinic. BR J Obstet Gynaecol 88, No. 4:421–425, 1981

Fishbach F: A Manual of Laboratory Diagnostic Tests. Philadelphia, JB Lippincott, 1980

Freidman SG, Rose JG, Winston MA: ultrasound and nuclear medicine evaluation in acute testicular trauma. J Urol 125, No. 5:748–749, 1981

Genitourinary Ultrasonography, Vol 2, Clinics in Diagnostic Ultrasound. New York, Churchill Livingstone, 1979

Gibowski M, Neumann, E: Non-specific positive test results to syphilis in dermatological diseases. Br Vener Dis, 56, No. 1:917–19, 1980

Green TH Jr: Gynecology: Essentials of Clinical Practice, 3rd ed. Boston, Little, Brown & Co, 1977

Greenhill JP: Office Gynecology, 9th ed. Chicago, Year Book Medical Publishers, 1971

Guyton AC: Textbook of Medical Physiology, 5th ed. Philadelphia, WB Saunders, 1976

Hansman, M: Sonar in early pregnancy. J Perin Med 9, Supplement 19:20–25, 1981

Hogan K, Tchenz D: The role of the nurse during amniocentesis. JOGN 7, No. 1:24–27, 1978

Jessup S, Botha P: False positive test results for syphilis in relatives of a patient with systemic lupus erythematosus. Br J Vener 55, No. 4:292–294, 1979

Jones, JE, Harris RE: Diagnostic evaluation of syphilis during pregnancy. Obstet Gynecol 54, No. 5:611–614, 1979

Jouppita P: Prognosis of threatened early pregnancy. J Perin Med 9, Supplement 1:72–74, 1981

Kawada CY, An-Foraker SH: Screening for endometrial carcinoma. Clin Obstet Gynecol 22, No. 3:713–728, 1979

Kistner RW: Gynecology: Principles and Practice, 3rd ed. Chicago, Year Book Medical Publishers, 1979

Kozlowski P, Terinde R, Schmidt J, Herberger J, Bender HG: Analysis of placental structures by ultrasound in normal and complicated pregnancies. J Perin Med 9, Supplement 1:138–139, 1981

Kratochwil A: Estimations of fetal age by means of ultrasound. J Perin Med 9, Supplement 1:25–32, 1981

Laing FC: Ultrasound. Human Nature 50–56, 1978

Low AC, Young H: Modern trends in the laboratory diagnosis of gonorrhea. Med Lab Sci 36, No. 3:275–281, 1979

Luckmann J, Sorensen KC: Medical-Surgical Nursing: A Psycho-Physiologic Approach, 2nd ed. Philadelphia, WB Saunders, 1980

Marchang DJ: Screening for breast cancer. Clin Obstet Gynecol 22, No. 3:759–776, 1979

Parmley TH: Screening techniques for vulvar and vaginal lesions. Clin Obstet Gynecol 22, No. 3:683–688, 1979

Perotti ME, Gioria M: Fine structure and morphogenesis of "headless" human spermatozoa associated with infertility. Cell Biology International Reports 5, No. 2:133, 1981

Phipps WJ, Long BC, Woods NF: Medical-Surgical Nursing: Concepts and Clinical Practice. St. Louis, CV Mosby, 1979

Pritchard JA, MacDonald PC: Williams Obstetrics, 16th ed. New York, Appleton-Century-Crofts, 1980

Richart RM: Screening techniques for cervical neoplasia. Clin Obstet Gynecol 22, No. 3:701–712, 1979

Sabbagha RE (ed): Diagnostic Utrasound: Applied to Obstetrics and Gynecology. New York, Harper & Row, 1980

Spermatozoa, Antibodies and Infertility: Proceedings of a Symposium on Infertility. Oxford, Blackwell Scientific Publications, 1978

Strax P (ed): Control of Breast Cancer Through Mass Screening. Littleton, Ma, PSG Publishing, 1979

Tamm J, Volkwein U, Tresquerres JA: Plasma testosterone glucosiduronate: a reliable indicator of female hyperandrogenism. Clin Endocrino (Oxf) 13, No. 5:431–435, 1970

Tannebaum M: Urologic Pathology: The Prostate. Philadelphia, Lea & Febiger, 1977

Tilkian SM, Conover MB, Tilkian AG: Clinical Implications of Laboratory Tests, 2nd ed. St Louis, CV Mosby, 1979

Toshach S, Coull J, Sigurdson S, Dublenko S, Grocholski J, Linarez L: Evaluation of five serologic tests for antibody to Neisseria gonorrheae. Sex Transm Dis 6, 214–217, 1979

Twinem FP: You and Your Prostate. Springfield, Ill, Thomas Books, 1980

Valle RF, Sciarra JJ: Current status of hysteroscopy in gynecologic practice. Fertil Steril 32, No. 6:619–632, 1979

Vandenberghe K: Ultrasonography of placenta. J Perin Med 9 Supplement 1:75–77, 1981

Vorher H: Breast Cancer: Epidemiology, Endocrinology, Biochemistry and Pathobiology. Baltimore, Urban & Schwarzenberg, 1980

Werch A, Acosta A, Besch PK: The roles of amniotic fluid analysis. JOGN Nurs 3:43–46, 1974.

Widmann FK: Clinical Interpretation of Laboratory Tests, 8th ed. Philadelphia, FA Davis, 1979

Young, H, Henrichsen C, McMillan A: The diagnostic value of a gonococcal complement fixation test. Med Lab Sci 37, 2:165–170, 1980

9

Tests Related to Immunology

Mary Ellen Schweitzer

OVERVIEW OF PHYSIOLOGY AND PATHOPHYSIOLOGY

The immunological system of man is a defensive mechanism that consists of three levels of defense response: local barriers, inflammation, and the immune response.

The *local barriers* include intact skin, mucous membranes, and normal flora, which protect the body surfaces.

The *inflammatory defense response* acts through phagocytic cells of the blood, reticuloendothelial system, and lymphatic system. The inflammatory response has the important defense function of ingesting and digesting foreign substances that have passed through the local barrier defense level.

The *immune response* is a physiologic reaction of the body to factors that the body considers threatening and foreign.

ANTIGEN–ANTIBODY REACTION

A factor that evokes the immune response is referred to as an antigen. An antigen is a foreign protein. When antigens are introduced into the body they cause the formation of specific antibodies by specialized sensitized lymphocytes. This characteristic of "specificity" makes particular antibodies or lymphocytes responsive only to particular antigens. Commonly occurring antigens are bacteria, viruses, toxins, and foreign tissue.

Haptens

Certain molecules or substances by themselves cannot induce the formation of antibodies or sensitized lymphocytes because of their low molecular weight. These molecules are known as haptens. However, when coupled with high molecular weight molecules, haptens do cause the antibody to be produced.

Haptens are important in the development of hypersensitivities to certain drugs such as antibiotics.

MECHANISMS OF IMMUNITY

Two mechanisms are involved in the immune response, which protects an individual from invading foreign substances, infectious disease, or the development of cancer. One of the mechanisms is referred to as humoral immunity and the other as cell-mediated immunity.

- The humoral system (B system) consists of protein molecules called antibodies and is effective against bacteria and some viruses.
- The T system or cell-mediated immune response combats fungi and most viruses and initiates the process by which organ transplants are rejected.

HUMORAL IMMUNITY

The humoral immune response involves the production of antibodies. Antibodies are protein molecules that are secreted by specialized plasma lymphocytes called beta (β) lymphocytes.

β Lymphocytes

β lymphocytes are originally derived from lymphocytic stem cells in the bone marrow in the embryo. These stem cells migrate to a yet unidentified area in the body, thought to be the lymphoid tissue of the gastrointestinal tract (Peyer's Patches), and mature under a thymic-independent source.

After maturation, β lymphocytes are capable of producing and secreting immunoglobulin molecules (antibodies). Antibodies react only with antigen which was responsible for the production of the antibodies.

Primary Response

When a mature β lymphocyte encounters an antigen, it is stimulated to divide and differentiate into a plasma cell, which in turn starts an assembly line production of antibodies. This is called the primary response and occurs in about 6 days. β lymphocytes have an immunologic memory.

Secondary Response

There are a number of antigen-stimulated β lymphocytes that do not make the transformation to antibody-producing cells, but remain in the circulation and are referred to as "memory cells." The next time the same antigen is present, these cells remember, transform to plasma cells, and then begin specific antibody production. This is called a secondary response.

TYPES OF IMMUNOGLOBULINS

All immunoglobulins or antibodies consist of four polypeptide chains, two heavy chains and two light chains that are linked together by disulfide bonds. The two light chains are common to all immunoglobulins and are called *Bence Jones proteins.*

Differences in the heavy chains are the basis for the division of immunoglobulins into five classes:

- *IgG* comprises about 75% of the total immunoglobulins. It is the only immunoglobulin that crosses the placental barrier, thereby protecting the infant during the first few weeks of life. It is found in the plasma and interstitial fluid. IgG produces antibodies against bacteria, viruses, and toxins and activates the complement system. IgG is the major immunoglobulin to respond in a secondary response.

- *IgA* comprises about 15% of the total immunoglobulins and is found in large quantities in tears, saliva, milk, and other exocrine secretions. IgA provides protection of the mucosal surfaces of the respiratory, digestive, and genital tracts from pathogenic invasion.

- *IgM* comprises about 10% of the total immunoglobulins and is found in the serum. IgM is the largest of the immunoglobulin molecules and the first to be synthesized in life. IgM functions in combination with IgG. IgM has specific antitoxin action and thus is capable of neutralizing toxins produced by bacteria. IgM also provides the natural antibodies, such as antibodies present without antigen stimulation, the rheumatoid factor, and the ABO blood group antibodies. IgM also activates the complement system.

- *IgD* comprises less than 1% of the total immunoglobulins and is found in the serum. IgD function is unknown.

- *IgE* also comprises less than 1% of the total immunoglobulins and is found in the serum and interstitial fluid. It is known as the anaphylactic (reagenic) antibody. IgE serves to mediate the severe allergic reactions. These include anaphylactic shock, allergic asthma, and hay fever.

TYPES OF ANTIGEN-ANTIBODY REACTIONS

Reactions between antigens and antibodies may take many forms. The reactions that may occur, and the system by which antibodies may be classified, include the following:

- *precipitation:* antibodies cause the separation of antigens from their fluid medium (precipitans)

- *limpis:* antibodies cause the disintegration of antigens (lipins)

- *agglutination:* antibodies cause a clumping of antigens (agglutinins)

- *opsonization:* antibodies make the antigens more susceptible to phagocytosis (opsonins)

- *neutralization:* antibodies neutralize the toxic products of the antigens (antitoxins)

COMPLEMENT SYSTEM

The humoral immune response cannot be separated from another system in the body called the complement system. The complement consists of nine serum proteins (enzyme precursors) that are designated C–1 through C–9. The antigen is the target of the complement system.

These serum proteins (enzymes) are naturally found in the plasma and other body fluids. These serum proteins are normally inactive. When an antibody combines with an antigen, the antigen–antibody complex becomes an activator of the complement system.

The activated enzymes attack the invading antigen in several different ways. They also initiate local tissue reactions that provide protection against damage by the invading organism. The following important effects occur:

- *Lysis:* The enzymes of the complement system digest portions of the cell membrane, thus causing rupture of the invading cells.

- *Opsonization and phagocytosis:* The complement enzymes attack bacterial and other invading antigen surfaces. This makes them more susceptible to phagocytosis by neutrophils and tissue macrophages. This process is called opsonization. Opsonization enhances by many hundred fold the number of antigens that can be destroyed.

- *Chemotaxis:* The complement enzymes cause chemotaxis (attraction) of neutrophils and macrophages. This increases the number of phagocytes into the region of the antigen.

- *Agglutination:* The complement enzymes can change the surface of some of the antigens, causing them to adhere to one another. This causes antigen agglutination.

- *Viral neutralization:* Complement enzymes attack the molecular structures of viruses, rendering them harmless.

- *Inflammatory effect:* The complement system causes a local inflammatory reaction. This reaction prevents movement of the invading antigen through the tissues.

CELLULAR IMMUNITY
T Lymphocytes

Cellular immunity is mediated by T lymphocytes. T lymphocytes are also originally derived from lymphocytic cells in the bone marrow of the fetus. These lymphoid stem cells migrate to the thymus gland and under thymic influence are modified and mature into T lymphocytes. Mature T cells emerge from the thymic medulla into the blood circulation.

When not circulating, T cells reside in the lymphoid tissues. T cells are the major type of cell found in the lymph nodes, spleen, Peyers patches, bone marrow, and intestinal mucosa.

Sensitized Lymphocytes

T lymphocytes are responsible for the production of sensitized lymphocytes. The presence of an antigen stimulates T lymphocytes, which become sensitized lymphocytes. These sensitized lymphocytes are specific for each antigen and capable of neutralizing only that antigen.

The sensitized lymphocytes neutralize antigens by releasing the chemical *lymphokines*, which either kills target cells or stimulates other cells, such as macrophages, to participate in the immune response. These particular lymphocytes are known as killer T cells.

The T lymphocyte also assists the β lymphocyte to synthesize antibodies.

Seconary Response

T lymphocytes, like β lymphocytes, have an immunologic memory. Instead of forming sensitized cells, some T lymphocytes divide into new lymphocytes and remain in the lymphoid tissue until the antigen is again reintroduced. Reintroduction of the antigen results in a stronger and longer secondary response.

Functions

Functions of the sensitized lymphocyte include delayed hypersensitivity reactions, graft-versus-host rejection, autoimmune responses and preservation of immunologic tolerance. The sensitized lymphocytes are also active against fungi and most viruses and may be responsible for the early recognition and destruction of cancer cells.

Sensitized lymphocytes persist in tissues for months, possibly years, while humoral antibodies survive only days.

IMMUNOLOGIC DEPRESSION

Immunocompetence exists when an individual's immune system is able to identify and destroy invading antigens. Unfortunately the immune process does not always function exactly as it should. Some individuals experience increased infection rates and possibly increased cancer occurrence rates because of a depressed immunological system.

Immunologic depression can result from 6 conditions, according to Burkhalter and Donley (1978). These conditions are as follows:

- *Age-related defects.* Infants and older individuals have a greater potential for immunologic depression than do individuals in other age groups. Infants have not yet developed the capacity for antibody production. Older individuals may begin to experience errors in the copying mechanism of DNA and RNA with resultant mutations. With increasing numbers of mutations, the immune system cannot "keep up" with the errors. Transformed cells are allowed to proliferate and cancer may result.

- *Congenital abnormalities.* Common abnormalities include absence of the thymus gland, the stem cell, or gamma globulins. Disorders that result from these abnormalities include Di George's syndrome and Swiss-type immunodeficiency syndrome.

- *Malnutrition.* Malnutrition can result from inadequate intake of essential nutrients or poor absorption of ingested nutrients. The nutrients referred to as essential include vitamins (especially B_6, B_{12}, folic acid, A and C), amino acids (particularly phenylalanine and tryptosine), and minerals (iron, magnesium, and phosphates). Decreased antigen recognition and decreased antibody production may result from these nutritional deficiencies.

- *Disease conditions.* Two common disorders associated with a depressed immunologic system are viral infections and cancer.

- *Drug-induced immunosuppression.* Certain drugs have a negative effect on the production of antibodies and can also cause hypoplastic bone marrow. Examples of such drugs include antineoplastic agents, antibiotics (chloramphenicol), antipsychotics (Thorazine), corticosteroids, barbiturates, heroin, colchicine, and excessive alcohol consumption.

- *Iatrogenically induced immunosuppression.* This includes treatments such as certain types of chemotherapy (and other previously listed drugs), radiotherapy, and surgery. All of these treatment modalities have varying degrees of immunosuppression. Radiation therapy and chemotherapy can destroy the cells of the bone marrow and cause bone marrow depression. Surgery acts to depress the immune system by acting as a stressor to the body. Stressors stimulate the adrenal cortex to secrete cortisol.

GAMMOPATHIES

Other conditions related to immunologic disorders are gammopathies, hypersensitivities, and autoimmune diseases.

Gammopathies are disorders in which there is an abnormal antibody formation as a result of a malignant proliferation of plasma cells.

- Gammopathies are serious disorders because high serum levels of dysfunctional gammaglobulins depress the synthesis of normal immunoglobulins.

- The hypergammaglobulinemic individual is susceptible to infections.

If multiple clones are involved, the disorder is termed *polyclonal gammopathies*. If a single clone is involved, the disorder is termed *monoclonal gammopathy*. Polyclonal gammopathies are the more common of the two.

- Polyclonal gammopathies involve the overproduction of all classes of immunoglobulins in response to inappropriate antigenic stimulation. Polyclonal gammopathies can develop from a variety of diseases including liver disease, systemic lupus, rheumatoid arthritis, and cancers.

- Monoclonal gammopathies occur most frequently in older individuals.

- Multiple myeloma, which is a skeletal destroying cancer, results from an abnormal clone of precursor cells in the bone marrow.

- Macroglobulinemia is another form of monoclonal gammopathy, which involves the overproduction of immunoglobulin M (IgM). This disease results in increased blood viscosity (due to the increased number of immunoglobulins) which can result in circulatory problems with resultant tissue hypoxia and tissue death.

HYPERSENSITIVITY / ALLERGY

Hypersensitivities and allergies are two terms that are used interchangeably. These terms indicate that the response of the body to an antigen is altered. Immune responses are usually beneficial, but in hypersensitive persons the response becomes harmful. The antigen evoking the reaction is referred to as an allergen.

Hypersensitivities are classified into two categories based on the components of the immune system involved:

1. humoral response or β lymphocyte mediated, known as immediate hypersensitivities, and
2. cellular or T lymphocyte mediated, known as delayed hypersensitivities.

Immediate hypersensitivity reactions include Type I, Type II, and Type III reactions.

TYPE I HYPERSENSITIVITY

Type I reactions result from an antigen reacting with a sensitized antibody of the IgE class. Type I reactions are termed immediate hypersensitivity reactions because the antibody-mediated response occurs within 10 to 15 minutes or less following exposure to the allergen.

- Some potential allergens that can cause immediate hypersensitivity reactions are pollens of grasses, trees and weeds, foods, dust, stinging insect venom, and drugs (especially antibiotics).

- Reactions that may occur include anaphylactic shock, skin reactions, atopic disorders (urticaria, hayfever, and extrinsic asthma) and drug reactions.

Anaphylactic Shock

In anaphylactic shock, IgE antibodies are attached to cells throughout the body, particularly to mast cells and basophils.

- Antigen exposure results in an antibody reaction that causes cellular rupture of these cells and release of the mediator substances—histamine, serotonin, kinins, slow-reacting substance of anaphylaxsis (SRS–A), and prostaglandins.
- These mediator substances cause vasodilatation, increased capillary permeability, and smooth muscle contraction.
- Smooth muscle contraction most severely affects the respiratory tract resulting in bronchospasm and laryngeal edema.
- Anaphylactic shock can be fatal if emergency medical measures are not instituted.

Skin Reactions

Skin (cutaneous) reactions are mediated by IgE antibodies. The reaction is seen as a wheal and flare. The wheal is the raised area of skin caused by edema and the flare is the reddened area surrounding the wheal, which is caused by capillary dilatation.

Atopic Disorders

In atopic disorders, the mechanism and mediator responsible for the symptoms is the same as described for anaphylactic shock, but the symptoms are less severe.

Drug Reactions

In drug reactions, the drugs are haptens which, when coupled with a protein molecule, bring about antigen–antibody reactions. An allergic reaction to a drug is similar to other hypersensitivity reactions, and can be cutaneous or systemic.

TYPE II SENSITIVITY (Cytotoxic Reactions)

Type II reactions, or cytotoxic reactions, result in cellular destruction in which IgG and IgM antibodies attach to an antigen on the surface of a cell. This antibody attachment to a cell marks it for destruction by phagocytosis. The type of cells involved in these reactions are blood cells. Blood incompatibility reactions are examples of Type II reactions.

TYPE III SENSITIVITIES

In Type III reactions, (immune complex hypersensitivity reactions) there is a union of soluble antigens and antibodies of the IgM and IgG class, to form complexes (microprecipitans) in the circulatory and interstitial fluids. These complexes are not destroyed by the reticuloendothelial system because their minute size tends to defy phagocytosis. The complex moves into the blood vessels in body tissues. Once in the tissues, these complexes bind with complement and result in an intravascular inflammatory response or vasculitis.

The disorders associated with these reactions are Arthus lesions and serum sickness.

TYPE IV REACTIONS

Delayed hypersensitivity reactions are referred to as Type IV Reactions. These reactions are referred to as delayed, because no immediate response is seen.

- Examples of delayed hypersensitivity reactions are tuberculosis, fungal diseases, and contact dermatitis.
- These reactions involve the union of a specific antigen with a sensitized T lymphocyte. This union results in tissue damage that is caused either by means of lymphokines (a chemical released by lymphocytes) or by direct T lymphocyte-mediated cell destruction (killer T-cell action).

AUTOIMMUNE DISORDERS

Autoimmunities are disorders in which the immune system has failed to recognize "self" from "non-self." In these cases antibodies against one's own tissues (auto-antibodies) develop, which leads to the destruction of body tissues and organs.

- Diseases of probable autoimmune origin include autoimmune hemolytic anemia, Hashimoto's thyroiditis, systemic lupus erythematosus, rheumatoid arthritis, myasthenia gravis, glomerulonephritic disease, Sjogren's syndrome, lupoid hepatitis, and autoimmune thrombocytopenia purpura.

BLOOD TESTS

Serology tests are used to diagnose some of the diseases and disorders of the immunological system (infections, hypersensitivities, autoimmune diseases, gammopathies, and cancer). In a serological test, either the antigen or antibody is known. The antigens and antibodies that are used as the known component of a serological test are commercially available. A known antigen can be tested with an individual's serum to find a specific antibody, or serum containing known antibody may be tested against antigens isolated from the individual's serum.

All serology tests have a qualitative aspect and most serology tests have a quantitative aspect. The qualitative aspect refers to the identification of the unknown antigen or antibody. The quantitative aspect refers to the ability of the test to determine the amount of antibody that is present. The quantitative aspect is also known as titer.

Serology tests are based on how antibodies react with antigens. These tests include the following:

- precipitation tests
- cytolytic tests
- agglutination tests
- opsonization tests
- neutralization tests
- complement fixation tests

Complement fixation tests are included in the study of antigen–antibody reactions because of the close association of the complement system to the humoral (antibody) system.

ALPHA₁ ANTITRYPSIN TEST

Alpha₁ antitrypsin is a serum protein produced by the liver that inhibits protease, a protein-splitting enzyme. A deficiency of this protein makes individuals more susceptible to tissue destruction. Conditions commonly associated with lowered alpha₁ antitrypsin levels are pulmonary emphysema and liver disease. This test is most frequently performed to diagnose emphysema and metabolic disorders in susceptible individuals.

Elevated levels are seen in the following conditions:

Adults

- acute and chronic inflammatory disorders
- cancer
- thyroid infections
- use of contraceptives, estrogen
- stress
- hematologic abnormalities
- maternal serum at term is elevated to levels of 200% of normal adult mean-declines to normal levels within 2 weeks.
- pregnancy

Decreased levels are associated with the following conditions:

Adults

- pulmonary emphysema and other respiratory diseases
- hepatic disease
- nephrotic syndrome
- malnutrition

Infants/Children

- premature infants with respiratory distress syndrome have markedly decreased levels, with levels rising during recovery.
- cirrhosis in children

Laboratory Results

Normal Adult

Average normal level is 160 to 400 mg/dl.

Infants

Found in fetal serum as early as 4th week of gestation

Adult levels reached at about 26 weeks of gestation

At birth, cord level is 70 to 150% of adult level.

Procedure for Collection/Storage of Specimen

1. The laboratory test is performed on a venous blood sample of 5 ml.
2. Fasting is required for individuals with elevated cholesterol or triglyceride levels.

Possible Interfering Factors

- pregnancy
- drug therapy such as contraceptives or estrogen therapy

Patient Education

1. Explain the test procedure to the patient.
2. Individuals with lowered alpha$_1$ antitrypsin levels should be taught proper pulmonary hygiene:

   - avoid smoking
   - avoid environments with increased pollution
   - air condition home (if living in high pollution area)
   - avoid persons with upper respiratory infection

ANTINUCLEAR ANTIBODIES (ANA)

This test detects antibodies that have been formed in response to one's own nuclear material.

Antinuclear antibodies can be found in individuals with the following diseases: systemic lupus erythematosus, systemic sclerosis, rheumatoid arthritis, polyarteritis nodosa, myasthenia gravis, liver cirrhosis, ulcerative colitis, infectious mononucleosis, acute and chronic leukemia, and diabetes mellitus. These antibodies may be found also in some nonsymptomatic relatives of persons with systemic lupus erythematosus.

Systemic lupus erythematosus (SLE) is the only disease of those listed, in which antinuclear antibodies are always present. Therefore this test is used to rule out SLE. If this test is negative, then the diagnosis of SLE is unlikely. Conversely, if the test is positive, it does not necessarily indicate SLE, as ANA can occur in so many conditions.

Laboratory Results

Normally there are no antinuclear antibodies in the serum.

Nursing Implications

Procedure for Collection/Storage of Specimen

The laboratory test is performed on a venous blood sample of 10 ml.

Possible Interfering Factors

Drugs that may cause a false-positive are the following:

- PAS
- chlorothiazide
- oral contraceptives

- hydralazine
- isoniazid
- procainamide
- sulfonamides
- thiouracil
- methyldopa
- streptomycin

Patient Care

1. Observe and record patient's symptomatology to aid in the diagnosis of systemic lupus erythematosus.
2. Assess the patient for any drugs being taken that might interfere with test results.
3. Positive antibody patterns may also be seen in elderly patients and in normal adults.

Patient Education

Explain the test procedure to the patient.

Signed Consent

Not required

CARCINOEMBRYONIC ANTIGEN (CEA) TEST

The carcinoembryonic antigen is a normally occurring glycoprotein that is secreted into the gastrointestinal tract by the mucosal cells. According to recent theories, disruption of the gastrointestinal mucosa by an invading cancer allows CEA to be released into the underlying connective tissue and to be absorbed into the lymphatic and circulatory systems.

This is a nonspecific test and cannot be used for the definite diagnosis of gastrointestinal tract carcinomas, because the carcinoembryonic antigen level is elevated in other conditions.

Other conditions that can cause elevated CEA levels include: cholecystitis, pancreatitis, cirrhosis, ulcerative colitis, heart disease, emphysema, bronchitis, and heavy smoking. Highest titers have been found in colon and pancreatic tumors.

Although the CEA test cannot be used to definitely diagnose cancer, it has been proven to be valuable in determining the success of cancer management. Following successful treatment of a tumor (*e.g.,* surgery, chemotherapy or radiation therapy) the initially elevated CEA level decreases. Any subsequent tumor growth or recurrence will be demonstrated by a rise in the CEA level. This rise in the CEA level can precede the development of symptoms by weeks or months.

Laboratory Results

Normal

A titer of 2.5 ng/ml or less, except in heavy smokers; titers above this level are considered diagnostic.

Nursing Implications

Procedure for Collection/Storage of Specimen

1. The laboratory test is performed on fresh venous blood serum.
2. The specimen requires an anticoagulant in the test tube.
3. The specimen requires immediate attention of laboratory personnel.

Possible Interfering Factors

None reported

Patient Care

1. Assess the patient for history of smoking.
2. Observe and record the patient's symptomatology to aid in the diagnosis of cholecystitis, pancreatitis, cirrhosis, heart disease, ulcerative colitis, emphysema, bronchitis, colon, and pancreatic tumors.

Patient Education

Explain the test procedure.

Signed Consent

Not required

COLD AGGLUTININS (Cold Hemagglutinin)

Cold agglutinins is an agglutination test used primarily to diagnose cases of atypical viral pneumonia. Cold agglutinins is a normally present antibody that causes agglutination (clumping) of red blood cells at refrigerator temperatures, when the serum is not diluted or only moderately diluted. In cases of atypical viral pneumonia, however, the cold agglutinins increase in quantity and cause agglutination even with the serum highly diluted.

Positive titers are associated with the following conditions:

- atypical viral pneumonia
- congenital syphilis
- cirrhosis
- lymphatic leukemia
- malaria
- peripheral vascular disease
- anemia
- elderly individuals

Laboratory Results

- An antibody titer of 1:32 to 1:64 is positive.
- To diagnose atypical viral pneumonia, there must be a four-fold or greater increase in antibody titer between a blood serum sample obtained during the acute phase of illness and a second sample obtained during the convalescent period.

Nursing Implications
Procedure for Collection/Storage of Specimen
1. The laboratory test is performed on a venous blood sample of 10 ml.
2. Do not refrigerate the blood specimen.
3. Send the specimen immediately to the laboratory.

Possible Interfering Factors
1. Refrigeration of blood sample before separation of serum
2. Antibiotic therapy
3. Exposure of the patient to cold, such as frostbite

Patient Care
1. Assess the patient's respiratory status for pulmonary involvement.
2. Assess the patient for clinical manifestations of atypical viral pneumonia.
3. Assess the patient for clinical manifestations of other conditions associated with a positive antibody titer.

Patient Education
1. Explain the test procedure to the patient.
2. There is no specific patient instruction regarding the test.
3. Patient teaching is directed toward the treatment of the underlying disorder.

Signed Consent
Not required

C-REACTIVE PROTEIN (CRP)
C-reactive protein is a nonspecific indicator of the presence of inflammation that is of either an infectious or a noninfectious nature. It is used to determine the progress of previously diagnosed diseases and it is positive in myocardial infarctions, acute rheumatic fever, widespread cancer, malaria, and bacterial infections.

The test is termed C-reactive protein because inflammation elicts the formation of a protein in the body (not an antibody) that forms a precipitate with the C-polysaccharide of streptococcus pneumonia. The presence of C-reactive protein in the blood serum can be detected 18 to 24 hours after the onset of tissue injury.

Laboratory Results
Normal
None present in the serum.

Nursing Implications
Procedure for Collection/Storage of Specimen
1. The laboratory test is performed on a venous blood sample of 5 ml.
2. Fasting 8 to 12 hr may be required. (Check the policy of the laboratory.)

Possible Interfering Factors

None reported

Patient Care

In situations where the patient is demonstrating vague symptomatology, observe for signs and symptoms of inflammation, such as fever.

Patient Education

Explain the test procedure to the patient.

Signed Consent

Not required

DIRECT COOMBS TEST (Direct Antiglobulin)

This test is used to detect autoantibodies against red blood cells. The autoantibodies become attached to the red blood cells. The autoantibodies do not cause visible agglutination of the red cells, but they do increase cell fragility or damage the cells in some other way.

A positive direct Coombs test indicates that antibody is attached to the red blood cells, but it does not indicate the class of antibody involved. Positive reactions are seen in hemolytic diseases of the newborn, hemolytic transfusion reactions, and autoimmune hemolytic anemia.

This test is called "direct" because only one laboratory procedure is required to detect the presence of antibodies. There is a related test procedure called indirect Coombs, which requires two laboratory steps in identifying the antibodies. In this procedure the antibodies can be specifically identified.

Laboratory Results

Normal

The test should be negative in adults and children.

Diagnostic

Positive results are reported from 1+ to 4+.

Nursing Implications

Procedure for Collection/Storage of Specimen

The laboratory test is performed on fresh venous blood.

Possible Interfering Factors

Common drugs that can cause a false-positive Coombs are the following:

- levodopa
- methyldopa
- aminopyrine
- cephaloridine
- cephalothin
- penicillin
- chlorpromazine
- diphenylhydantoin
- isoniazid
- mephalan
- procainamide
- quinidine
- rifampin
- streptomycin
- sulfonamides
- tetracycline

Patient Care

1. Treatment is related to symptomatology and diagnosis.
2. There is no special preparation of the patient.

Patient Education

Explain the test procedure to the patient.

Signed Consent

Not required

HEMAGGLUTINATION INHIBITION (HI) TEST

This is an agglutination test that demonstrates the presence or absence of antibodies against the rubella virus, which is the causative organism of German measles. The test is used to determine susceptibility to or immunity to the disease.

Laboratory Results

- A titer of 1:10 indicates that the individual is susceptible to rubella infection.
- A titer of 1:20 indicates immunity from rubella infection, either from active infection or immunization.

Nursing Implications

Procedure for Storage/Collection of Specimen

The laboratory test is performed on a venous blood sample of 5 ml.

Possible Interfering Factors

None reported

Patient Care

Nurses should encourage the following populations to be tested:

- women considering pregnancy
- persons who might expose pregnant women and infants to the disease, such as doctors, nurses, teachers
- pregnant women in the first trimester who have been exposed to the rubella virus
- individuals with a rash, to determine the diagnosis of German measles

Patient Education

1. Explain the test procedure to the patient.
2. In susceptible individuals, explain the importance of immunization, as the rubella virus can damage the fetus, especially in the first trimester of pregnancy.

Signed Consent

Not required

IMMUNOGLOBULINS (Immunoelectrophoresis)

This test uses the technique of electrophoresis to determine the quantity of the immunoglobulin fractions IgA, IgG, IgM, IgD, and IgE. A variety of diseases are associated with changes in one or more levels of the immunoglobulins. Changes in the levels of immunoglobulins A, G, and M seem to be responsible for the major diseases.

IgA

Increased levels are seen in the following diseases:

- liver cirrhosis
- collagen and autoimmune diseases
- chronic infections
- IgA gammopathies
- Wiskott–Aldrich syndrome

Decreased levels are seen in the following disorders:

- malabsorption syndromes
- ataxia telangiectasia
- immunologic deficiency disorders, such as agammaglobulinemias, and hypogammaglobulinemias

IgG

Increased levels are associated with the following diseases:

- infections of all types
- chronic granulomatous infections
- liver disease
- malnutrition
- dysproteinemia
- disease associated with hypersensitivity granulomas, dermatologic disorders and IgG gammopathy

IgM

Increased levels are associated with the following diseases:

- actinomycosis
- Carrion's disease
- infectious mononucleosis
- malaria
- trypanosomeasis
- Waldenstrom's macroglobulinemia

Decreased levels are seen in the following disorders:

- agammaglobulinemia

- IgG and IgA myeloma
- dysgammaglobulinemia
- lymphoid aplasia

  IgD
  Increases are associated with the following:

- chronic infections
- IgD gammopathies

  IgE
  Increases are associated with the following diseases:

- atopic skin diseases
- asthma
- anaphylactic shock
- IgE gammopathies

  Decreased levels are associated with the following:

- congenital agammaglobulinemia
- hypogammaglobulinemia

Laboratory Results

Normal Range

Adults	IgA 160 to 400 mg/dl
	IgG 800 to 1500 mg/dl
	IgM 50 to 110 mg/dl
	(IgD very small amount)
	(IgE very small amount)
Children	Newborn levels of IgG are similar to adults, but IgA and IgM levels are much lower.
	By age 6 months the IgG levels have decreased and the IgA and IgM levels have risen.
	In childhood, all levels gradually rise until adulthood.

Nursing Implications

Procedure for Collection/Storage of Specimen

The laboratory test is performed on 10 cc fresh blood serum.

Possible Interfering Factors

1. Recent active and passive immunizations may produce confusing results for a variable period of time.
2. Recent blood transfusion or transfusion of blood components will also result in varied test results.

Patient Care

1. Obtain history for possible interfering factors.
2. Carefully record patient's signs and symptoms to assist in the diagnosis.

Patient Education

Explain the test procedure to the patient.

Signed Consent

Not required

RADIOALLERGOSORBENT TEST (RAST) FOR REAGINIC IgE

In persons suffering from allergies (allergic asthma, atopic eczema, and hay fever) it is important to find the allergen (antigen) that is responsible for their symptoms. Many substances have been found to be potential allergens. These include pollens of weeds and grasses, cosmetics, and drugs, especially antibiotics. It is known that the antibodies of the IgE class are responsible for allergic reactions. In this test, a person's serum containing IgE antibodies is tested against specific allergens to determine the cause of the allergy. This is generally a safer procedure for determining allergens than skin testing.

Laboratory Results

Results of the test are recorded from class 0 to class 4.

Significance of Results

Class 0:	No detectable specific IgE antibodies
Class 1:	Borderline
Class 2:	
Class 3:	Increasingly positive for specific IgE antibodies
Class 4:	

Nursing Implications

Procedure for Collection/Storage of Specimen

1. The laboratory test is performed on fresh blood serum.
2. The allergens to be tested must be listed on the laboratory slips.

Possible Interfering Factors

None reported

Patient Care

Interventions are directed toward the specific symptoms produced by the allergens. Assess the patient for symptoms of:

- Asthma — wheezing and dyspnea when the bronchial muscles are constricted.
- Atopic eczema — hives, urticaria and skin rash.
- Hay fever — sneezing, tearing of the eyes and a watery discharge from the nose.

Patient Education

1. Give the patient a list of the positive allergens so that contact with these can be minimized or avoided.

2. Provide patient teaching in regard to other treatment modalities that may be prescribed by the physician.
3. Describe how to prepare an environmentally controlled room.
4. Explain to the patient measures to be taken during periods of high pollen counts (remain indoors, air conditioned environment).
5. List signs and symptoms that require immediate medical attention (*e.g.*, respiratory distress not relieved by usual methods during an asthma attack).
6. Explain the importance of follow-up medical care.

Signed Consent

Not required

RHEUMATOID ARTHRITIS (RA) TESTS FOR RHEUMATOID FACTOR

Persons with rheumatoid arthritis may develop a dissimilar group of the IgM class of immunoglobulins to form the rheumatoid factor. The rheumatoid factor is an autoantibody (IgM), which is directed against the person's own IgG class of immunoglobulins. In these tests the fraction of immunoglobulins studied is the IgM. Tests are based on agglutination of either sensitized sheep red blood cells or latex particles coated with an IgG fraction.

Test results vary in relation to the stage of the disease. The most evident titers are seen in persons with advanced RA, those having the classical symptoms such as systemic RA, deforming arthritis and subcutaneous nodules. In early RA positive reactions are found in about 50% of the cases. Approximately 5% of nonaffected adults have rheumatoid factor and low titers are found in the elderly as well as in persons with other connective tissue diseases.

Laboratory Results

Titers of 1:20 and greater are considered diagnostic of rheumatoid arthritis.

Nursing Implications

Procedure for Collection/Storage of Specimen

The laboratory test is performed on a fresh venous blood sample.

Possible Interfering Factors

1. Diseases such as systemic lupus erythematosus, dermatomyositis, and chronic infections give false positives.
2. False positives may occur in unaffected individuals and in the elderly.

Patient Care

1. Observe and record the patient's symptomatology to aid in the diagnosis of rheumatoid arthritis.
2. If test results are positive, implement nursing measures for the patient with rheumatoid arthritis. Treatment is directed at relief of symptoms.

Patient Instruction

1. Explain the test procedure to the patient.
2. Instruct the patient on the treatment plan for rheumatoid arthritis if this diagnosis has been made.

Signed Consent

Not required

ROSETTE TEST

This test is used to evaluate the effectiveness of the immune system by identifying the number of T and β lymphocytes involved in the immune response.

T and β lymphocytes are distinguishable from one another by surface marks called rosettes. T cells have smooth surfaces, whereas β cells have projections (rosettes) on the cell surface. An electronmicroscope is used to determine the number and type of lymphocytes present in the serum.

β lymphocytes are increased in systemic lupus erythematosus. They are decreased in x-linked agammaglobulinemia, multiple myeloma, and chronic lymphocytic leukemia. T lymphocytes are increased in Grave's disease and decreased in De George's syndrome, Hodgkin's disease, chronic lymphocytic leukemia and long-term immunosuppressive drug therapy.

Laboratory Results

Normal	β lymphocytes: 10% to 30% of the total lymphocytes
	T lymphocytes: 70% to 90% of the total lymphocytes

Nursing Implications

Procedure for Collection/Storage of Specimen

The laboratory test is performed on a venous blood sample of 10 ml.

Possible Interfering Factors

None reported

Patient Care

1. Treatment and care is related to the patient's symptomatology and diagnosis.
2. Precautions to protect the patient from infection are indicated when the T lymphocytes are decreased, as in immunosuppressive drug therapy.

Patient Education

1. Explain the test procedure to the patient.
2. The patient with decreased T-lymphocytes should be taught to take extra precautions against infections, such as avoiding persons with viral or bacterial infections.
3. The patient should also be taught to report signs and symptoms of infection, such as low grade fever and malaise.

Signed Consent

Not required

THYROID ANTIBODIES

This test detects autoantibodies that have been formed against one's thyroid gland. The autoantibodies attack the normal cells of the gland and combine with the thyroglobulin produced by the thyroid, resulting in an enlargement of the gland and hypothyroidism. This test is used in the diagnosis of Hashimoto's thyroiditis (autoimmune thyroiditis).

Hashimoto's thyroiditis is associated with other possible autoimmune diseases such as pernicious anemia, rheumatoid arthritis, systemic lupus erythematosus, lupoid hepatitis, and idiopathic adrenal insufficiency.

Laboratory Results

Adults: No diagnostic titer has been established.

Children: This test is not usually performed on children.

Nursing Implications

Procedure for Collection/Storage of Specimen

The laboratory test is performed on a venous blood sample of two ml.

Possible Interfering Factors

1. Other thyroid diseases may result in the production of thyroid antibodies.
2. Approximately 10% of normal adults may have some detectable thyroid antibodies.

Patient Care

1. Nursing interventions are directed toward administration of medicine, which decreases the size of the thyroid gland and prevents systemic effects of hypothyroidism.
2. Assess for symptoms of hypothyroidism.
3. Treatment consists of replacement therapy, usually with thyroxine.
4. Assess family members for presence of thyroid disease symptoms.

Patient Education

1. Explain the test procedure to the patient.
2. Patient teaching is related to diagnosis and treatment modality.

Signed Consent

Not required

URINE TEST
BENCE JONES PROTEIN

This urine test is most frequently used to diagnose multiple myeloma. Bence Jones protein may also be found in the urine in other skeletal-destroying diseases, renal diseases, and some nonrenal disorders.

Bence Jones protein has diagnostic potential because of its low molecular weight. This protein is more easily excreted in the urine than are other serum proteins (albumin and globulin). This protein is called Bence Jones after the individual who first discovered the compound.

Diagnostic values. A trace of 1+ reaction indicates significant proteinuria. Positive values are found in the following disorders:

Musculoskeletal diseases
- multiple myeloma
- osteomalacia (adult rickets)
- tumor metastasis to bones

Renal diseases
- nephritis
- nephrosis
- polycystic kidney diseases
- tuberculosis of the kidney
- kidney tumors
- kidney stones

Nonrenal diseases
- severe anemias
- lymphocytic leukemia
- amyloidosis
- macroglobulinemia
- fever
- trauma
- abdominal tumors and intestinal obstruction
- cardiac diseases
- lead, phosphorus, mercury poisoning

Laboratory Results
Normal

None present in urine.

Nursing Implications
Procedure for Collection/Storage of Specimen

1. A single-voided urine specimen is tested. The specimen required is the second morning voiding. The patient voids at bedtime and again upon arising. These specimens are discarded. The second morning voided specimen is collected after the patient has been ambulating.
2. Use a standard specimen container.
3. If a 24-hour urine specimen is desired, obtain appropriate containers from the laboratory, and keep specimen refrigerated or iced during the collection period. Inform the patient that all of his urine must be collected for 24 hours.

Possible Interfering Factors
1. The following drugs may result in a false-positive reaction:
   - gold
   - arsenic
   - sodium bicarbonate
   - sulfisoxazole
   - thymol
   - chlorpromazine
   - radiopaque contrast media for 3 dy prior to the test
   - penicillin (large doses)
   - outdated tetracycline
2. Conditions that result in renal vasoconstriction such as the following:
   - severe emotional stress
   - exercise
   - cold showers or baths
3. Other conditions that can result in a false-positive reaction such as the following:
   - increased dietary consumption of proteins
   - pregnancy and immediate postpartum period
   - newborn infants
   - premenstrual period
   - immobility

Patient Care
1. Assess the patient for possible interfering factors.
2. Observe and record the patient's symptomatology to aid in the diagnosis of multiple myeloma.

Patient Education
1. Explain the test procedure and the method of urine collection.
2. Patient teaching is related to diagnosis and treatment modality.

Signed Consent
Not required

DIAGNOSTIC TESTS
SKIN TESTS

Skin tests are used to detect the antigen (allergen) responsible for hypersensitivity reactions. There are three types of skin tests: patch test, scratch test, and intradermal test.

Prior to skin tests, the patient should avoid taking medications that may inhibit the skin reaction. These drugs include antihistamines, subcutaneous epinephrine and isoproterenol (Isuprel). Patients receiving corticosteroids, aminophylline, and ephedrine should notify the physician of these drug uses prior to skin testing.

THE PATCH TEST

The patch test is used most often to diagnose contact dermatitis and determine the causative allergens.

Nursing Implications

Preprocedure

1. Explain the procedure to the patient.
2. Answer any questions the patient or family may ask.
3. Cleanse the skin:
   Wash the site where the test is to be given with alcohol and allow it to dry thoroughly. Be sure the skin is free of cuts or abrasions. The anterior forearms and upper back are frequent test sites. The back is the preferred site if large numbers of patches are necessary. It is also the preferred site for children.

Procedure

1. Prepare impregnated patches.
   A drop or two of the specified allergen is applied to a 1 cm gauze dressing. The gauze should have a plastic backing to avoid leaking or wetting of the dressing.
2. Apply the patches:
   Patches are placed in rows on the skin 2 to 3 in. apart. Write test numbers or allergen names on the patches, or on the skin above or below the patch to correspond with the allergen numbers. The patches are held in place with tape.

Postprocedure

1. Instruct the patient on the following self-care items:
   - The patch must be kept in place for the specified time—usually 48 hr. (The patch may be removed earlier if intense itching or burning occurs. The patient should wash the area with soap and water and report the incident to the doctor or nurse for further instruction.)
   - The patient should avoid wetting or scratching the test site.
   - After the specified 48 hr, the patient should return to have the test read.
2. Read the test.
   The center of the patch of skin is read with the following interpretations.

+ (1+)	mild erythema
+ + (2+)	severe erythema—smooth skin
+ + + (3+)	erythema with papules
+ + + + (4+)	erythema with papules and vesicles

3. Instruct the patient. Share with the patient the positive reactions so that exposure to those allergens can be avoided or minimized. Instruct the patient on other treatments, such as medications that may be prescribed by the physician.

CAUTION: Patients with contact dermatitis lesions and patients receiving corticosteroids should not be tested. If the patch test is performed on persons with lesions, a false-positive reaction could occur and the lesions could get worse.

THE SCRATCH TEST

The scratch test is used primarily for detecting the causative allergen in inhalant allergies, such as dusts, danders, molds, and pollens. Scratch test kits are available, containing varying types of allergens. Multiple dose vials are also available for testing use. The scratch method has a low level of sensitivity and will detect only the stronger and more obvious reactions.

Testing may be restricted on the basis of patient history. If it is known that the patient has a severe allergy to an allergen, the patient should not be exposed to the risk of being tested with that allergen. Partial allergy testing (testing with two or three allergens) may be indicated, based on the patient's history.

Nursing Implications
Preprocedure
1. Assess the patient for history of allergies, including allergic symptoms.
2. Explain the procedure to the patient.
3. Answer any questions the patient or family may ask.
4. Cleanse the skin.
   Wash the site with alcohol and allow to dry thoroughly.
   The back or forearm are preferred sites.

Procedure
1. Write test numbers on the skin to correspond with the antigen numbers.
   Use washable ink. Each antigen has a number and this should correspond with the number marked on the skin to prevent incorrect readings. The numbers should be placed about 2 in. apart.
2. Make a scratch approximately ⅛ in. in length. Use a separate sterile needle for each scratch. A 26 gauge, ½ in. needle with an intradermal bevel is preferred. Penetrate only the epidermal layer.
3. Place a drop of the allergen on the scratch. If the solution is in a capillary tube, break the tube and let the solution drop onto the scratch. If the solution is in a multiple vial, use a medicine dropper to draw up a small amount and let one drop fall onto the scratch. Use a different medicine dropper for each allergen.
4. Allow the solution to remain on the scratch for approximately 30 min. Do not cover the test site during this time. Immediate reactions may

occur, causing itching. The patient should be instructed of this and avoid scratching.

5. Read the results.

Negative: No change in the skin.

Positive: A wheal appears, and is designated as slight (1+), moderate (2+), or marked (3+).

Postprocedure

1. Instruct the patient.
2. Share with the patient positive results so that exposure to those allergens can be avoided or minimized.
3. Instruct the patient on other treatments that may be prescribed by the physician.

THE INTRADERMAL TEST

The intradermal method of skin testing is used for two purposes: (1) to detect specific allergens and (2) to diagnose certain infectious diseases.

INTRADERMAL TESTING FOR ALLERGENS

The allergens frequently tested are pollens of trees, weeds and grasses, dust, foods, stinging insect venom, and drugs.

Nursing Implications

Preprocedure

1. Assess the patient for history of allergies, including allergic symptoms.
2. Explain the procedure to the patient.
3. Answer any questions the patient or family may ask.
4. Cleanse the skin. Wash the site to be tested with alcohol and allow to dry thoroughly. The arm is the preferred site so that a tourniquet can be applied at the first sign of an anaphylactic shock.
5. Emergency cart should always be present when skin testing. Intradermal skin tests are 100 times more sensitive than the scratch test. The emergency cart should contain an airway, ambu bag, oxygen, IV fluids and the following medications: benadryl, sodium bicarbonate, epinephrine, and aminophylline.

Procedure

1. Write test numbers on the skin to correspond with the antigen number. Use washable ink. Each antigen has a number and this should correspond with the number marked on the skin to prevent incorrect readings. The numbers should be placed about 2 in. apart.
2. Prepare the intradermal injection.
   Using a sterile disposable allergist syringe with a 26 gauge ½ in. nondetachable needle, draw up .02 ml of the allergen solution. The nurse must be certain to check the strength of the allergen solution, since solution may vary in strength.

3. A control substance is injected also to determine the patient's possible allergy to the base compound of the solution, such as egg.

4. Insert the needle and inject the solution. With the bevel of the needle facing upward, insert the needle at an angle parallel to the skin. Insert the needle so only the bevel penetrates the skin. If you have inserted the needle correctly, when you inject the solution a small bleb (looks like a blister) will appear.

5. Observe the patient for signs of anaphylactic shock. Epinephrine is the drug of choice in an anaphylactic reaction. Epinephrine 0.5 ml. 1:1000 strength should be administered subcutaneously or intravenously every five to ten minutes, according to the physician's standing orders. Observe the test site for a wheal and flare reaction. The absence of a bleb indicates that some of the test solution escaped into underlying tissue and the reliability of the test is diminished. A false negative reaction could occur in these cases.

6. Read the results. Ten to fifteen minutes following the injection, the diameter of the wheal is measured with a millimeter ruler. (Wheals from 7 to 10 mm in diameter are usually considered diagnostic). To assist in reading the results, a nurse may use a pen. The nurse can draw a line lightly toward the induration, stopping at the first feeling of resistance from the wheal. This is done in all four directions. The distance between these lines is measured.

Postprocedure

1. Instruct the patient. Share with the patient positive results so that exposure to those allergens can be avoided or minimized. Instruct the patient on other treatments that may be prescribed by the physician.

CAUTION: Both false-negative and false-positive reactions can occur in intradermal allergen testing.

INTRADERMAL TESTS FOR DIAGNOSING INFECTIOUS DISEASES*

The reagents used in these skin tests are not the pure antigen (microorganism) but a mixture of potentially reactive substances. Both immediate and delayed skin reactions may occur with some test reagents, but the delayed reaction is the significant reaction in diagnosing a specific infectious disease.

To perform these tests usually 0.1 ml of the test preparation is given intradermally. A bleb should appear following the injection. The absence of a bleb indicates that some of the test solution escaped into the underlying tissue and the reliability of the test is diminished. A false-negative reaction could occur in these cases.

In most cases, the test is read in 48 hours. Readings at 24 and 72 hours may be helpful in diagnosing some diseases. In positive reactions, there will be an indurated area (hardened area) surrounded by an area of redness (erythema). The size of the induration (which is measured with a millimeter ruler) is the only criterion for a positive reaction, erythema is not diagnostic. To assist in reading the results, the nurse may use a pen. The nurse can draw a line lightly toward the induration, stopping at the first feeling of

*Note: Individual skin tests and interpretations appear on pages 344–349.

resistance from the wheal. This is done in all directions. The distance between these lines is measured.

A positive reaction indicates that the individual has, at some time in the past, been exposed to the organism. It does not necessarily indicate a present infection, unless the individual has recently converted from a negative to a positive skin test.

Positive reactions should be explained to the patient and the patient should be instructed on the treatments prescribed by the physician.

TISSUE TYPING

Tissue typing tests are performed to determine the extent of compatibility of the donor and the recipient for organ transplantations. Because both the humoral-mediated and cell-mediated components of the immune system are involved in rejection reactions, both donor and recipient leukocytes and antibodies are tested for compatibility. The most commonly employed tissue used in typing prospective donors and recipients is the lymphocyte.

The three tests performed are the following:

1. Detection of Histocompatibility (HL-A)

    The tissue cells possess histocompatibility (H) antigens. The antigenic system is highly specific for each individual and the antigenic profile (system) is genetically determined. The histocompatibility system is referred to as the human leukocyte antigen (HL-A) system. The human leukocyte system consists of 51 identified distinctive antigens. HL-A antigens are the chief human tissue antigens. They are composed of large glycoproteins. They are found in all tissues except red blood cells. They are especially found in the liver, spleen and lymphoid tissues. The lung, kidney, and adrenals contain HL-A antigens. HL-A antigens are located on the surface of the cell. Each antigen contains one or more antigenic sites, each capable of eliciting a separate immunologic response. The HL-A locus is located on an unidentified pair of autosomal chromosomes. Each locus contains two alleles or genes. One allele or gene of each locus is found on each chromosome. Since there are two alleles at each of the two HL-A loci, the tissue of every normal person contains two to four HL-A antigens.

    In HL-A typing, the serum of both the donor and recipient (both of which contain the HL-A antigens) are tested against antisera of human origin (serum containing HL-A antibodies) to determine which of the 51 antigens the donor and recipient have in common. The greater the number of like antigens, the closer the tissue match.

2. Cytotoxic–Antibody Test

    This test is used to detect antibodies in the recipient's serum that are directed against HL-A antigens in the donor's serum. It is important to detect these antibodies prior to transplantation, because if a patient receives an organ transplant, and has cytotoxic antibodies directed against the donor's cells, an immediate acute rejection will occur.

3. Mixed Leukocyte Culture (MLC)

    This test is another method of detecting the degree of histocompatibility between the donor and recipient. Lymphocytes from the serum of both the donor and recipient are cultured together for 5 days, during which the stimulator cells die, leaving only the responding cells. On the 5th day, the lymphocytes in the culture are labeled with a radioactive material (thymidine). This radioactive material will then be incorporated into any new DNA that is synthesized by the leukocytes. Thus, the level of radioactivity will increase in response to increased cellular stimulation (DNA formation). DNA formation increases as a result of exposure to antigens, which are recognized as foreign. The greater the difference in the donor and recipient cells, the greater the cellular stimulation and the greater the level of radioactivity.

4. MLR (one-way Mixed Leukocyte Reaction) HLD-D antigens are detected through their stimulatory capacity in the MLR. The test is performed by mixing leukocytes from the donor and recipient in tissue culture for several days and noting the amount of DNA synthesis. The one-way MLR is used in intrafamiliar typing to confirm that siblings, who appear HLA identical by serologic typing, are also identical at the D locus.

Nursing Implications
Preprocedure
1. Explain the purpose of the blood tests to the patient.
2. Answer any questions the donor or recipient may ask.

Procedure
Tests are performed on blood samples drawn in the laboratory.

Postprocedure
Donor and recipient teaching will depend on test results.

Signed Consent
Not required

DIAGNOSTIC TESTS FOR IMMUNOCOMPETENCE

To determine if an individual is immunocompetent (the ability to detect and respond to foreign antigens), delayed hypersensitivity tests are used. Individuals who have an unresponsive cellular immune system (referred to as anergic) will have little or no reaction to the test antigen despite previous exposure or sensitization to the antigen. Immunocompetence must be assessed in cancer patients before immunotherapy can be initiated.

DNCB (Dinitrochlorobenzene) Skin Test

DNCB is a chemical that is topically applied to the skin. DNCB is a hapten that binds to skin carrier proteins and results in sensitization of the cellular immune system in competent individuals (sensitized T lymphocytes are formed in response to the drug [antigen]).

Nursing Implications
Preprocedure
1. Explain the procedure to the patient.
2. Answer any questions the patient or family may ask.

Procedure

The test consists of two applications of the chemical. The first application is referred to as the primary sensitization.

The second topical application of DNCB follows 7 to 10 days after the sensitizing dose. The second application is of a lower concentration of the chemical. Failure to see a response (induration and erythema) 48 hours after the second application indicates an unresponsive immune system.*

Postprocedure

Patient teaching and care will depend on test results, for example, if the patient is immunocompetent, immunotherapy might be helpful in treatment of certain types of cancer.

Intradermal skin tests

Intradermal injections of antigens may also be used to determine immunocompetence. The antigens used are candida, mumps, and streptococcal extracts as well as intermediate PPD.†

BIBLIOGRAPHY

Barrett T: Basic Immunology and Its Medical Application. St Louis, CV Mosby, 1976

Bio-Science Laboratories: The Bio-Science Handbook, 11th ed. Main Laboratory 7600 Tyrone Ave., Van Nuys, California 91405, 1975

Blake PJ, Perez RC: Applied Immunological Concepts. New York, Appleton-Century-Crofts, 1978

Boyd RF, Hoerl BG: Basic Medical Biology. Boston, Little, Brown & Co, 1977

Burkhalter PK, Donley Diane L: Dynamics of Oncology Nursing. New York, McGraw–Hill, 1978

Fischbach F: A Manual of Laboratory Diagnostic Tests. Philadelphia, JB Lippincott, 1980

Garb S: Laboratory Tests in Common Use, 6th ed. New York, Springer, 1976

Jones DA, Dunbar CF, Jirovec MM: Medical–Surgical Nursing. New York, McGraw–Hill, 1978

Luckman J, Sorensen KC: Medical–Surgical Nursing. Philadelphia, WB Saunders, 1974

Peacock J, Tomar, RH: Manual of Laboratory Immunology. Philadelphia, Lea & Febiger, 1980

Phipps WJ, Long BC, Woods NF: Medical–Surgical Nursing. St Louis, CV Mosby, 1979

Weir DM: Immunology, 4th ed. Edinburgh, Churchill Livingston, 1977

Wilson ME, and Mizer HE: Microbiology in Patient Care, 2nd ed. New York, Macmillan, 1974.

Winner HI: Microbiology in Patient Care, 2nd ed. London, Hodder and Stroughton, 1978

Wood L: Nursing Skills for Applied Health Services, Vol 3. Philadelphia, WB Saunders Company, 1975

*See Patch Test for the procedure technique.
†See Intradermal Test for procedure technique.

Skin Tests of Diagnostic Value for Infectious Diseases

Disease	Test	Antigen	Procedure	Interpretation	Nursing Implications
Bacterial Diseases					
1. *Undulent fever*	Brucellosis test	One of two antigens may be used: 1. Sterile broth culture filtrate 2. Extract of bacterial nucleoproteins	0.1 ml of antigen is injected intradermally	Test read in 48 hours. Positive reaction is characterized by an area of induration and erythema. Careful interpretation is required. Serologic test is more specific.	In persons with an active infection, an exacerbation of symptoms may occur with skin testing. Observe for malaise, weakness, muscular aches, chills and fever. Positive cases are treated with tetracycline or streptomycin.
2. *Cat-scratch fever*	Cat-scratch fever test	Treated pus from another active infection	0.1 ml of the antigen is injected intradermally	Test is read in 48 hr. Positive reaction is characterized by an area of induration.	This test is used to confirm the clinical diagnosis. Clinical symptoms are regional lymphadenopathy associated with a scratch wound—usually inflicted by a cat. There is often a recurring fever with chills and malaise. Positive cases are treated with broad spectrum antibiotics.
3. *Chancroid*	Ducrey Test	Treated suspension of Haemophilus ducreyi	0.1 ml of the antigen is injected intradermally	Test is read in 72 hr. Positive: An area of induration of at least 8 mm.	A positive test indicates a previous or current infection. Signs and symptoms indicative of a current infection are: a soft chancre with ragged edges that appears on the genitalia. The ulcer is swollen and painful as are the regional lymph nodes. Positive cases are treated with sulfonamides and tetracycline.

4. *Diphtheria*	Schick Test	Active diphtheria toxin and heated toxin for control	0.1 ml of the antigen and 0.1 ml of the control are injected intradermally. A control is used in diphtheria testing to rule out a hypersensitive reaction to the culture proteins.	Test is read at 24-hr, 48-hr and 72-hr intervals. Positive reaction is characterized by erythema and flaking of skin around the test site.	A positive test indicates absence of antitoxin and therefore susceptibility to the disease.
5. *Lympho-granuloma venereum* (LGV)	Frei Test	Virus suspension	0.1 ml of antigen is injected intradermally. NOTE: antigen is incubated in yolk sac of chicken embryos; therefore, allergies to either eggs or chickens could result in a false-positive or an allergic reaction.	Test is read at 48-hr and 96-hr intervals. Positive reaction: a raised papule of at least 6 mm in diameter. A positive reaction will occur within 1 to 6 wk following infection. A positive test result will remain positive for the life of the individual.	A positive result indicates a previous or current infection with LGV (trachoma group). A sign of a current infection is a small painless primary lesion on the genital mucosa. Clinical evidence of a systemic infection begins in approximately two weeks after infection with enlargement of regional lymph nodes, fever, and malaise. Treat with broad spectrum antibiotics for systemic involvement. Determine if the patient has any allergies to eggs or chicken.

(Continued)

Skin Tests of Diagnostic Value for Infectious Diseases *(Continued)*

Disease	Test	Antigen	Procedure	Interpretation	Nursing Implications
6. *Scarlet Fever*	Dick Test	Diluted erythrogenic toxin and heated toxin for control	0.1 ml of the antigen and 0.1 ml of the control are injected intradermally. A control is used to rule out a hypersensitivity reaction to the culture proteins.	Test is read in 24 hr. Positive reaction is characterized by erythema and swelling at the test site of at least 3 mm in diameter.	A positive test indicates absence of antitoxin and therefore susceptibility to the disease.
7. *Tuberculo-sis*	1. PPD	Purified Protein Derivative	0.1 ml of antigen is injected intradermally. Three concentrations are available.	Test should be read in 48 hr—no later than 72 hr. Positive reactions: tests are interpreted as positive if the injection site shows an area of induration of at least 10 mm diameter. Edema and erythema may also be present, and intense reactions lead to central necrosis. Strong positive reactions may persist for several days, but weak ones disappear quickly after 72 hr.	A positive test indicates a previous or current infection. A false-negative reaction can occur in the presence of an overwhelming tuberculosis infection, or during the course of the illnesses such as Hodgkin's Disease, measles, fever or pleural effusion. Therefore, hospitalized patients should not be tuberculin tested. Persons who have had positive skin tests in the past should not be retested, as these individuals can experience severe reactions. Persons vaccinated with BCG become tuberculin positive and should not be skin tested. Severe reaction may result after
	2. Heaf Test	Old Tuberculin (OT)	A gun device is used to inject the antigen from 6 spring-released needle points that enter only the epidermal layer. This method is convenient and safe for mass surveys but accuracy is not quantitative.		
	3. Mantoux Test	PPD or OT	0.1 ml of antigen is injected intradermally.	Nonspecific reactions may appear during the first 24 hr, but do not persist beyond 48 hr.	
	4. Tine Test	OT	This test employs dried OT on multiple		

Test	Antigen	Method	Reading / Positive Reaction	Comments
		metal tines. Tines are pressed against the skin for intracutaneous insertion of antigen. Each unit is used once. Advantages and limitations similar to Heaf Test.	Tuberculin reactivity begins 3 to 6 wk after infection/exposure.	skin testing. A current infection is commonly characterized by fever, malaise, easy fatigue and weight loss. Active tuberculosis is treated with a combination of the following antituberculosis drugs: Streptomycin, Isoniazid (INH), Para-aminosalicylic acid (PAS), Ethambutol, and Rifampin. Newly infected persons without evidence of active disease are treated prophylactically for 1 yr with 1 drug, usually INH.
5. Vollmer Patch Test	Same as above	OT on a gauze strip (with lanolin) is applied to the surface of the skin. Least accurate but safest.	Same as above	

Viral Diseases

Test	Antigen	Method	Reading / Positive Reaction	Comments
1. Mumps	Mumps vaccine	0.1 ml of antigen is injected intradermally	Test read in 48 hr. Positive reaction: Area of erythema and a lesion at least 10 mm in diameter.	Negative test identifies susceptible individual. Positive reaction indicates resistance to the mumps virus.

Mycotic Diseases

Test	Antigen	Method	Reading / Positive Reaction	Comments
1. Blastomycosis	Concentrate of broth culture filtrates	0.1 ml of antigen is injected intradermally	Test read in 48 hr. Positive reaction: Area of induration at least 5 mm in diameter.	Cross-reaction frequently occurs with these fungal antigens in systemic fungal diseases. Positive skin tests may be obtained in persons who have had previous subclinical or clinical infections or those individuals with current infections.
2. Coccidio-mycosis	same as above	same as above	Test read in 48 hr. Positive reaction: Area of induration at least 5 mm in diameter.	

(Continued)

Skin Tests of Diagnostic Value for Infectious Diseases (Continued)

Disease	Test	Antigen	Procedure	Interpretation	Nursing Implications
3. *Histoplas-mosis*		same as above	same as above	Test read in 48 hr. Positive reaction: Area of induration at least 5 mm in diameter.	*(Continued from p. 347)* Clinical manifestations of mycotic diseases are fatigue, dizziness, fever, cough, dyspnea, anorexia and weight loss. The individual may have anemia, thrombocytopenia, splenomegaly, hepatomegaly, and malignant lymphoma. Other possible problems include ulcerations at mucocutaneous junctions, such as lips or perianal area. Histoplasmosis may produce bleeding, gastrointestinal ulcers, and Addison's disease. Fungal infections mimic symptoms of many other diseases. Fungal diseases may be localized in the lungs or disseminate systemically. Amphotericin B is the therapy of choice. (Extremely nephrotoxic)
Parasitic Diseases					
1. Echino-coccosis		Inactivated hydatid fluid	0.1 mg of antigen is injected intradermally	Test read in 15 min. Positive reaction: Immediate swelling and erythema at test site.	Positive skin test indicates an infection. Symptoms depend on size and location of cysts. No specific chemotherapy for this disease.

| 2. *Toxoplasmosis* | Suspension of dead organisms | same as above | Test read in 48 hr. Positive reaction: an area of induration at least 10 mm in diameter. | Positive skin test indicates previous or current infection. Symptoms are mild and localized to lymph nodes. Sulfonamides combined with pyrimethamine are treatment of choice. |
| 3. *Trichinosis* | Antigens extracted from parasite | same as above | Test read in 15 min. Positive reaction: Immediate wheal and flare. | Positive skin test indicates previous or current infection. This may be a mild or serious disease depending upon the number of larvae ingested. Initially there is gastrointestinal discomfort as the larvae migrate. There is fever, periorbital edema. This is followed in several days by chills, weakness, and muscle pain. There is a marked eosinophilia. Other tissue injury results from localization of the larvae. Cardiac and respiratory involvement are the most serious complications and can result in death. |

10

Tests Related to Neuromuscular Function

Cathy C. Jones

OVERVIEW OF PHYSIOLOGY AND PATHOPHYSIOLOGY

Pathological changes may occur at any point in the neuromuscular system, from the brain and spinal cord to the end organs and muscles, which the peripheral nerves innervate. These changes may have their origin in the nervous or muscular tissue. Alterations in the associated bony structure or systemic imbalances may also cause these changes.

THE SKULL

The eight bones of the skull intersect at rigid joints called sutures. In the infant, these sutures are still separated by spaces called fontanels, but gradually become ossified by the time the child is two years old. *Craniosynostosis* is a disorder in which the fontanels close prematurely, cramping the normally growing brain. This condition can be diagnosed readily by observation of the skull, head measurements, and skull x-rays that will show closed suture lines.

Skull Fractures

Trauma to the head may produce one or several types of skull fracture. Since the bones of the skull bear no weight and are not movable, fractures are not in themselves a problem. It is only damage that is done to underlying structures from the edges of broken bone or from the force of the blow itself that produces problems.

- *Linear fractures* appear as lines on the skull films. If a group of linear fractures radiate out from the point of impact, they may be called "stillate." The chief danger from these fractures is that they can lacerate one of the arteries beneath the skull on the surface of the dura. The resultant arterial bleeding forms an epidural hematoma, which may rapidly accumulate causing the brain to be pushed to the opposite side.

- *Depressed fractures* appear on skull films as indentations of variable size on the smooth, rounded surface of the skull. If the skin is broken, they are compound fractures. The brain and dura may be damaged. Ping-pong fractures, which occur in children, are very small, simple depressions of pliable bone.

- *Basilar skull fractures* are breaks in the fragile ethmoid and sphenoid bones beneath the brain at the base of the skull. The fracture lines may tear the dura at the base of the brain allowing cerebrospinal fluid (CSF) to escape through the torn dura into the nose or ears. Cerebrospinal fluid (CSF) may also leak into the sinuses, which are air-filled spaces, causing the air-fluid level in these sinuses to appear on the skull films. The basilar fractures are usually obscured on skull films by the multiple bones of the face.

INCREASED INTRACRANIAL PRESSURE

After the fontanels have closed, the skull becomes a rigid structure enclosing the intracranial contents. These contents are divided into four compartments: the brain, its blood supply, extravascular fluid, and cerebrospinal fluid.

If any of the four compartments begin to increase in size, it occupies more of the limited intracranial space. Initially the other compartments can compensate for the increased intracranial pressure. Compensatory mechanisms will eventually reach their limits, and increased intracranial pressure results.

Herniation Syndromes

Focal lesions may be referred to simply as a "mass"; the damage they produce is called their "mass effect." Mass lesions are frequently laterally placed and so produce lateral shift of the midline structures and a lateral herniation syndrome. If the lesion becomes very large and expands rapidly enough, it will displace the brain from the side of the lesion and down through the opening in the tentorium. The edge of the temporal lobe (the uncus) is pushed over the rim of the opening in the tentorium.

If a mass lesion is located in the midline, or if the pressure in the head is caused by a more generalized process, a central herniation syndrome or "pressure cone" will result as the diencephalon is displaced through the tentorial opening down on the brain stem.

- Mass lesions may be caused by hematomas, abscesses, tumors, or cerebral vascular accidents.
- The more generalized processes that cause mass lesions include meningitis, hydrocephalus, generalized brain edema, pseudotumor cerebri, and Reye's syndrome.

Other Causes

Small, unexplained increases in intracranial pressure may be caused by increased intrathoracic pressure.

- Since venous drainage from the head is a large determinant of intracranial pressure, such diseases as chronic obstructive pulmonary disease, congestive heart failure or pericardial effusion may impede venous return and elevate the intracranial pressure.
- Jugular venous obstruction or abdominal compression from improper positioning for lumbar puncture will have the same result.
- The cerebral vasculature is exquisitely sensitive to arterial carbon dioxide, and hypercarbia will dilate cerebral vessels and elevate intracranial pressure.

VASCULAR DISEASE OF THE BRAIN

The two internal carotid arteries anteriorly, and the vertebrals which become the basilar artery posteriorly, supply most of the blood to the brain. The external carotid may also supply additional blood to the brain if one internal carotid is blocked. Any part of the arterial or venous system may occlude or hemorrhage. This interrupts the blood supply to a given area of brain tissue and may damage the tissue immediately next to the vessel.

- Systemic diseases such as systemic lupus erythematosus, polyarteritis nodosa, amyloidosis, thrombocytopenic purpura, syphilis, and many other inflammatory and infective processes may produce widespread cerebrovascular lesions.

Stroke (CVA)

Stroke, or cerebrovascular accident (CVA), is caused by thrombosis, embolism or hemorrhage of a branch of the cerebrovascular system. The internal carotid artery is most commonly affected by arteriosclerosis. The pathologic process causing stroke is identical to atherosclerotic changes that occur elsewhere in the body. High degrees of blockage or even total occlusion of large arteries may not produce infarction of brain tissue owing to good collateral circulation.

Emboli may come from many sources. The plaque from the carotid artery is a common source, but subacute bacterial endocarditis and atrial fibrillation are other common sources of cerebral emboli.

Aneurysms

Aneurysms are bulges in the arterial wall. There are several types of aneurysms:

- Berry (or saccular) aneurysms are congenital defects in the muscular wall of a vessel, usually at its juncture with another artery. They may rupture at times of physical stress or in the presence of hypertension.

- Giant (fusiform) aneurysms are large tubular swellings that may cause a mass effect. They are usually seen in older, hypertensive patients.

- Mycotic aneurysms may be caused by septic emboli.

- Charcot–Bouchard aneurysms are microscopic and seen in the basal nuclei or brain stem of hypertensive individuals.

- Traumatic (sacculated) aneurysms are due to a weakening on one side of the artery. These aneurysms may arise following head injury or surgery.

Aneurysms may not produce any signs or symptoms unless they become quite large or rupture. If rupture occurs, the free blood may spread through the subarachnoid space and cause a *subarachnoid hemorrhage*. These can be detected by the neck stiffness they cause, by blood in the cerebrospinal fluid obtained at lumbar puncture, or seen on CT scan. There are other causes of subarachnoid hemorrhage, such as trauma and hemorrhagic stroke. The vessels adjacent to the bleeding aneurysm may respond by constricting. This vasospasm will produce a stroke syndrome.

Angiomas

Angiomas of the central nervous system are congenital vascular malformations of at least five types.

- *Capillary telangiectases* are groups of dilated capillaries that are not usually clinically significant.

- *Cavernous angiomas* are larger capillary lesions that may hemorrhage or cause neighboring infarction.

- *Venous angiomas* are tangled masses of thin-walled vessels most common in the spinal cord.

- *Arteriovenous malformations* (AVM) are masses of tangled arteries and arterialized veins without the connecting capillaries.

- *Sturge–Weber disease* is a combination of a portwine nevus on the face and capillary-venous malformation on the cortex.

Intracranial Hematomas

Intracranial hematomas may be caused by many of the previously described lesions, or by direct trauma to the head. There are three types of hematomas.

- *Epidural hematomas* are collections of blood between the skull and dura usually caused by a tear of an artery on the surface of the dura. The force of the bleeding may cause rapid accumulation of blood and the mass effect of the clot may cause abrupt neurological deterioration. The underlying brain may be undamaged and recover completely if the clot is promptly removed.

- *Subdural hematomas* are clots that form between the dura and surface of the brain. They are usually caused by tearing of the veins. Accumulation of blood may occur more slowly, but may cause more severe damage to the underlying brain. Subacute subdural hematomas take from two days to two weeks to cause symptoms; chronic subdurals may take weeks to months for symptoms to develop. Subdural hematomas are commonly seen in alcoholics, patients on anticoagulant therapy, or others with impairments in coagulation.

- *Intracerebral hematomas* are located within the substance of the brain and may contain strands of neural tissue.

Carotid Sinus Fistula

Carotid sinus fistula is a vascular disorder in which the internal carotid artery develops a communication with the venous cavernous sinus. This communication may be caused by blunt or penetrating trauma or rupture of an aneurysm. The high pressure causes retrograde flow in the ophthalmic vein, and exophthalmus and blindness may result. There may also be a stroke syndrome to the cerebral hemisphere if the blood flow is sufficiently decreased.

DISORDERS OF CEREBROSPINAL FLUID CIRCULATION

Under normal circumstances, about 500 ml of cerebrospinal fluid (CSF) are produced each day by the choroid plexus in the two lateral and the third ventricles. The fluid flows slowly through these ventricles, down the cerebral aqueduct and through the fourth ventricle between the cerebellum and brain stem. The fluid exits the central nervous system through the three openings called the foramina of Luschka, Magendie, and Magna. Cerebrospinal fluid then circulates up over the cerebellum and cerebral hemispheres and down and around the spinal cord. The fluid is eventually reabsorbed into the venous system by the arachnoid granulations on the top of the brain.

There are three problems that can arise with the cerebrospinal fluid system:

- overproduction of cerebrospinal fluid,
- blockage of flow, and
- impaired reabsorption.

Any of these problems can produce a type of *hydrocephalus,* in which the pressure in the head builds, the ventricles become enlarged, and eventually the brain may become shrunken and atrophic from the pressure. In an infant, the head will enlarge dramatically from the building pressure. In an adult, early signs of increased intracranial pressure will call attention to the problem.

Overproduction of Cerebrospinal Fluid

Overproduction of cerebrospinal fluid occurs only in the presence of a type of tumor called choroid plexus papilloma.

Blockage of CSF Flow

Obstruction of cerebrospinal fluid circulation is the most common cause of hydrocephalus and may occur at any site along the path of flow. Congenital malformations and inflammation caused by subarachnoid infections or hemorrhage are the most common causes of hydrocephalus in infants. After that age, neoplasia is a more common cause of obstructive or noncommunicating hydrocephalus. Tumors in the area of the third and fourth ventricles are the most frequent culprits.

Impaired Reabsorption of CSF

In addition to overproduction of cerebrospinal fluid, the other variety of communicating or nonobstructive hydrocephalus is caused by blockage of the arachnoid granulations so that cerebrospinal fluid cannot be reabsorbed. Subarachnoid hemorrhage secondary to trauma, ruptured aneurysm, or hemorrhagic stroke will frequently clog the arachnoid granulations with blood and produce an acute hydrocephalus.

A similar variant that occurs chiefly in middle-aged women is benign intracranial hypertension. It is thought to result from decreased cerebrospinal fluid reabsorption, which causes intracranial pressure to rise.

INTRACRANIAL NEOPLASMS

Tumors inside the skull may arise from the brain, meninges, and other supporting structures. Tumors originating elsewhere in the body may also metastasize to the central nervous system. Tumors of the central nervous system almost never metastasize outside the central nervous system. Intracranial tumors may produce symptoms through hormonal or neurological changes, by initiating seizures, by obstructing cerebrospinal fluid flow, or by mass effect. The noninvasive types may be considered malignant and may cause a great deal of damage as a result of their size and location.

Metastatic Tumors

Metastatic tumors generally occur in multiple sites in the brain. These tumors metastasize most often from a primary site in the lung, breast, bowel, or kidney.

Gliomas

Gliomas are tumors that arise directly from the glia. Glia are the cells that support and surround the neurons in the brain. Glial cells are histologically classified as astrocytoma, oligodendroglioma, and ependymoma. Astrocytomas are the most common gliomas.

Meningiomas

Meningiomas arise from the meninges. They are usually noninvasive, although the skull overlying the tumor may either increase in thickness or erode. Meningiomas may become quite large before the tumor produces symptoms by mass effect.

Neuromas

Neuromas are the third most common form of primary intracranial tumors. The eighth cranial nerve is the most common site of tumor growth. Acoustic neuromas may distort the brain stem and obstruct cerebrospinal fluid flow. Bilateral acoustic neuromas or multiple spinal neuromas may indicate Von Recklinghausen's disease (neurofibromatosis).

Pituitary Tumors

The pituitary gland is not a part of the central nervous system, but pituitary tumors may extend above the sella turcica and invade the hypothalamus, the third ventricle, cavernous sinus, or frontal or temporal lobes.

Childhood Tumors

In childhood, most intracranial tumors ocur in the posterior fossa, below the tentorium around the brain stem and cerebellum.

- The most common tumor type is the *cerebellar astrocytoma*, which tends to be a noninvasive slow growing tumor.
- *Medulloblastomas* are the second most common type. Medulloblastomas may seed along the cerebrospinal fluid pathways to the ventricles or spinal cord.
- *Ependymomas* arise from the ependymal cells lining the ventricles and usually are benign.
- *Brain stem gliomas* are most commonly found in the area of the pons where they cause progressive cranial nerve impairment and paralysis. The pneumoencephalogram will reveal pontine enlargement.
- *Craniopharyngiomas* are tumors that also occur in childhood and may compress the optic chiasm or tracts, pituitary or hypothalamic areas, or cause increased intracranial pressure.

CONGENITAL MALFORMATIONS

Congenital neurological malformations are usually caused by intrauterine trauma (*i.e.,* toxins) rather than by hereditary factors. The fetal age at the time of exposure to the trauma will determine the character of the defect.

Midline Defects

The most common malformations are caused by midline defects so that the developing central nervous system is not posteriorly enclosed. These malformations may occur at any site from the skull to the base of the spine.

- *Spina bifida* or *cranium bifidum* is a condition in which there is some covering of skin, connective tissue, and dura over the bony defect.

- *Rachischisis (spinal cord)* or *cranioschisis* are defects in which skin, connective tissue, and bone are all absent and the central nervous system is completely exposed. These defects may occur together and in severe cases the underlying central nervous system is partly absent or deformed. These infants may die shortly after birth.

Cranium bifidum are less severe lesions consisting of a bony opening with herniated central nervous system tissue, usually at the back of the skull (encephalocele).

- *Meningoceles* are hernias in which the meninges protrude through an opening in the skull or spinal column.
- *Myelomeningoceles* are sacs overlying the spinal defect containing the herniated spinal cord.
- Most cases of myelomeningocele are also associated with *Arnold–Chiari malformation,* which consists of a herniation of part of the medulla and cerebellum through the foramen magnum.
- The *Dandy-Walker* malformation consists of a cystic dilation of the fourth ventricle from which cerebrospinal fluid cannot exit.

Other Congenital Malformations

Other congenital malformations are not associated with midline closure defects.

- *Prosencephaly* or *holotelencephaly* is the result of failure of the brain to divide into two hemispheres.
- *Arhinencephaly* is absence of the olfactory lobes and other structures.
- In *hydroencephaly* the cerebral hemispheres are largely replaced by large cystic sacs.
- *Porencephaly* is presence of a cavity between a lateral ventricle and subarachnoid space.
- *Diastematomyelia* is division of the spinal cord into two longitudinal structures.
- *Hydromyelia* is dilatation of the central canal, often associated with hydrocephalus, myelomeningocele, and the Arnold–Chiari malformation.

MOVEMENT DISORDERS OF THE EXTRAPYRAMIDAL SYSTEM AND CEREBELLUM

The coordination of movement is a highly complicated and intricate process. Paralysis of varying degrees may result from damage to the corticospinal tract anywhere between the motor cortex and the final motor neuron.

Damage to the extrapyramidal pathways in the basal ganglia, brain stem, and cerebellum can produce bizarre types of movement disorders, such as Parkinsonism, choreas, hemiballismus, athetosis, and dystonias. Movement disorders are largely either metabolic or degenerative disorders.

Cerebellar ataxias may be caused by lead poisoning or maple syrup urine disease. They may be caused by a number of other disease entities and by tumors in or near the cerebellum.

SEIZURE DISORDERS

Seizures are sudden attacks of involuntary muscle contractions and relaxations. Seizures are caused by excessive cortical neuronal discharges. The causes of seizures are numerous.

- *Petit mal epilepsy* (seizures) usually begin in childhood, and generally cease before the age of 30. In a petit mal seizure, the child may pause and be still for a few seconds, and then continue activities, unaware of the episode.

- *Grand mal*, or tonic–clonic epilepsy, is a more serious form of generalized seizure. The grand mal seizure is characterized by recurrent episodes of sudden loss of consciousness with associated major motor activity.

- *Status epilepticus* or convulsive grand mal attacks are either continuous grand mal convulsions or convulsions that occur so frequently that each attack begins before the postictal period of the previous one ends. These seizures may be precipitated by withdrawal of anticonvulsants, metabolic imbalances, or by head injury or tumor.

- *Myoclonus* is a seizure disorder in which there is involuntary single or multiple jerks of all or part of the body. Some instances of myoclonus, like that experienced by persons falling asleep, are completely normal. A few types are thought to represent a form of epilepsy. Infantile spasms and childhood myoclonic epilepsy are usually related to severe underlying neurologic disease.

- *Febrile seizures* are generalized seizures in a young child. The child has a fever but no central nervous system infection.

- *Focal seizures* arise from a particular part of the brain. They may be restricted to that part, spread to other parts (Jacksonian) or proceed to a generalized convulsion. They may be caused by old strokes, birth injury, congenital anomalies, remote infections, head injury, cranial surgery, and primary or metastatic neoplasms.

DEMYELINATING DISEASES

Myelin is the lipid–containing material that insulates many nerve axons in both central and peripheral nervous systems. It greatly increases the conduction speed of those fibers. Myelin gives nerves a white appearance.

There are three diseases in which nerve fibers become demyelinated.

- *Multiple sclerosis (MS)* is the most common demyelinating disease. It is a disease of young adulthood characterized by acute exacerbations and remissions. Multiple lesions in the white matter of the central nervous system may produce disorders of the visual or brain stem pathways, disorders in the spinal cord, or anywhere in the central nervous system.

- *Optic neuritis* is an acute demyelinating disease that results in acute loss of vision, and frequently accompanies multiple sclerosis.

- *Acute disseminated encephalomyelitis* is an uncommon demyelinating disease of the brain and spinal cord, which occurs several days after exposure to such viral diseases as measles, chickenpox, smallpox, rubella, or after a rabies vaccination.

DISEASES OF THE SPINAL COLUMN AND SUPPORTING STRUCTURES

The spinal cord has 30 segments. Each segment has four nerve roots that are named by the segments in which the nerve root enters or exits (cervical 1–8, thoracic 1–12, lumbar 1–5, and sacral 1–5). The last spinal cord segment usually is found in the adult at about the lumbar 1 or 2 vertebral level. The spinal canal below this level does not contain any spinal cord, but only the nerve roots passing down to their exit foramina. Lumbar puncture may be performed at any of the lower lumbar interspaces without danger of damaging the spinal cord.

Herniated Disc

Between each vertebra is a disc that allows flexibility and cushioning of the spine. Many factors may lead to herniation or rupture of the disc. Herniated discs occur most frequently in the lumbar area and in the cervical vertebrae. Nerve root compression usually occurs as a result of the herniated disc.

Spondylosis

Spondylosis is a degenerative disease of the spine that occurs in the elderly. Spondylosis may be found in either the cervical or lumbar areas and consists of calcified lips or spurs. Those spurs develop from atrophic discs and impinge upon the roots in the intervertebral foramina.

- *Spondylolysis* and *spondylolisthesis* involve fractures or displacements of the vertebrae, usually in the lumbar spine, which result from earlier birth trauma or degenerative disease.

Bone Disorders

Diseases of the bone may affect the spine, and some produce neurological deficits.

- *Ankylosing spondylitis* is a condition in which the vertebral joints become fused.
- *Rheumatoid arthritis* may result in serious complications from displacement (subluxation) of one vertebra onto another.
- *Paget's disease* may also affect the spine and cause cord compression.
- *Metabolic bone diseases,* such as osteoporosis, hyperparathyroidism, and osteomalacia may also affect the spine.

Trauma

Trauma to the spine may result in fractures of the bone, and displacement of the vertebrae. Spasm of the supporting muscles will usually occur, but neurological deficit may or may not appear.

DISEASES OF THE SPINAL CORD

The spinal cord may be affected by metabolic, infective, vascular, developmental, and neoplastic diseases. The most common disease of the spinal cord is progressive cervical myelopathy.

Motor Neuron Diseases

Multiple sclerosis is also a frequent cause of spinal cord disease. Motor neuron disease is a degeneration of the neurons in the motor tracts from the cerebral cortex and pyramidal tracts or the ventral horns in the cord. Amyotrophic lateral sclerosis (ALS) is the most common form of motor neuron disease. Brain stem nuclei and motor nerves may be involved. Rare forms of motor neuron disease may occur in infancy (Werdnig–Hoffman disease) or in juveniles (Kugelberg–Welander syndrome). Poliomyelitis is now a rare viral infection of the anterior horn cells (lower motor neuron).

Subacute combined degeneration of the spinal cord is a gradually progressive metabolic disease of the cord, caused by pernicious anemia. Subacute combined degeneration of the spinal cord is now rare. Tabes dorsalis is a disease caused by the effects of syphilis on the spinal cord. Radiation myelopathy may occur when the cord receives radiation that is directed toward a lesion in the thorax.

Spinal Cord Compression

Spinal cord compression may be caused by lesions of the vertebral column, the nerve roots (neurofibroma), or the meninges (meningioma). Epidural and subdural hematomas and abscesses may also occur at any cord level and produce compression.

Spinal Cord Tumors

Tumors such as ependymomas or gliomas occur in the cord just as they do in the brain. Syringomyelia is a progressive degeneration of the cord that produces a cavity in the center of the cord. It will produce an enlarged, swollen cord that may block cerebrospinal fluid flow. Syringomyelia may progress upward into the brain stem (syringobulbia).

The cord may be damaged by interruption of its vascular supply. Damage to a feeder vessel may produce an infarction. Trauma to the cord may cause an acute vascular occlusion and infarction, contusion to the cord, or transection of the cord.

PERIPHERAL NEUROPATHIES

The peripheral nerves carry sensory information into the central nervous system or carry information from the central nervous system to the skeletal muscles. When a muscle loses its peripheral nerve innervation, the muscle cannot be controlled by the central nervous system. The muscle will gradually atrophy until it is almost completely wasted. If the nerve should regenerate, the process of muscle wasting will halt.

There are a vast number of systemic diseases, deficiencies, toxins, and drugs that commonly cause permanent or transient damage to the peripheral nerves. There are also several primary neurologic disorders that affect the peripheral nerves or roots. Trauma or a mass may impinge on the nerve pathway.

Inherited Peripheral Neuropathies

Some peripheral neuropathies are inherited. Charcot–Marie-Tooth disease produces wasting and weakness of the distal muscles with accompanying loss of sensation. Dejerine's–Sottas disease involves diffuse thickening of all the peripheral nerves, even the cranial nerves and also begins with atrophy of the distal muscles of the legs. Sensory neuropathies may also be inherited.

Leprosy and Guillain–Barré Syndrome

Leprosy, an infective neuropathy, is caused by a viral infection of the nerve. Leprosy produces patches of total sensory loss. Guillain–Barré syndrome is a more common response of the central nervous system to a variety of infective processes, particularly viral infections. It begins with painful peripheral paresthesia and advances to weakness of the proximal muscles.

Other Causes

- Lead, arsenic, and organic solvents are a few of the toxic chemicals that may cause peripheral nerve damage.
- Alcohol and the secondary vitamin B deficiencies are a cause of a painful neuropathy that may advance.
- Diabetes mellitus is a very common cause of a mild neuropathy that results from small vessel disease.
- Chronic renal failure also produces a peripheral neuropathy.

DISEASES OF THE NEUROMUSCULAR JUNCTION
Myasthenia Gravis

Myasthenia gravis is the most common neuromuscular junction disease. The underlying pathology involves failure of depolarization of the end-plate region of the muscle fiber. This results in decreased excitation and contraction of skeletal muscles. Myasthenia gravis may be caused by insufficient acetylcholine (ACH) release from the nerve ending, insensitivity of the muscle end-plate, or reduction or blockage of the acetylcholine receptors in the muscle end-plates. Eaton–Lambert syndrome is similar to myasthenia. It is usually associated with oat-cell carcinoma of the lung.

Botulism and Tetanus

Botulism is caused by the exotoxin of *Clostridium botulinum,* which is a powerful presynaptic blocker of acetylcholine release. Tetanus is caused by tetanus toxin from *Clostridium tetani,* which causes generalized neuromuscular excitability.

DISEASES OF THE MUSCLE
Muscular Dystrophy

Muscular dystrophy is a chronic, inherited disease of skeletal muscle characterized by progressive muscular weakness and loss of muscle mass. The pathologic process involves a decrease in number of muscle fibers. There are four varieties of dystrophy:

- Duchenne or pseudohypertrophic muscular dystrophy
- Limb–girdle dystrophy
- Facio scapulohumeral dystrophy
- Myotonic dystrophy

Myopathies

Congenital myopathies produce a "floppy infant" syndrome, which takes a variety of forms. Cerebral palsy from birth trauma, early peripheral neuropathy, or early myotonic dystrophy may also cause a floppy infant syndrome.

Abnormal muscle metabolism can produce a variety of myopathies. There are four glycogen storage disorders that are associated with myopathies. These are: Pampe's disease (a fatal disease of infancy), McArdle's syndrome, debranching enzyme disease, and Tarui's disease.

Hyperkalemia

Muscle disease can also be due to abnormal cellular levels of potassium.

- Dangerous hyperkalemia may occur in the presence of rhabdomyolysis, which results in the breakdown of muscle cells and the release of myoglobin and other muscle protein into the plasma.

- Hyperkalemia can be caused by many conditions, including trauma, strenuous exercise, heat stroke, alcohol, or diabetic acidosis.

Trichinosis

Trichinosis is an infestation caused by a nematode. The nematode is usually contracted by eating undercooked pork. The parasite moves through the gastrointestinal tract, lymphatics, bloodstream, and ends as an encapsulated embryo in the muscle.

TOXIC AND METABOLIC DISORDERS

Systemic Diseases

Most systemic diseases eventually produce neurologic changes. Cerebral hypoxia may be caused by pulmonary or cardiac disease. Virtually all endocrine disorders and collagen disease have associated neurologic changes. Liver disease and renal failure may produce encephalopathies. Acute intermittent porphyria (AIP) is an inherited metabolic disease.

Toxins and Drugs

There are also many toxins and drugs that affect the central nervous system. Lead, mercury, arsenic, and thallium (rat poison) are the most common industrial toxins. Alcohol is probably the most commonly taken central nervous system depressant. Withdrawal may also precipitate dangerous neurologic dysfunction (delirium tremens). Prolonged use will damage the liver and lead to hepatic encephalopathy. The thiamine deficiency associated with alcoholism and other malnutrition disorders can cause Wernicke's encephalopathy.

Barbiturate overdose can cause depression of all bodily functions. Barbiturates do not damage the central nervous system.

Other central nervous system depressants commonly abused are opiates, glutethimide, chloral hydrate, diazepam, and chlordiazepoxide. Central nervous system stimulants that may be abused include amphetamines and tricyclic antidepressants. Salicylate from aspirin is a common cause of intoxication.

BLOOD TESTS
BARBITURATE LEVELS

Serum blood levels of a variety of barbiturates can be measured. Phenobarbital is the most commonly used barbiturate. Phenobarbital is primarily used for the control of seizures in all age groups.

Normal range drug	Therapeutic level	Toxic level
Phenobarbital	15 to 40 μg/ml	>40 μg/ml
Most other barbiturates	0.5 to 3.0 μg/ml	>10 μg/ml

Nursing Implications
Procedure for Collection/Storage of Specimen

A 5 ml specimen of whole blood is collected.

Possible Interfering Factors

None reported

Patient Care
1. Notify the physician of toxic or less than therapeutic blood levels.
2. The chief side effect of barbiturates is sedation. Observe for signs of an overdosage that may lead to fatal respiratory depression.
3. In patients with seizure disorders, withdrawal of the drug may precipitate the onset of seizures.
4. If a specific barbiturate level is needed, request the laboratory to differentiate the total barbiturate level.

Patient Education
1. Phenobarbital may be taken at bedtime since the drug will produce sedation.
2. The drug may produce paradoxical hyperactivity and irritability in children.

Signed Consent
Not required

DILANTIN SERUM LEVEL

Serum Dilantin levels are done to determine the therapeutic levels or toxic levels of Dilantin. Phenytoin sodium (Dilantin) is the most effective of the anticonvulsants which are used in the treatment of generalized grand mal convulsions.

Laboratory Results

Therapeutic level	10–20 μg/ml
Toxic level	>20 μg/ml

Nursing Implications
Procedure for Collection/Storage of Specimen

Collect 3 ml of whole blood.

Possible Interfering Factors

The following drugs interfere with phenytoin metabolism, increasing the serum levels and increasing the risk of toxicity:

- isoniazid
- coumarin anticoagulants
- disulfiram
- chloramphenicol
- Librium
- Valium
- Ritalin
- phenothiazines
- estrogens
- Zarontin
- phenylbutazone
- alcohol

Patient Care

1. Notify the physician of toxic levels or less than therapeutic blood levels.
2. Observe for nystagmus, ataxia, and lethargy. Nystagmus is frequently present at 10 to 20 µg/ml. Ataxia (staggering) begins at 30 µg/ml. Lethargy develops at 40 µg/ml.

Patient Education

1. Gingival hypertrophy may be prevented by meticulous oral and dental hygiene, including use of a soft toothbrush, and dental floss.
2. Phenytoin may be taken with milk to prevent occasional gastric upset.

Signed Consent

Not required

SERUM ELECTROLYTES

Altered potassium levels may result in periodic paralysis or acute weakness. Hypocalcemia may cause weakness, tetany, convulsions, and cataracts. Hypercalcemia may cause weakness or psychosis. (For details related to these tests, see pages 92 and 96.)

ERYTHROCYTE SEDIMENTATION RATE

The ESR is used as a quick screen in many neurologic disease entities. The ESR is the first test ordered in suspected cases of temporal arteritis. ESR is almost always elevated in collagen vascular diseases that may cause seizures, strokes, neuropathies, or cord lesions. (For details related to this test, see page 72.)

FASTING BLOOD SUGAR

Diabetes mellitus is a frequent contributor to stroke and peripheral neuropathy. Any patient experiencing stroke or peripheral neuropathy will be screened for diabetes mellitus. Trauma may cause a transient rise in blood sugar. Profound hypoglycemia is also a cause of coma. (For details related to this test, see page 238.)

LEPROSY

Leprosy is rare in the United States but is very common in many of the underdeveloped countries of the world. *Mycobacterium leprae* is found in large, nodular lesions, or in peripheral blood smears during a reaction period.

TESTS FOR SYPHILIS

Late (tertiary) syphilis may infect the central nervous system in several ways: meningitis, meningovascular disease, tabes dorsalis, and general paresis. All of these conditions have a positive serologic test in the CSF and in the blood. In asymptomatic CNS lues, there is a negative blood test and a positive CSF serologic test. The VDRL may be negative in late syphilis. (For details related to this test, see page 286.)

BLOOD TOXICOLOGY SCREEN

A toxicology screen is performed on comatose patients to help identify the cause of coma. The test may be done to help differentiate between coma caused by drugs or other toxic substance ingestion or coma caused by other cerebral pathology such as head injury.

Normal range	Therapeutic level	Toxic level
Ethanol	None	Marked intoxication 0.3 to 0.4%
		Alcoholic stupor 0.4 to 0.5%
		Coma >0.5%
Barbiturates		
Amobarbital (Amytal)	0.5–3.0 µg/ml	>10 µg/ml
Butabarbital (Butisol)	0.5–3.0 µg/ml	>10 µg/ml
Glutethimide (Doriden)	0.5–3.0 µg/ml	>10 µg/ml
Meprobamate (Miltown)	0.5–3.0 µg/ml	>10 µg/ml
Methaqualone (Quaalude)	0.5–3.0 µg/ml	>10 µg/ml
Methyprylon (Noludar)	0.5–3.0 µg/ml	>10 µg/ml
Pentobarbital (Nembutal)	0.5–3.0 µg/ml	>10 µg/ml
Phenobarbital	15–40 µg/ml	>40 µg/ml
Secobarbital (Seconal)	5–3.0 µg/gml	>10 µg/ml
Lithium	0.5–1.5 mEq/l	> 2 mEq/L
Bromides		>17 mEq/L (150 mg/dl)
Salicylate	20–25 mg/dl	>30 mg/dl >age 10
	(35–40 mg/dl	>45 mg/dl ≤age 10
	≤age 10)	>20 mg/ml >age 60

Normal range	*Therapeutic level*	*Toxic level*
Carbon monoxide	None	>30% COHb marks the beginning of coma
Lead	None	>40 µg/dl

Nursing Implications

Procedure for Collection/Storage of Specimen

1. The amount of whole blood varies with the study. The use of preservative or anticoagulant varies with the study.
2. In addition to blood studies, urine and gastric specimens may be analyzed.

Possible Interfering Factors

Blood should be drawn immediately after admission in emergency cases; delay may result in decreased blood levels.

Patient Care

The patient's care may vary depending upon the toxic substance and the patient's reaction. Care may include: (1) questioning of patient or witnesses about the types, amount, and time of the consumed substance, (2) protecting the airway and respiratory function of the patient if impaired level of consciousness is present, and (3) performing gastric lavage in emergency cases.

Patient Education

The patient or parent may require instructions about drug regimen, and avoidance of toxic substances (*i.e.*, lead paint). Psychiatric counseling may be indicated for cases of street drug usage or intentional overdose.

Signed Consent

Not required

VITAMIN B$_{12}$

Vitamin B$_{12}$ deficiency can lead to spinal cord lesions. Vitamin B$_{12}$ is frequently associated with the peripheral neuropathy found with pernicious anemia. (For details related to this test, see page 179.)

DIAGNOSTIC STUDIES
AUDIOMETRY

Hearing may be impaired by a lesion at any point along the external auditory canal, tympanic membrane, organs of hearing, eighth cranial nerve, or brain stem pathways. Vertigo may result from damage to the vestibular system. To diagnose the location of the lesion, audiometry may be performed. Audiometry is a noninvasive test. The patient listens to tones and voices through earphones and indicates when sound is heard. The test is not painful or tiring. The patient must be cooperative in order to obtain valid results. The results usually differentiate between lesions in the mechanical conduction structures, the cochlea, or the eighth nerve going to the brain stem. Audiometry is used to determine hearing loss in suspected cases of acoustic neuroma and in head-injured patients.

Normal Results

Normal response to auditory stimuli

Nursing Implications
Preprocedure

Inform the patient of the purpose of the test and of the need to cooperate.

During the Procedure

1. Have the patient sit comfortably with the earphones in place.
2. Instruct the patient to respond as quickly as possible when a sound is heard.

Postprocedure

There are no special care instructions.

Signed Consent
Not required

AUDITORY-EVOKED RESPONSES

The auditory-evoked response test measures the response of the auditory system to sounds (usually clicks) which are delivered through earphones. The test does not depend upon patient cooperation. An electroencephalogram (EEG) is used to record the patient's response to sound. The intensity of sound is measured along with the presence of the response on the EEG to test the acuity of hearing. Changes in the waveforms of the EEG indicate damage at points along the auditory pathways and in the brain stem. Auditory-evoked response changes can indicate brain stem damage after a head injury. The test is also useful in studying hearing deficits in infants and patients who are suspected of being malingerers.

Normal Results

Normal group of waveforms on the EEG

Nursing Implications
Preprocedure

1. Explain the procedure to the patient and family.
2. Wash the patient's hair to facilitate electrode attachment to the scalp.
3. Sedate infants or agitated patients if prescribed by the physician.

During the Procedure

Instruct the patient to sit or lie quietly, with as little movement as possible.

Postprocedure

1. There are no special care instructions.
2. If the patient was sedated prior to the procedure, institute safety precautions such as side rails.

Signed Consent
Not required

CEREBRAL ANGIOGRAM

Cerebral angiography is a test used to visualize intracranial or extracranial circulation. During the cerebral angiography, a dye is injected into an artery. The carotid, vertebral, brachial, axillary, subclavian, or femoral arteries are used. The femoral artery is usually the route of choice. A catheter is threaded through the femoral artery and the dye is injected. The carotid arteries and vertebral arteries can be injected with the dye directly. A complication of the direct method is dislodging of a thrombus that may cause a stroke. After injection of the dye, a rapid series of x-rays is taken to demonstrate the arterial, capillary, and venous phases of filling. X-rays may be repeated several times.

A cerebral angiography is done to demonstrate vascular lesions, and to define the blood supply of a tumor. Many tumors may be diagnosed by their characteristic vascular supply. (For details related to this test, see page 76.)

Normal Results

Normal arterial filling and vascular pattern

Nursing Implications

Preprocedure

1. Explain the procedure to the patient.
2. Inform the patient that a warm sensation will occur in the neck and face when the dye is injected.
3. The patient may be kept NPO several hours before the procedure. However, many doctors prefer that the patient drink fluids prior to the test in order to be well hydrated. Instruct the patient according to the policy of the hospital or physician.
4. Administer a preoperative medication if prescribed.
5. Instruct the patient to empty the bladder prior to the test.
6. Remove jewelry, dentures, or prosthetic devices. Provide a hospital gown for the patient to wear.
7. Record a base-line neurological assessment on the patient's chart.
8. Shave the femoral area if ordered.
9. Inquire about any allergies the patient may have.
10. Start an intravenous infusion or check patency of existing intravenous line.

During the Procedure

1. Monitor the patient's vital signs including neurological signs.
2. Observe the patient for untoward reaction to the dye or to the procedure. An untoward reaction to the dye may cause: flushing, hives, laryngeal stridor, seizures, or cardiovascular collapse and arrest. Observe for increased neurologic deficit such as blindness, weakness, or loss of consciousness.

Postprocedure

1. Monitor the neurological signs every hour for 4 hr, then every 4 hr for 24 hr.
2. Keep the insertion site straight for 6 hr.

3. Supply an ice bag to the injection sites. Check the site for hematoma formation or bleeding every 30 min for 2 hr, then every hour for 4 hr.
4. Elevate the patient's head if desired.
5. Observe the extremity distal to the insertion site for color, temperature, and pulse.
6. Resume the patient's normal diet.

Signed Consent

Required

CEREBRAL BLOOD FLOW

Cerebral blood flow studies measure the total or regional cerebral blood flow. This test is used to detect increased and deficient areas in the cerebral circulation. This test is still experimental in some hospitals. The test is used to evaluate vasospasm following an aneurysm rupture, regional blood flow during carotid procedures, vascular malformations during a craniotomy, and for the presence of tumors, or aneurysms. The test may also be used postoperatively to predict the effectiveness of an operative procedure.

Several techniques can be used to perform the cerebral blood flow test. Some techniques involve inhalation of nitrous oxide or Xenon 133, or intracarotid injection of Xenon 133 or Krypton 85. Blood sampling is done by peripheral arterial, central venous, or jugular bulb cannulation. Some techniques also use external scintillation detectors to record passage of the radioactive isotopes.

Normal Results

Normal total or regional cerebral blood flow

Nursing Implications

Preprocedure

1. Explain the procedure to the patient. The test may be performed under general or local anesthetic.
2. Prepare the patient for a surgical procedure.
3. Do a baseline neurological assessment of the patient.

During the Procedure

Reassure the patient, if the patient is awake during the procedure.

Postprocedure

1. Perform routine postoperative care.
2. Observe cannulation sites for bleeding or hematoma formation.
3. Perform periodic neurological checks.

Signed Consent

An experimental consent form must be signed by the patient.

COMPUTED AXIAL TOMOGRAPHY (CT Scan)

A CT scan is a technique in which pictures are produced of the contents of the skull (for head scans). These pictures appear in black and white, with higher density areas being lighter than lower density areas. Bone and collections of blood appear lighter than brain tissue, while areas of edema or infarction appear darker than surrounding brain tissue. Hematomas, subarachnoid hemorrhage, cortical atrophy, tumors, hydrocephalus, abscesses, and shifts of the midline are also visible. Infarctions of brain tissue may show a decreased density after 24 to 48 hours. An iodine-containing contrast material can be given intravenously to emphasize areas of increased vascularity or a defective blood–brain barrier.

Normal Results
Normal density and structure of brain tissue is observed. Air appears black, bone appears white, soft tissue appears in shades of gray. There is no evidence of tumor or other pathology.

Nursing Implications
Preprocedure
1. Explain the procedure to the patient. The patient will be required to lie quietly for about 30 min.
2. Inquire about patient allergies, especially to iodine.
3. Administer sedation if prescribed. Sedation may be ordered for children or uncooperative patients.
4. Remove earrings or other metal from the patient's head or neck.
5. Start an intravenous infusion or check the present infusion for patency.

During the Procedure
1. The patient lies quietly with his head resting on a stationary box. A moveable frame rotates around the head.
2. Observe the patient for allergic reaction to the contrast material. Benadryl may be prescribed by the physician to relieve itching or rash.
3. The contrast material may cause vomiting. Instruct the patient to take slow, deep breaths. Have an emesis basin ready.

Postprocedure
1. If sedation has been given, provide safety measures to protect the patient.
2. Observe the patient for signs of reaction to iodine, such as dyspnea, tachycardia, nausea, vomiting or diaphoresis.

Signed Consent
A written consent form must be signed if a contrast material is used.

ECHOENCEPHALOGRAM
A Sonar A or echo scan is used to detect midline shift when a calcified pineal is not visible on skull films and a CT scan is not available. The echo scan is a noninvasive test. A probe that is placed on the side of the head emits a sonic beam and reabsorbs those beams that are reflected back to the probe.

Normal Results
Normal size of ventricles. Midline structure of the brain in normal position.

Nursing Implications

Preprocedure

1. Explain the procedure to the patient.
2. Instruct the patient to lie still during the test.

During the Procedure

Explain to the patient that pictures of the brain may be seen on a screen.

Postprocedure

There are no special patient care implications if the test results are normal. If a midline shift is detected, observe for impending neurological deterioration by frequent neurological assessment.

Signed Consent

Required

ELECTROENCEPHALOGRAPHY (EEG)

EEG is the recording of brain electrical activity from electrodes that are placed on the scalp. A permanent record of the tracing is made. There are several methods of electrode placement all of which use varying numbers of electrodes. The International 10–20 system with 21 standard sites is probably the most widely used method. Two nasopharyngeal leads may be passed through the nares. This allows for recording of electrical activity from the temporal lobes deep in the brain.

The primary use of the EEG is to evaluate possible seizures. The EEG is not always accurate. Many patients without seizures have abnormal EEGs, and many with confirmed seizures have normal EEGs. The EEG is of greatest value in localizing or ruling out a focal seizure location. Areas of tumor, infarct, or hematoma may frequently be seen as areas of focal slowing on the EEG. Brain death may be diagnosed by an isoelectric (flat) EEG. EEG is also used for routine screening in psychiatric disorders. A form of EEG monitoring may be used during surgeries, such as carotid endarterectomy, to assess adequacy of cerebral blood flow.

Normal Results

Normal symmetrical pattern of alpha, beta, and delta waves

Nursing Implications

Preprocedure

1. Explain to the patient that no electrical shocks will be given, however electrodes will be applied to the patient's head.
2. Wash the patient's hair.
3. Observe the physician's special orders—the test may require sleep deprivation or withholding of anticonvulsants, coffee, tea.
4. Carefully note any sedatives (phenobarbital) or diagnostic tests that the patient has recently had, as these may affect the EEG.

During the Procedure

1. Have the patient sit comfortably.
2. Instruct the patient not to move, if possible.

3. Some special instructions for the patient may include opening and shutting eyes, relaxing and sleeping, watching a strobe light, or breathing deeply and rapidly. These activation techniques are used in an attempt to elicit a seizure.

Postprocedure

1. Wash the patient's hair to remove the electrode paste.
2. Discuss the findings of the test with physician and patient. Use simple and easily understood terminology.

Signed Consent

Not required

ELECTROMYOGRAPHY (EMG) AND NERVE CONDUCTION TIMES

EMG and nerve conduction studies are used in the diagnosis and management of peripheral nerve and muscle diseases. These studies are of limited use in myasthenia gravis since the muscles which are usually affected are inaccessible. The EMG is used to diagnose disease of the spinal nerve roots which occur from disc disease, peripheral nerve injury, and plexus injuries. The EMG assesses the electrical characteristics of the muscle. A needle electrode is inserted into the muscle. The electrical potential is heard on an amplifier and observed on an oscilloscope. The electrical potential is measured during insertion of the needle, with the muscle at rest, and during full contraction of the muscle. The electrical patterns can indicate if there is a lesion of the nerve innervating the muscle or damage to the muscle fibers themselves.

Nerve conduction studies include the following:

- Motor conduction studies measure the speed of conduction between two electrodes that are placed along a motor neuron. Conduction is decreased in Guillain–Barré syndrome, diphtheria, and Charcot–Marie–Tooth disease.
- Sensory conduction times record the speed of conduction along sensory nerves. Conduction times are prolonged in demyelination neuropathies.

There is no standard examination for any patient who is undergoing EMG and conduction studies. The protocol will be determined by the neurologist who performs the test based on the presenting symptoms and physical examination.

Nursing Implications

Preprocedure

1. Assess the patient's reflexes and response to sensation.
2. Explain the basic procedure and its purpose to the patient.
3. Explain to the patient that the patient will feel pricks when the needle is inserted, some deeper aching pain when the needles are manipulated, and some small electrical shocks.

During the Procedure

Instruct the patient to slowly flex certain muscles when requested and then to contract the muscles to their maximum when requested.

Postprocedure

There are no special patient care considerations.

Signed Consent

Required

ELECTRONYSTAGMOGRAPHY

Nystagmus is involuntary, rhythmic movements of the eye. Nystagmus may be normal, drug induced, or caused by lesions in the vestibular system. To record these movements accurately, electrodes are placed on the skin around the eyes and various tests are performed. The electronystagmogram records the changing electrical field as the eye moves. Analysis of the results may locate a lesion in the central or peripheral vestibular pathways.

Nursing Implications

Preprocedure

1. Explain the procedure and reason for the study to the patient.
2. Place the patient NPO for 3 hr prior to the test.
3. Hold any unnecessary medications for 24 hr prior to test.
4. Send the patient's eyeglasses with the patient to the test.

During the Procedure

1. Inform the patient to follow instructions during the procedure. The patient will be asked to
   a. gaze at lights
   b. watch a moving pattern
   c. watch a moving point
   d. sit with eyes closed
2. Explain to the patient that he will be sitting during the procedure. The patient will be rotated clockwise and counterclockwise and upside down during the procedure.
3. Explain to the patient that it will be necessary to irrigate the ears with cool and warm water.
4. Observe the patient for nausea and vomiting.
5. Reassure the patient frequently since the test is long and tiring.

Postprocedure

1. Place the patient on a regular diet.
2. Allow the patient to rest.

Signed Consent

Some hospitals may require the patient to sign a written consent.

LUMBAR PUNCTURE

Lumbar puncture (LP) is performed by insertion of a hollow-bore needle into the spinal canal at the L2–3, 3–4, or 4–5 vertebral interspaces. Lumbar puncture may be performed to obtain a specimen of CSF, to measure CSF pressure, as part of other diagnostic studies, or to therapeutically decrease CSF volume. Lumbar puncture is strongly contraindicated in most cases of increased ICP, since removal of CSF can cause the brain to herniate down through the foramen magnum. The lumbar puncture is also contraindicated in suspected spinal cord compression or if there are infected areas in the skin around the puncture site.

Examination of CSF: In addition to the tests given below, additional tests may be done on CSF. Serologic tests for syphilis, cryptococcal, or coccidioidal antigens or antibodies may be performed on CSF. Viral isolation studies or antibody titers may be performed also.

Laboratory values are as follows:

Parameter	Normal Range	Interpretation
Glucose	20 mg/ml < blood level (blood determination should be made simultaneously)	Elevated—merely reflects systemic hyperglycemia. Decreased—bacterial, fungal, tuberculous meningitis or meningeal neoplasm.
Protein	15 to 45 mg/dl	May be increased by presence of cells or by degenerative processes or blockage of spinal CSF circulation.
Gamma globulin	5% to 12% of total protein	Elevated in 75% of patients with multiple sclerosis.
Color	Clear	Cloudy—increased WBC Dark—metastatic melanoma Pale yellow—increased protein Yellow—subarachnoid hemorrhage, occurring several hours previously Bloody—new subarachnoid hemorrhage
Cell count	No RBC's; <5 lymphocytes per cu mm	RBC's indicate a traumatic tap or bleeding into the subarachnoid space. Neutrophils are indicative of bacterial infection
Colloid gold	Not more than 1 in any tube	Changes classified by zones: Zone 1—syphilis, multiple sclerosis Zone 2—tubercular meningitis, polymyositis, tabes dorsalis Zone 3—purulent meningitis
Chloride	20 mEq/L higher than serum value	
Potassium	2.2 to 3.3 mEq/L	

(Continued)

Parameter	Normal Range	Interpretation
Carbon dioxide	25 mEq/L	
pH	7.35 to 7.40	
Transaminase (GOT)	7 to 49 u	
Lactic dehydrogenase (LDH)	15 to 71 u	
Creatinine phosphokinase (CPK)	0 to 3 IU	
Bilirubin	0	
Urea nitrogen	5 to 25 mg/dl	
Amino acids	30% of blood level	
Culture	No growth	Presence of bacteria, fungi, or amebae indicates pathology
CSF pressure	Normal: 80 to 180 mm H_2O	

Nursing Implications

Preprocedure

1. Explain the procedure to the patient and answer any questions.
2. Instruct the patient to void if necessary.
3. Sedation may be prescribed for anxious patients.
4. Obtain a LP tray, physician's sterile gloves, and table.

During Procedure

1. Position the patient on his side with his back flush with the edge of his mattress, which should be firm. Hips are flexed 90°, pillow between knees and to chest, held by patient. The head may be on a low pillow, the neck does not need to be forcibly flexed.
2. The patient may be asked to sit if this position facilitates the insertion of the spinal needle.
3. If CSF pressure is to be obtained, pressure will be measured by attaching a stopcock and manometer to the spinal needle. This "initial pressure" reading should be taken before any CSF is removed. The fluid level in the manometer should fluctuate with respirations. The pressure may be temporarily elevated if the abdomen is compressed by improper positioning or if the patient is very tense.
4. The patient may be asked to cough, breathe deeply, or strain as if for stool to demonstrate pressure fluctuation.
5. Jugular compression may be performed digitally or with a cuff as requested by the physician.
6. Instruct the patient to report any pain radiating to either leg.
7. Offer comfort and reassurance to the patient.
8. Fill 3 tubes with 1 to 2 ml each of CSF. The first tube is examined for cells and chemistries. The second tube is examined for cultures and

sensitivities. The third is saved, or the cells in it are counted and compared with the first tube. This comparison serves to distinguish a fresh subarachnoid hemorrhage from a traumatic puncture.

9. Note the color and clarity of the fluid.

Postprocedure

1. Monitor the patient's level of consciousness, pupillary reactivity, and vital signs every 30 min, for two hr, then every hour for 4 hr.
2. If CSF pressure is elevated, observe for acute deterioration of neurological status. Prepare to administer osmotic diuretics as prescribed.
3. Keep all patients flat for 12 to 24 hr, to decrease the incidence of headache.
4. Encourage the patient to drink fluids to replenish the CSF and to decrease the incidence of headache.
5. Observe the puncture site for leakage of clear fluid or development of a hematoma.
6. Send the CSF specimens to the laboratory immediately.

Signed Consent

Required

MYELOGRAM

A myelogram is a fluoroscopic examination of the spinal cord and neural foramen. Contrast media is injected into the spinal subarachnoid space. The contrast media may be air, an oil-based substance (Pantopaque), or a water-based preparation (Metrizamide). A lumbar or cervical puncture is performed. Contrast media is injected. The patient lies prone and is tilted. This causes the contrast media to flow around the cord. As much as possible of the oil-based media is usually removed after the study is completed. Air- or water-based media will be reabsorbed by the body.

A myelogram is used to search for cord or root compression in disc disease, lesions within the cord, tumors within the dura and occasionally lesions of the foramen magnum, basal cisterns, and cerebello–pontine angle.

Normal Results

Normal lumbar or cervical structures

Nursing Implications

Preprocedure

1. Explain the procedure and its purpose to the patient.
2. Explain that the procedure should not be very painful. However, preexisting pain or spasm may make the patient unable to lie comfortably in the prone position.
3. Inquire about allergy to iodine or seafoods.
4. Administer sedation if prescribed.
5. Place the patient in a hospital gown. No jewelry should be worn by the patient.
6. Have the patient empty the bladder.
7. Establish a baseline neurological assessment.

During the Procedure

Inform the patient that a lumbar puncture (spinal tap) will be performed, CSF removed, and contrast media injected. The table is tilted and x-ray films are taken. Tell the patient before the test why it is necessary for the table to be tilted. Reassure the patient that he will be securely fastened to the table.

Postprocedure

1. Check vital signs every 4 hr for 24 hr post examination.
2. Assess the patient for headache, which may be severe. The patient should remain flat and drink fluids to replenish spinal fluid and hasten reabsorption of contrast media.
3. Observe the patient for nausea and vomiting.
4. Institute routine seizure precautions. If any contrast liquid reaches the middle fossa, seizures may result.
5. If raised ICP was present prior to the procedure, observe for signs of tentorial herniation.
6. If spinal block was found, increasing neurological deficit may occur. Prepare the patient for immediate surgery.
7. If multiple sclerosis is the diagnosis, rapid deterioration may occur after myelography.
8. Observe muscle strength, sensory function, and other neuro-vital signs frequently.
9. Observe for normal bladder function.

Signed Consent

Required

PNEUMOENCEPHALOGRAM AND VENTRICULOGRAM

Pneumoencephalogram involves the injection of air into the lumbar subarachnoid space. A lumbar puncture is performed. Ventriculography is the direct injection of air or contrast media into a lateral ventricle. A cannula is inserted through a burr hole in the skull. Both studies have been largely replaced by CT scanning for diagnosis of hydrocephalus and mass lesions. Pneumoencephalography (PEG) is now used for examination of the area around the pituitary gland and the brain stem. Ventriculography is used to examine the third and fourth ventricles and Aqueduct of Sylvius. It is also used during stereotaxic surgery so that the air in the ventricles can be used to visualize key landmarks. They are highly invasive procedures and are usually performed only when absolutely necessary, such as in the preoperative evaluation of a pituitary tumor.

Normal Results

Normal ventricles and subarachnoid spaces

Nursing Implications

Preprocedure

1. Explain the procedure and reason for the study to the patient.
2. Place the patient NPO past midnight before the test.

3. Prepare the patient as for surgery. The patient may wear pajama bottoms and elastic hose.
4. Inquire about allergy to iodine or seafood.
5. For a ventriculogram, shave the hair over the cannulation site.

During the Procedure

1. Place the patient in the revolving chair. An alternative position for the patient is to sit upright. The patient's head is placed in a sling.
2. If nausea or agitation occur, administer antiemetics or barbiturates as prescribed.

Postprocedure

1. Neuro assessment should be done every half hour or as the patient's response indicates.
2. Place the patient on bedrest for 24 to 48 hr. Instruct the patient to move his head slowly and to remain flat in bed.
3. Encourage fluids.
4. Place the patient in a dark, quiet room.
5. Medicate for severe headache. An ice bag may be used after ventriculostomy.
6. Observe for transtentorial herniation, seizures, hypotension, hemorrhage.

Signed Consent

Required

RADIOISOTOPE BRAIN SCAN

Radioisotope brain scans involve the intravenous injection of a small amount of a radioisotope to visualize vascular lesions in the brain. The scan is most successful in cases of abscesses and highly vascular tumors such as meningiomas and metastases. Many other lesions will not be discernible.

Normal Results

Normal distribution and uptake of the radioisotope

Nursing Implications

Preprocedure

1. Explain the procedure and the purpose of the test to the patient/family. The test is not painful.
2. Inquire about allergies to iodine or seafoods.
3. Check for patency of the IV or start an intravenous line.

During the Procedure

Ask the patient to remain still. The patient will be placed in several positions with large, heavy instruments near his head.

Postprocedure

1. Discontinue the intravenous line, unless ordered otherwise.
2. Observe for allergic reaction.

Signed Consent

Required

TENSILON TEST

The tensilon test is used to confirm a diagnosis of myasthenia gravis, to diagnose cholinergic crisis, or to evaluate oral anticholinesterase therapy. When tensilon is administered, it briefly blocks the activity of cholinesterase at the neuromuscular junction, allowing more neurotransmitter to accumulate in the synaptic cleft. This temporarily improves muscular strength in patients who have myasthenia gravis. This effect can only be evaluated if there is an easily observed weakness, such as grip strength, extraocular muscles, or swallowing. The test may also be performed with neostigmine, a longer-acting anticholinesterase.

Normal Results

A positive test is strengthening in weak muscle groups in myasthenia gravis patients.

Nursing Implications

Preprocedure

1. Explain the test and its purpose to the patient.
2. Evaluate respiratory status of the patient.
3. Establish weak muscle groups.
4. Have the patient empty the bowel and bladder.
5. Atropine may be administered if prescribed to prevent side effects.
6. Start an IV line or check for patency of the present intravenous line.

During the Procedure

1. Tensilon will be given IV slowly. Observe for the side effects of sweating, salivation, nausea, cramping, diarrhea, incontinence, hypotension, small pupils.
2. Observe the patient for improvement in strength. If strength is improved, the effect will last 5 to 30 min.
3. In cholinergic crisis, Tensilon may cause apnea. Have an emergency tracheostomy setup at hand.

Postprocedure

1. Observe the patient for effects of the test. All effects are gone in 2 hr (3 to 4 hr for neostigmine).
2. Instruct the patient about increased or decreased oral drug dose as prescribed by physician.

Signed Consent

Not required

VISUAL-EVOKED RESPONSES (VER)

VERs are similar to brain stem- or auditory-evoked responses. A stimulus is delivered to the brain. The brain's response to each stimulus is taken from surface electrodes and averaged. The stimulus in this case is usually a flickering checkerboard pattern. The stimulus-locked EEG is recorded over the occipital poles. Although it is not known exactly what the parts of the characteristic waveforms mean, it is known that slowing of the pattern indicates damage to one or the other optic nerve. Since only minimal patient cooperation is required, the test is suitable for visual evaluation of infants, patients recovering from head injury or suspected hysterical blindness, and malingerers. It is particularly useful in multiple sclerosis because it can detect lesions in the visual pathways that are not yet symptomatic. VER has also been used in evaluating the damage to the visual pathways in hydrocephalus.

Normal Results

Normal speed of waveform characteristics

Nursing Implications

Preprocedure

1. Explain the test and purpose to the patient or family.
2. Wash the patient's hair.

During the Procedure

Instruct the patient to fix his gaze on a central light, while the checkerboard changes about it.

Postprocedure

There are no special nursing care considerations.

Signed Consent

Not required

X-RAYS OF THE SKULL AND SPINE

Roentgenographic films or x-rays of the skull or spine are routinely ordered in most neurological evaluations. They are used as an initial screening test or as a definitive study. X-rays will only show calcified structures. In the infant, skull films will show premature closure of suture lines in craniosynostosis, separation of sutures in hydrocephalus, or bony abnormalities associated with congenital malformations. Skull fractures are found on skull films, and several views (PA, Townes and lateral) are usually ordered after head injury. Tangential views may be ordered to illustrate depressed skull fractures. Basilar skull fractures may be detected by an air-fluid level in a paranasal sinus partly filled with leaking CSF. Long-standing increased intracranial pressure will cause the inner table of the skull to have a "beaten silver" appearance on x-ray, and the thin bony surface of the sella turcica may be eroded. Laterally placed mass lesions may be detected by a shift of the calcified pineal gland. Some intracranial tumors such as meningioma, craniopharyngioma, and oligodendroglioma will become calcified and appear on skull films.

Films of the spine may be used to assess the bony structure of the vertebrae or to evaluate the spinal canal which contains the cord. Congenital deformities and scoliosis are detected on spinal films. After spinal cord injury, plain films and tomograms are used to identify fractures, dislocations, and assess the effectiveness of realignment. After head injury, spinal films are always obtained since some head-injured patients also have cervical fractures. Spondylosis and spondylolysis are visualized in oblique views of the spine that show the neural foramina. In disc disease, bony abnormalities are not usually found unless it is an acute scoliosis caused by spasm. Tumors on nerve roots may be visible by erosion of the neural foramina. Tumors in and on the cord may erode the entire canal at the level of the tumor. Progress of vertebral fusion operations is followed by observing osteophyte formation on spine films. Metabolic or metastatic diseases, which destroy the spine, may be seen on x-ray.

Normal Results

Normal bony structure of the skull and spine

Nursing Implications

Preprocedure

1. Explain the test and purpose to the patient. There is usually no danger to the patient from the levels of radiation absorbed in one series of skull or spine films. The exception might be in the case of spine films on a pregnant patient.
2. Remove jewelry or other metal from the patient.

During the Procedure

1. Ask the patient to lie very still during the x-ray.
2. Nursing and paramedical personnel should wear lead aprons.

Postprocedure

1. No special considerations postprocedure, unless the x-ray demonstrates pathology.

Signed Consent

Not required

BIBLIOGRAPHY

Clinical Oncology, published by the American Cancer Society for the University of Rochester, New York, 1978

Howe JR: Patient Care in Neurosurgery. Boston, Little, Brown & Co, 1977

Patten J: Neurological Differential Diagnosis. New York, Springer Verlag, 1977

Samuels MA: Manual of Neurologic Therapeutics. Boston, Little, Brown and Co, 1978

Slager UT: Basic Neuropathology. Baltimore, Williams and Williams, 1970

Wallach J: Interpretation of Diagnostic Tests. Boston, Little, Brown & Co, 1978

11

Tests Related to
Musculoskeletal Function

Connie L. Richardson

Gayle Deets Miller

OVERVIEW OF PHYSIOLOGY AND PATHOPHYSIOLOGY

The musculoskeletal system is responsible for movement of the body and body structure. This system is composed of muscles, ligaments, tendons, joints, and bones. The 206 bones of the skeleton serve five functions:

- protection
- manufacture of RBCs
- movement
- support of the tissues
- storage of minerals

MUSCLES
TYPES OF MUSCLES

All of the body's physical functions involve muscle activity. There are three types of muscles that are responsible for this activity: visceral, cardiac, and skeletal.

Visceral Muscles

The visceral or smooth muscles are responsible for all physical activity except skeletal movement and the pumping action of the heart. The characteristics of the smooth muscle will vary according to the function to be performed.

Cardiac Muscle

The cardiac muscle, similar in appearance to the smooth muscle, is responsible for the pumping action of the heart. The cardiac fibers, like the smooth muscle fibers, are arranged in a lattice-work pattern that permits rapid transmission of impulses through the myocardium and visceral muscles.

Skeletal Muscles

The skeletal muscles used to perform movement are called voluntary muscles because they can contract by conscious control. The skeletal muscles make up more than 40% of the body weight.

Muscle Structure

The muscle cells are striated, multinucleated, and arranged in bundles surrounded by sheaths of connective tissue. The muscles are controlled by nerve impulses that are transmitted from the brain to the bundles of muscle fibers.

The muscle fiber contains parallel bundles of myofibrils composed of filaments made of actin and myosin protein molecules. These protein molecules make up the contractile element of the muscle.

MUSCLE INNERVATION

In order for a skeletal muscle to contract, a stimulus must be applied. This stimulus is normally transmitted by nerve cells called neurons. The neurons that transmit stimuli to muscle tissue are called motor neurons.

After the nerve enters the muscle fascia, it divides into bundles that form a plexus of nerves. Gradually the nerve continues to divide until a single nerve fiber terminates on the muscle fibers. One nerve fiber may supply up to 150 muscle fibers. Within the muscle fiber, the nerve fiber terminates in the motor end plate. The motor nerve fiber and the muscle fibers it supplies are called a motor unit.

The neuromuscular junction is the area of contact between a myelinated nerve fiber and a skeletal muscle fiber. When a nerve impulse reaches the junction, *acetylcholine* is released by the axon terminal of the motor neuron. The acetylcholine acts to increase the permeability of the muscle fiber membrane. The increased permeability results in an enhanced flow of sodium ions into the fiber. This flow of ions causes a local electrical current flow. When the local electrical current flow is sufficiently strong, an *action potential* is initiated. This action potential travels in both directions along the fiber. The surface action potential causes the electrical current to flow toward the fiber interior by ionic conduction through special tubular structures.

There are two different types of tubular structures. The longitudinal tubules are found along the border of the muscle fiber. The tubules contain endoplasmic fluid in which calcium is stored. The longitudinal tubules end in large chambers called cisterns. The cisterns lie against the transverse or T tubule. The T tubule connects to the fiber exterior and contains extracellular fluid.

When an action potential occurs on the muscle fiber surface, the resulting electrical current flows to the fiber interior through the T tubule's extracellular fluid by ionic conduction. This current flow also passes through the walls of the T tubules and enters the cisterns. The flow into the cisterns causes the release of calcium ions into the myofibrils. Some of the calcium combines with the myosin filaments to form activated myosin. The activated myosin functions as an enzyme that releases energy from the adenosine triphosphate (ATP), which is bound with the actin and myosin filaments. In addition, the activated myosin causes an attractive force to develop between the actin and myosin filaments. The actin filaments then slide inward along the myosin filaments. The result is a muscle contraction.

To summarize, in order for a contraction to occur, an interaction must occur between the actin and myosin filaments. Calcium ions are vital in creating this interaction and energy must be available to cause the contraction.

- The primary purpose of the *acetylcholine* mechanism is one of amplification. Acetylcholine permits a weak nerve impulse to stimulate a large muscle fiber by amplifying the electrical current generated by the nerve impulse. This causes the muscle to elicit its own impulse.

- The enzyme *cholinesterase* is released by the muscle fibers to destroy the acetylcholine. Cholinesterase splits acetylcholine into acetic acid and choline. This destruction of acetylcholine permits repolarization of the membranes and prepares the fibers to receive a new stimulus.

TENDONS AND LIGAMENTS
TENDONS
The voluntary muscle consists of a fleshy belly and ends in a cordlike band of dense fibrous connective tissue called a tendon. The tendon attaches the

muscle to the periosteum of the bone. When the muscle shortens during contraction, the tendon is pulled and movement occurs at the joint.

Tendons are composed of collagen and elastin. The amount of elastin present determines the "stretchability" of the tendon. Tendons vary in shape and length and are flexible, relatively inelastic, and resistant to the friction caused by the movement of the bone and joint.

LIGAMENTS

Ligaments are also examples of dense fibrous connective tissue. Ligaments connect the articular ends of bones and serve to bind bones together, while reinforcing the joint capsule by restraining movement.

BONES
BONE STRUCTURE AND PRODUCTION

The bone is also a connective tissue consisting of various cell types and an extracellular matrix. The extracellular matrix of the bone is composed of protein fibers that prevent the bone from breaking when tension is applied. Deposited within this matrix are salts, primarily calcium and phosphorus, which make the bone hard and nonbendable.

There are three cell types found in bone: osteoblasts, osteoclasts, and osteocytes.

Osteoblasts

Osteoblasts are the cells active in bone formation. They are uniform, spindle-shaped cells found on the bone surface. Osteoblasts secrete an enzyme, *alkaline phosphatase,* that polymerizes to form strong collagen fibers. These fibers form the basis of the matrix. Calcium phosphate salts are deposited within this matrix and give the bone its hardness.

Bone production is regulated by the amount of strain and trauma applied to a bone. At the injury site, osteoblastic activity greatly increases in order to deposit large amounts of the matrix in the bone.

Osteocytes

Osteocytes are the mature, primary cells of formed bone. They are formed by osteoblasts, which become surrounded by matrix material in small pockets called lacunae. The osteocytes maintain indirect communication with one another by way of small canals called canaliculi, which run from the lacunae. The osteocytes send protoplasm into the canaliculi.

The haversian system is the unit of compact bone. The system consists of osteocytes, their lacunae, matrix, and canaliculi, which surround the haversian canal. The canal carries lymph, blood vessels, and nerves to the bone.

Osteoclasts

The osteoclasts are giant multinucleated cells found in nearly all cavities of the bone and are capable of causing bone resorption. Bone resorption occurs when these cells secrete enzymes that dissolve the protein matrix and split bone salts, thus releasing calcium and phosphate into the extracellular fluid.

This resorption of the bone is a continual process that is offset by the activity of the osteoblasts. The strength of a bone relates directly to the balance between production and resorption of bone.

Parathyroid Hormone

Bone resorption is also stimulated by the parathyroid hormone, which causes the number and size of osteoclasts to increase. This proliferation of osteoclasts causes increased osteoclastic activity, which removes both calcium and phosphate from the bone. Parathyroid hormone secretion is regulated by the calcium ion concentration of extracellular fluid.

Calcium

Ninety-nine percent of the body's calcium stores are found in the bone. Calcium is needed for muscle contraction, nerve conduction, the clotting mechanism and certain cellular enzyme systems. An adequate dietary intake of Vitamin D is necessary for proper calcium absorption in the intestine.

Other Regulatory Substances

Calcitonin, a hormone released by the thyroid gland in response to calcium elevations, is responsible for decreased bone resorption.

Bone growth is further stimulated by *thyroxine, somatropin, estrogens,* and *androgens.*

Vitamin C is needed for the proper formation and maintenance of the collagenous fibers of the matrix, and *Vitamin A* is needed for bone resorption.

BONE TISSUE

There are two forms of bony tissue: cancellous and compact. Cancellous tissue is spongy and found in the interior of the bone. Compact tissue, on the other hand, is found on the exterior surface. Compact tissue is dense, feels like ivory, and forms the cortex.

Endosteum

Lining the marrow cavities and haversian canals is a loosely woven vascular membrane called the endosteum. The endosteum is active in the healing of fracture sites. The endosteum also has a role in osteogenesis and hemopoiesis.

Periosteum

The periosteum is the tough fibrous membrane that covers all other bone surfaces except the joints. The periosteum in children is thick, loosely attached to the cortex and produces new bone easily. In adults, the periosteum is thinner, more adherent, and regenerates slower. As a result, as a person matures, fractures heal more slowly.

BONE MARROW

Bone marrow, also a form of connective tissue, fills the cavities of all bones. It is highly vascular. Yellow marrow is composed primarily of fat cells and is found in the modullary cavities. Red marrow is more prominent in membranous bones such as the skull, vertebra, ribs, sternum, and ilia. It is found in the shafts of long bones only during preadolescence.

Red marrow is responsible for the production of red blood cells which form hematocytoblasts. These cells mature from stem cells under the influence of *erythropoietin*. The mature erythrocyte squeezes through the capillary wall into the marrow vessels. Both Vitamin B-12 and folic acid are needed to form RBCs.

CIRCULATION

Bone is an active metabolic substance that requires an adequate blood supply. A large network of blood vessels are found in the periosteum and these vessels supply compact bone. These vessels are distributed through Volkmann's and haversian canals. Blood is also supplied to the medullary cavity of long bones by way of nutrient arteries that enter through foramens found near the center of the bone.

NERVE SUPPLY

An abundant nerve supply to the periosteum and interior of the bone provides both sensory and motor capabilities. Synovial joints have both myelinated and nonmyelinated nerve fibers within their capsules. The myelinated nerve fibers are sensitive to increased fluid pressures within the joint, twisting and stretching.

JOINTS

A joint is the junction between two or more bones. Joints are composed of fibrous connective tissue and cartilage. They prevent rigidity by permitting motion and weight bearing. The articulating bone ends vary in shape according to the degree of motion needed.

TYPES OF JOINTS

Joints are classified by the degree of movement permitted:

- synarthrosis: no movement, thin layers of fibrous tissue continuous with the periosteum
  example: cranial sutures
- amphiarthrosis: some movement
  example: symphysis pubis
- diathrosis: free movement (also called synovial)
  example: hip, knee

  Diathrotic joints can be further classified by type:
- pivot–rotation movement (atlas–axis)
- ball and socket—widest range of motion (hip, shoulder)
- gliding (vertebral, sternoclavicular)
- hinge (elbow, knee, ankle)
- saddle (thumb)
- condyloid (wrist)

SYNOVIAL FLUID

The joint capsule is formed by surrounding ligaments and hyaline carti-lage, which covers the ends of the bones. In specialized synovial joints, the synovial membrane produces a fluid to lubricate the joint. In addition to lubrication, this synovial fluid nourishes the articular cartilage lining.

MUSCULOSKELETAL DISORDERS

The structure and function of the musculoskeletal system can be altered by congenital abnormalities, acquired disease processes, and trauma.

- *Congenital disorders* may result from chromosomal abnormalities, intra-uterine conditions including fetal positioning, and maternal–fetal and fe-tal–placental circulatory disturbances. Environmental influences such as exposure to viral infections, drugs, alcohol, cigarettes, and environmental pollutants may also cause congenital disorders.

- *Disease processes* that affect other body systems, such as the immune system or metabolic processes, can result in temporary or permanent factors that alter the musculoskeletal system's ability to function normally. In addition, this system may be altered by inflammatory, infectious, degenerative or neoplastic conditions.

- *Trauma* to the musculoskeletal system can result in multiple injuries lead-ing to prolonged and repeated hospital admissions. Trauma is the leading cause of death in the young adult today.

FRACTURES

A fracture is an interruption or disruption in the normal continuity of a bone owing to direct or indirect violence, muscle contraction, or a pathologic condition. Fractures can involve the surrounding soft tissue, muscle, tendon, ligament, joint, and joint capsule. The type of fracture will vary according to the direction of the external force and internal forces of the muscle.

Types of Fractures

Type of fracture	Definition
Avulsion	Bone fragment is torn away with muscle damage
Capillary	Hairline
Comminuted	Bone is broken or splintered into fragments
Complete (transverse)	Bone is broken across the diameter of the bone at a right angle to the axis of the bone
Compound	A complete fracture of the bone with a wound extending through the mucous membranes to the skin
Compression	One bony surface is forced against an adjacent one compressing the bone, seen with vertebral fractures

Type of fracture	*Definition*
Depressed	Fracture site is driven in (seen with facial and skull fractures)
Greenstick	An incomplete fracture in which the bone is broken and bent but remains intact or hinged on one side
Incomplete	Fractures involve only a portion of the bone
Impacted	One bone segment is firmly driven into the other by the force causing the fracture
Intracapsular	Fracture occurs inside the joint
Linear (longitudinal)	Fracture extends lengthwise along the bone
Displaced	Dislocation of bony fragments
Oblique	Fracture occuring at angle across the bone
Pathological (spontaneous)	Fracture occuring in an area of diseased bone
Simple (closed)	A fracture without an external wound
Spiral	Fracture twists along the axis of the bone
Undisplaced	No dislocation of fragments

Fracture Healing

Fracture site repair occurs in four stages and can be monitored by x-ray.

1. Procallus—7 to 60 days after the injury the blood clot, osteoblasts, and chrondoblasts form the procallus between the fracture segments.
2. Fibrocartilaginous callus—fibrous connective tissue that promotes ossification and calcification at the injury site.
3. Ossification and calcification—occurs in fibrocallus when the site becomes immobile and the site is clinically united, x-ray findings at this stage reveal healing fracture sites.
4. Consolidation—cortical mature bone replaces callus, osteoclasts absorb excess callus in cancellous bone.

Improper Healing

Fracture sites may not heal properly. If the bone repairs itself but the alignment is improper, it is called *malunion*. Fractures that take longer than normal to heal are called *delayed unions*. Nonunion refers to fractures that heal without bone formation. In this instance, a fibrous repair takes place, which results in a false joint or pseudoarthrosis.

SPRAINS/STRAINS/DISLOCATIONS

The soft tissue surrounding the bone is subject to trauma from excessive use or misuse.

Strains

A strain is caused by trauma to the musculotendenous unit, although strains may also involve other tissues.

Sprains

A sprain is similar to a strain but involves a partial or complete tear of the ligament. In addition to ligament injury, there may be tearing of the synovial membrane and joint capsule with subsequent bleeding into the joint.

Sprains may result from dislocations or cause avulsion fractures.

Sprains and strains are classified by the degree of injury as first, second, or third degree.

Dislocations

A dislocation results when a bone is temporarily moved from its normal position in a joint. A subluxation is an incomplete dislocation. This movement causes all the ligaments to be disrupted and degeneration of the cartilage may result from the loss of the synovial nourishment.

CONGENITAL DISORDERS
Dysplasia of the Hip

Dysplasia of the hip(s) has no known cause, although there are numerous contributing factors such as familial tendencies, fetal position in utero, and maternal hormonal influences.

This disorder occurs more commonly in the female, with the left hip affected more often than the right. The femoral head of the affected hip is subluxated or dislocated and has a shallow acetabular cup.

Clubfoot

Talipes equinovorus, or clubfoot, also has no known cause but may be the result of familial tendencies, arrested fetal growth, or a defect of the ovum. Clubfoot is usually bilateral and is two times more common in males.

Spina Bifida

Spina bifida is a malformation of the posterior vertebral segments of the spine.

- *Spina bifida occulta* results when only the vertebrae is involved.
- *Spina bifida cystica* is a malformation of the posterior vertebral segments with displacement of the intraspinal contents.

There are two types of spina bifida cystica: meningocele and myelomeningocele.

- *Meningocele:* the cord membranes protrude through the defect with cerebrospinal fluid into a sac covered by skin.
- *Myelomeningocele*: protrusion of the spinal cord, cord membranes, and cerebrospinal fluid into the external sac.

Spina bifida is of unknown etiology, but is the most common developmental defect seen in the newborn. Although it is more common in females, it is generally more severe in the male.

Osteogenesis Imperfecta

Osteogenesis imperfecta is a congenital defect that is demonstrated by abnormally soft and brittle bones, thin skin, blue sclera, hypermobile joints, and multiple pathological fractures. It is thought to be a hereditary connective tissue disorder resulting from a lack of osteoblasts.

Muscular Dystrophy

Progressive muscular dystrophy, a disorder of unknown cause, is thought to be an inherited degenerative disorder resulting in muscular degeneration and weakness that affects all muscles of the body.

ACQUIRED DISORDERS
Legg–Calve–Perthes Disease

Legg–Calve–Perthes disease is a nonmalignant, idiopathic, avascular, aseptic necrotic lesion of the epiphyseal center of the bone. It is four times more common in the male and is most often seen in the three to eleven year old. The disease is usually unilateral.

ARTHRITIS

Arthritis is a chronic, systemic rheumatoid disorder that affects more than 2% of the adult population but which can affect all ages.

Arthritis can be classified as an inflammatory or degenerative process.

- Inflammatory arthritic conditions include rheumatoid arthritis and Marie–Strumpell arthritis.

- Degenerative arthritis includes osteoarthritis and traumatic arthritis.

- Juvenile rheumatoid arthritis is an inflammatory condition with onset following trauma or an acute systemic infection. There is indication that this disorder may be an autoimmune response.

Ankylosing Spondylitis

Marie–Strumpell arthritis or ankylosing spondylitis is a chronic progressive inflammatory disease of unknown cause that affects the spine. It is most common in males. The disease is often seen in the sacro-iliac joints and spreads up the spine. Peripheral joints, most often the hips, may be involved. The spinal ligaments calcify, which results in a rigid spine and loss of thoracic expansion.

RHEUMATOID ARTHRITIS

Rheumatoid arthritis (RA) is the most common cause of chronic disability and limitation of function. Females are more often afflicted than males. There is growing evidence that supports alterations in the immune mechanism as the causative agent of rheumatoid arthritis.

The initiating factor has yet to be identified, however, the result is a persistent immune stimulus in the synovial tissues. One theory suggests the gamma globulin IgG becomes altered and in the altered form is antigenic. The altered IgG stimulates the production of an antibody in the joint tissue. This antibody, usually an IgG, reacts with the altered IgG. This macroglobulin antibody is known as the rheumatoid factor.

Pathophysiologic Changes

The persistent immune stimulus leads to thickening of the synovial membrane. As the synovium thickens it begins to fold. The increased surface area created by the folds has numerous villi and is highly vascular. Synovial lining cells then multiply to cover this increased surface area. In addition, the thickened synovial membrane is infiltrated by lymphocytes and plasma cells. As the membrane becomes infiltrated with these cells, edema, vascular congestion, and a fibrinous exudate appear. The synovial fluid increases in turbidity and amount as a result of the inflammatory process.

Clinical Manifestations

In the early stages of rheumatoid arthritis, the joints become warm, red, and swollen. A synovitis occurs. As the disease progresses, tenosynovitis and carpal tunnel syndrome may appear. Chronic inflammation of the periarticular structures, tendons, ligaments, and other supportive structures leads to joint instability or dislocation. Muscular atrophy results from disuse and systemic myositis. Joint destructive follows. Major systemic manifestations may occur with RA including rheumatoid granulomas, cardiopulmonary lesions and diffuse neuropathy.

Juvenile Rheumatoid Arthritis

Juvenile rheumatoid arthritis or Still's disease occurs following trauma or after an acute systemic infection. The joints are inflamed. X-ray findings include articular cartilage destruction, fibrous ankylosis, and bone fusion. The loss of the articular space in affected joints as well as destruction of the epiphyseal plate adjacent to the affected joint lead to deformity.

Osteoarthritis

Osteoarthritis, a degenerative arthritis disorder, affects the articular cartilage of all weight-bearing joints. Osteoarthritis is thought to arise from the wear and tear on the joint surfaces with resulting joint and bone alterations. Contributing factors are obesity, strenuous physical activity, trauma, and the aging process. The joints most commonly involved are the hips, knees, fingers, and the spine.

Traumatic Arthritis

Traumatic arthritis occurs secondary to previous injury from trauma, infection, overuse, or abnormal development. There is a loss of articular cartilage and joint malfunction. As the disease progresses joint changes resemble those of osteoarthritis.

NEOPLASTIC DISORDERS

Primary vs Secondary Tumors

The musculoskeletal system can be affected by primary or secondary bone tumors. Primary tumors are benign or malignant. Secondary tumors are metastatic and generally result from breast, lung, prostate, thyroid, or kidney malignancies.

Multiple Myeloma

Multiple myeloma is the most common malignant neoplasm occurring in the 40 to 60-year-old group, most often in the male. In this disease, the cancellous bone is replaced by cells similar to plasma cells.

Osteosarcoma

Osteosarcoma is a rapidly developing malignant bone tumor. Osteosarcoma erodes the cortex of the metaphyseal region of the long bone and thus predisposes to pathological fractures.

Paget's Disease

Osteitis deformans or Paget's disease is a chronic disorder of unknown etiology most commonly seen in adult males. The disorder results in an increase in bone resorption and repair. The bones become enlarged but are weaker and more sponge-like than normal. This inherent weakness results in pathological fractures, deformity, and degenerative disease.

METABOLIC DISORDERS

The two most common metabolic disorders affecting the musculoskeletal system are gout and osteoporosis.

Gout

Gout is a hereditary disorder of uric acid metabolism. The urate crystals are deposited in and around the peripheral joints causing acute arthritic flareups and eventually joint destruction. The most commonly affected joint is the great toe.

The attacks of gouty arthritis may be precipitated by stress from surgery, trauma, and emotional difficulties. Dietary factors such as obesity, excessive alcohol intake, and high purine diets may also cause an attack.

Recurrent attacks or uncontrolled gout result in deposition of the urate crystals in the kidney tubules and subsequent hypertension.

Osteoporosis

Osteoporosis is primarily a protein metabolism disorder that results in a loss of calcium from the bone matrix and the appearance of osteopenia on x-ray film.

There are two subtypes of osteoporosis: primary and secondary.

Primary osteoporosis or postmenopausal osteoporosis has no known cause, but is thought to result from an interruption in the maturity of bone cells.

Secondary osteoporosis may result from endocrine, nutritional, or disuse factors. Alterations in the hormonal secretions from the thyroid, parathyroid, adrenal cortex, anterior pituitary, and gonads have been cited as causative factors.

Disuse osteoporosis is a decrease in bone mass caused by lack of normal stress on the bones. Immobilization through bedrest, traction and casting can cause disuse osteoporosis.

Nutritional factors such as lack of the necessary vitamins and minerals needed for bone metabolism may also contribute to osteoporosis.

INFECTIOUS PROCESSES

Osteomyelitis

Osteomyelitis is an acute or chonic pyogenic infection of the long bones and marrow. Osteomyelitis may follow trauma, such as from a compound fracture with subsequent wound infection or from a systemic infection. In children osteomyelitis is sometimes seen secondary to acute otitis media, impetigo, and pyelonephritis. Osteomyelitis may also follow teeth abscesses. In most cases, the causative organism has been found to be *Staphylococcus aureus.*

IMMOBILITY

Any condition that restricts or impairs movement can have effects on all systems of the body. These restrictions of movement can result from treatment modalities such as casting or traction, loss of motor function owing to disease or trauma, and voluntary limitation of movement to control pain.

Systemic Effects

The possible systemic outcomes of immobility reflect functional and metabolic changes owing to a lack of use. These physiological changes affect even the healthy individual and may result in loss of bone mass, muscle atrophy, decreased muscle endurance, and increased urinary excretion of calcium, phosphorus, and the nitrogenous waste products of metabolism. When muscular activity is decreased, the functional reserves of the muscle diminishes. In addition to atrophy of the muscle, a loss of tone and strength occurs.

Contractures, Pathologic Fractures, and Venous Stasis

Bedridden patients will often assume a position of comfort, which places joints in positions of adduction and flexion. Without sufficient exercise, the connective tissue surrounding these joints becomes fibrosed. The result is a contracture and loss of function. Owing to the release of calcium and phosphorus from the bone secondary to immobilization, pathological fractures of the weight-bearing bones and joints may occur when muscle activity is resumed. Venous stasis and postural hypotension may result from the loss of muscle tone in the smooth muscles of the blood vessels.

Fat Embolism

Fat embolism may occur in patients who are immobilized because of their injuries. Although the cause is not known, fat emboli are suspected to arise from the fat of the marrow at the fracture site, or as a result of alterations in lipid metabolism following the stress of injury.

Pressure Sores

Prolonged pressure on vulnerable areas such as bony prominences of the sacrum, heel, back of the head, and shoulder blades will result in pressure sores or decubitus ulcers. This breakdown in skin integrity may further restrict movement, increases the risk of infection, and causes the loss of body fluids.

Disuse Osteoporosis

Disuse osteoporosis with its resulting loss of calcium and phosphorus from the bone may cause renal calculi in the immobilized patient. This problem is enhanced by the reduction of lactic acid production owing to decreased metabolic activity. The urine pH rises, predisposing the patient to urinary tract infections, stones, and stasis.

BLOOD TESTS
ACID PHOSPHATASE (ACP)

Acid phosphatase is an enzyme found in erythrocytes and platelets. Acid phosphatase enzymes are also present in prostatic tissue. The biologic roles of these enzymes is not clearly understood. Only elevations of ACP are considered relevant. Slight elevations occur in diseases involving the bone, such as multiple myeloma, Paget's disease, hyperparathyroidism, and bony metastasis from breast and prostatic cancer.

Laboratory Results
Normal

  Adult and children

  1.0 to 5.0 u (King Armstrong)

  0.5 to 2.0 u (Bodansky)

  0.2 to 1.8 IU

Nursing Implications
Procedure for Collection/Storage of Specimen

1. 5 to 10 cc whole blood by way of venipuncture is collected.
2. The blood sample should not be left to stand at room temperature, because as the pH increases the enzyme is inactivated.

Possible Interfering Factors

1. Hemolysis of the cells must be avoided. Lysis of the erythrocytes may cause false elevations.
2. Tartrates inhibit the prostatic enzyme.
3. Fluorides may also inhibit the enzyme activity.
4. Diurnal variations are normally 25% to 50% from 9 A.M. to 3 A.M.

Nursing Implications
None related to test

Patient Education
None related to test

Signed Consent

Not required

ALKALINE PHOSPHATASE (ALK-P)

Alkaline phosphatase is an enzyme found in granulocytes and osteoblasts. There have been five identified isoenzymes related to the liver, bone, intestine, kidney and placenta, but the primary sources are the bone and liver. Certain malignant tumors may produce an isoenzyme, Regan isoenzyme, similar to the placental isoenzyme.

Alkaline phosphatase will normally be elevated during periods of bone growth as a result of the increased activity of the osteoblasts in infancy, early childhood, and puberty. Elevations have also been noted during the last trimester of pregnancy.

Elevations in disease states relate primarily to bone and liver disorders. Hyperparathyroidism, Paget's disease, primary bony malignancies, osteomalacia, and healing fractures have been associated with ALK-P elevations. Certain inflammatory conditions, infectious mononucleosis, infectious hepatitis, pulmonary infarcts, and tissue rejection processes will also show rises in ALK-P. Low alkaline phosphatase is usually insignificant. If it persists, however, certain rare disorders, such as vitamin C deficiency and cretinism should be ruled out.

Laboratory Results

Normal Results

Adult	14 to 13 (King Armstrong) u/100 ml
	1.5 to 4.5 (Bodansky) u/100 ml
Children	15 to 30 (King Armstrong) u/100 ml
	5 to 14 (Bodansky) 100 ml

Nursing Implications

Procedure for Collection/Storage of Specimen

Obtain 5 to 10 cc whole blood by way of venipuncture.

Possible Interfering Factors

1. Medications

   Decreased alkaline phosphatase

   • fluorides

   • oral contraceptives

   Increased alkaline phosphatase

   • allopurinol

   • anticonvulsants

2. Hepatic toxicity secondary to coumarin, kanamycin and acetylsalicylic acid may elevate ALK-P levels.

Nursing Care

None related to test

Patient Education

None related to test

Signed Consent

Not required

ANTINUCLEAR ANTIBODIES (ANA)

Antinuclear antibodies are gamma-globulins that react to specific antigens. In the serum, these antibodies lead to the production of the LE cell.

Antinuclear antibody elevations are seen with connective tissue disorders such as systemic lupus erythematosus, rheumatoid arthritis, polyarteritis nodosa, juvenile arthritis, and polymyositis. Elevations may also be present in ulcerative colitis, infectious mononucleosis, and posthepatic cirrhosis.

Approximately 95% to 100% of patients with systemic lupus erythematosus have these antibodies present in their serum. These antibodies generally appear when clinical evidence of joint and skin involvement is present.

Laboratory Results

Normal

Less than 1:10 titer

Nursing Implications

Procedure for Collection/Storage of Specimen

Obtain fresh whole blood by way of venipuncture.

Possible Interfering Factors

1. Massive steroid therapy may result in false-negative reports.
2. Dilantin, procainamide, and smoking may have positive effects on serum levels.

Nursing Care

None related to test

Patient Education

None related to test

Signed Consent

Not required

ANTI-DNA ANTIBODY (Antideoxyribonuclease)

The serum measurement of this antigen is useful in determining a serologic response to streptococcus. There are four known isoenzymes of streptococcal desoxyribonuclease. The titer is comparable to the ASO titer.

Laboratory Results

Normal

Up to 250 u

Titers below 1:20 are considered negative

Nursing Instruction
Procedure for Collection/Storage of Specimen
Obtain fresh whole blood by way of venipuncture.

Possible Interfering Factors
None known

Nursing Care
None related to test

Patient Education
None related to test

Signed Consent
Not required

ANTI-STREPTOLYSIN O TITER (XR-C-V Chapter)
The anti-streptolysin O titer measures the antigen–antibody reaction resulting from the presence of an enzyme produced by group A streptococcus. The test is used to identify the recent occurrence of a streptococcus infection, but does not identify the strain, location, or the time the infection was present.

Laboratory Results
Normal
- 0 to 150 or 160 Todd units. Values over 500 Todd units are seen with acute rheumatic fever and glomerulonephritis.
- The titer generally peaks 4 to 6 weeks after a streptococcus infection.

Nursing Implications
Procedure for Collection/Storage of Specimen
Fresh whole blood is collected by venipuncture.

Interfering Factors
None reported

Nursing Care
1. Observe the patient for signs of acute illness, fever, joint pain, hematuria, or decreased urinary output.
2. The duration and elevation of the titer is not related to the cause of the disease.

Patient Education
None related to the test

Signed Consent
Not required

CALCIUM

Serum calcium levels may be elevated or decreased in diseases such as multiple myeloma, Paget's disease, metastatic bone cancer, sarcoidosis, hyperparathyroidism, vitamin D deficiencies, and pseudohypoparathyroidism. In addition, immobility, fractures, pregnancy, polycythemia, pancreatitis, rickets, and osteomalacia will alter serum levels. Normally 50% to 58% of the total calcium is ionized. (For details related to this test, see page 92.)

CREATININE

Creatinine is a catabolic end product of phosphocreatine metabolism. The production of creatine is related to the individual's muscle mass.

Synthesized by the liver, creatine is transported to the muscle where ATP, creatine, and creatine phosphokinase catalyze to form phosphocreatine, a high-energy compound.

Serum creatinase levels rise when muscle destruction occurs, such as in wasting disorders with increased tissue catabolism, severe strenuous muscular activity, and in early muscular dystrophy. Serum levels fall in the later stages of muscular dystrophy because of the loss of muscle mass.

Creatinine is excreted in the urine. Serum levels reflect renal function and primarily glomerular filtration. Urinary excretion levels reflect total muscle mass and the degree of muscular activity. It is unaffected by protein ingestion.

PHOSPHORUS (Phosphate)

Eighty-five percent of the phosphorus is combined with calcium in the skeleton to form calcium phosphate which gives bone its rigidity. Phosphorus is also involved in carbohydrate metabolism, the formation of ATP and the structure of RNA and DNA molecules.

Alterations in serum phosphorus levels reflect endocrine or bone metabolism disorders. Elevations in phosphate levels are seen during fracture healing, Paget's disease, multiple myeloma, metastatic disease, acromegaly, and chronic glomerular disease. Low phosphate levels are associated with osteomalacia, rickets, malabsorption syndromes, and hyperparathyroidism.

RHEUMATOID FACTOR

The rheumatoid factor is a serum measurement of the IgM immunoglobulin present in the patient with rheumatoid arthritis. This globulin IgM reacts with the gamma globulin IgG to form an immune complex. The incidence of a positive rheumatoid factor will vary with the severity of the disease state.

Laboratory Results

Using latex fixation method	<1:80
Using Bentonite method	<1:32

Possible Interfering Factors

Titers are normally higher in older patients.

Nursing Implications
Procedure for Collection/Storage of Specimen
A fresh serum specimen is collected by venipuncture.

Patient Education
None related to test

Patient Care
None related to test

Signed Consent
Not required

SEDIMENTATION RATE

The sedimentation rate measures the rapidity at which RBC's settle in uncoagulated blood during a one hour period. This test is a nonspecific indicator of an inflammatory response. Elevations in the sedimentation rate may be seen in general or localized inflammatory reactions, Marce-Strumpell arthritis, malignancy and renal disorders. Low sedimentation may be associated with sickle cell disease, polycythemia and congestive heart failure.

Serial studies are generally performed. A gradual decrease in the sedimentation rate indicates improvement of the patient's conditions. (For details related to this test, see page 72.)

TOTAL PROTEIN ALBUMIN–GLOBULIN RATIO

Plasma proteins serve four functions: (1) buffers in the acid–base balance, (2) in the transport of blood constituents such as enzymes, hormones, vitamins, copper, iron and lipids, (3) as a source of rapid replacement of tissue proteins lost during injury and disease, and (4) in blood coagulation. The gamma globulins contain the antibodies of the body. Approximately 52% to 68% of the total protein in the body is albumin, a fraction responsible for the maintenance of the colloid osmotic pressure in the serum.

The advent of serum electrophoresis is slowly replacing these studies since the different albumin and globulin fractions can be more clearly identified by that method. Electrophoresis will show protein elevation in multiple myeloma, rheumatoid arthritis, and osteomyelitis.

Laboratory Results
Normal Range

Globulin	2.3 to 3.5 gm/100 ml
Albumin	3.2 to 4.5 gm/100 ml
Protein total	6.0 to 7.8 gm/100 ml

Nursing Implications
Procedure for Collection/Storage of Specimen
1. Fresh blood is collected by venipuncture.
2. Many hospitals send blood samples out to centers for electrophoretic studies and reports will not return for 4 to 5 days.

Nursing Care

None related to test

Patient Education

None related to test

Signed Consent

Not required

URIC ACID

Uric acid is an end product of purine metabolism. It is cleared from the plasma by glomerular filtration. Serum levels of uric acid reflect the balance between production and excretion.

Elevations of uric acid are associated with gout. Clinically there may be acute arthritic flareups or tophi accompanying the gout. Chronic renal failure is another common cause of hyperuricemia. Serum uric acid levels may also be increased in CHF with decreased creatinine clearance, glycogen storage diseases such as Lesch–Nyhan syndrome, starvation, lympho and myeloproliferative diseases such as acute and chronic leukocytic and granulocytic leukemia, multiple myeloma, excessive ethyl alcohol intake, hypoparathyroidism, and following therapy with thiazide diuretics, chemotherapy, and radiation therapy.

Laboratory Results

Normal Serum

Male	2.1 to 7.8 mg/dl
Female	2.0 to 6.4 mg/dl

Normal Urine

250 to 750 mg/24 hr

Nursing Implications

Procedure for Collection/Storage of Specimen

1. 5 to 10 cc of fresh blood is collected by venipuncture.
2. Urine study requires a random 24 hr specimen. Results will vary with dietary intake. Notify the laboratory if more than one bottle will be sent. Label each bottle.

Possible Interfering Factors

Serum elevations

- thiazide therapy
- acetaminophen therapy may increase results on the SMA 12/60
- blind individuals have a tendency to have serum uric acid elevations of approximately 1.4 mg/dl. The cause is unknown.

Urine elevations

- cortisone therapy

Decreased

- low dose ASA therapy
- thiazide therapy

Nursing Care
None related to test

Patient Education
Instruct the patient to save all urine during the 24-hr period of collection.

Signed Consent
Not required

URINE TEST
BENCE JONES PROTEIN

The occurrence of the Bence Jones protein in the urine is associated with bone tumors, particularly multiple myeloma, hyperparathyroidism, and osteomalacia. This protein differs from other urine proteins because it coagulates upon heating to 45°C to 60°C and then redissolves if further heating occurs.

Laboratory Results
Normal

No Bence Jones protein is found in the urine.

Nursing Implications
Procedure for Collection/Storage of Specimen

1. A 4cc random urine specimen is collected. First morning specimen preferred.
2. The specimen should be taken directly to the laboratory. Refrigeration of the specimen is needed if the study cannot be done within an hour of the time the specimen was collected.

Possible Interfering Factors

The presence of albumin in the urine will mask the presence of the Bence Jones protein.

Nursing Care
None related to test

Patient Education
The patient should notify the nurse when the urine specimen has been collected.

Signed Consent
Not required

DIAGNOSTIC TESTS
ARTHROGRAM

An arthrogram is an x-ray examination that requires the injection of a radiopaque substance and air into the joint cavity. An arthrogram is done to inspect the joint capsule integrity and the shape and outline of the cartilaginous surfaces of the joint. The study is done on the major joints of the body.

Normal Results
Normal appearance of bony and cartilaginous structures

Nursing Implications
Preprocedure
1. Explain the procedure to the patient.
2. Explain to the patient that joint noise will occur for several days following the procedure. This noise is a result of the air injected into the joint. (Check with your radiology department. Some radiologists routinely remove this air after the procedure if the patient desires.)
3. Explain to the patient that minimal discomfort can be expected after the procedure and that pain medication will be available.
4. Have the patient verbalize understanding of the procedure and what to expect.

During the Procedure
None related to test

Postprocedure
1. Observe and record vital signs and the appearance of the injection site BID.
2. Report to the physician any increase in swelling or pain. Give pain medication as indicated.

Signed Consent
Required

ARTHROSCOPY
Arthroscopy is the visualization of a joint using a fiberoptic scope. This procedure enables the physician to see the ligaments, menisci, and articular surfaces of a joint. Arthroscopy is performed under local or general anesthesia.

The arthroscopic examination of the knee is accomplished by inserting a large bore needle into the suprapatellar pouch and injecting sterile saline to distend the joint. The fiberoptic scope is passed through puncture sites made lateral or medial to the tibial plateau for direct visualization of the joint cavity. The larger operating scopes permit the removal of articular debris or small loose bodies and the dissection of torn menisci. This study may be diagnostic. Further tests or surgery may be necessary.

Normal Results
Normal appearance of ligaments, menisci, and articular surfaces of the joints

Nursing Implications

Preprocedure

1. Reinforce explanation of the procedure as given by the physician.
2. Teach the patient about coughing, turning, and deep breathing exercises if a general anesthetic is to be given.
3. Instruct the patient on postoperative leg exercises. Explain to the patient about activity permitted, the possibility of pain and swelling occurring, and wound care, which will be done postoperatively.
4. Have the patient verbalize what to expect of the procedure and the postoperative care.
5. Prep the skin as ordered by the physician.

During the Procedure

None related to test

Postprocedure

1. Observe and record vital signs and the operative dressing BID.
2. Elevate the extremity and apply ice to the joint if ordered by the physician.
3. Give pain medication as prescribed.
4. Check the neurovascular status of the extremity by checking the pulse, and assessing pain, pallor, paresthesia, or paralysis. Notify the physician of any change in the neurovascular status, or of excessive swelling or drainage of the puncture site.
5. Obtain a physical therapy consult.
6. The physical therapist will instruct the patient on crutch walking and isometric quadricips exercises postoperatively.
7. Observe for signs and symptoms of possible complications such as infection or synovial cyst or sinus.

Signed Consent

Required

ARTHROCENTESIS

Arthrocentesis is a procedure in which synovial fluid is aspirated from a joint cavity. The test is used in differentiating various joint diseases. Synovial fluid may be obtained from the joint, bursa, or tendon sheaths.

All counts, smears, and cultures may be done on the fluid when there is suspicion of the presence of infection or gouty arthritis.

Normal Results

Synovial fluid is normally clear and serous in appearance.

	Noninflammatory	*Inflammatory*	*Septic*
WBC	≤500/cu mm	2,000 to 50,000	50,000 to 200,000
Neutrophils	≤25%	>50%	>75%
Viscosity	high	low	variable

(Continued)

	Noninflammatory	Inflammatory	Septic
Appearance	clear	yellow, turbid	turbid, yellow green
Culture	negative	negative	positive

Nursing Implications
Preprocedure

1. Prepare equipment and any medication for instillation in advance.
2. Explain the procedure to the patient.

During the Procedure

1. Assist the patient to the position of comfort.
2. Assist the physician as needed.

Postprocedure

1. Cover the puncture site with a bandaid.
2. Label specimens and take them to the laboratory at once.
3. Chart the procedure including the type, amount, and character of aspirated fluid. Chart the patient's tolerance to the procedure.

Signed Consent
Required

BIOPSY (Bone Marrow)
A bone marrow exam can be diagnostic for multiple myeloma if the sheath of the plasma cells can be visualized. (For details related to this chapter, see page 48.)

BIOPSY (Muscle)
A muscle biopsy is a diagnostic test involving microscopic examination of frozen muscle tissue. Muscles selected for the biopsy are usually the biceps, quadriceps, gastrocnemius, or the deltoid. The muscle tissue must be sampled from a site that was not previously the site of injections or needle EMG, since these would produce characteristic changes of inflammation in the muscle.

Normal Results

Normal appearance of muscle tissue

Nursing Implications
Preprocedure

1. Explain the procedure to the patient. The patient should be aware of:
   a. which muscle is to be biopsied
   b. possible postoperative complication, such as bleeding, infection, and slow healing

During the Procedure

1. Inform the patient that two painful points during the procedure will occur:
   a. when the anesthesia agent is injected
   b. when the muscle itself is cut

Postprocedure

1. Inform the patient that after the biopsy, use of the muscle may cause soreness.
2. Report signs and symptoms of infection or bleeding.

Signed Consent

Required

BONE SCANS

The bone scan is a diagnostic x-ray study that is used to detect bony metastasis. Bone scans are also used in the detection of benign disease, fractures, avascular necrosis and infection.

Following an intravenous injection of radioactive dye (Technetium–99m) is given to the patient, the bone scan is performed.

This particular isotope seeks out areas of increased bone activity or active bone formation.

Normal Results

No areas of increased uptake

Abnormal Results

Increased concentrations of isotopic uptake are considered positive areas.

Nursing Implications

Preprocedure

1. Explain the procedure to the patient.
2. Assess the patient for allergies, particularly to iodine or seafood.
3. Inform the patient that the duration of the procedure is dependent on the specific bone scan being done. A general bone scan takes about 1½ hr; a scan of the leg takes about 25 min.

During the Procedure

1. Inform the patient that he may be medicated prior to the completion of the scan (because of the length of the procedure, the hardness of the procedures table, and the need for immobility during the scan).
2. Following the injection of the isotopic agent in the nuclear medicine department, the patient will return to the room for approximately 2½ hr. During this time period, have the patient drink at least 1 quart of liquids (approximately 6 to 8 oz glasses).
3. The scan is then completed in nuclear medicine and will take 25 min to 1½ hr.

Postprocedure

Have the patient return to the same activity level as prior to scan.

Signed Consent

Not required

CRAIG NEEDLE BONE BIOPSY

The Craig needle bone biopsy is a closed-biopsy procedure that is done using fluoroscopy. Biopsies may also be obtained using an open surgical approach in the operating room.

The Craig needle bone biopsy is used in the diagnosis of suspected infection or tumor of the low thoracic or lumbar spine. The biopsy may be done under general or local anesthesia.

Normal Results

Normal appearance of tissue obtained.

Nursing Implications

Preprocedure

1. Implement routine preoperative teaching and preparation of the patient.
2. Reinforce explanation of the procedure as given by the physician.
3. Allow opportunities for the patient to verbalize fears and expectations.
4. Prepare the skin as ordered.
5. Have the patient verbalize understanding of the procedure.
6. Have the patient demonstrate cough-turn-deep breathing routine if a general anesthetic is to be used.

During the Procedure

1. The patient is placed in the prone position and a Steinman pin is inserted into the selected vertebrae. The position is checked by lateral views on x-ray film.
2. A cannulated guard is placed over the Steinman pin to maintain correct position and the pin is removed. A large serrated biopsy needle is inserted into the guard and tapped or twirled into the vertebrae to remove a plug of bone. The needle is removed and the plug of bone is placed in formalin.
3. Prior to removal of the guard, a second x-ray film is taken to verify the position of the biopsy.

Postprocedure

1. Observe the biopsy site for hemorrhage.
2. Medicate the patient for pain as prescribed by the physician.
3. Reinforce activity limits as ordered.

Signed Consent

Required

ELECTROMYOGRAM (EMG)

Electromyography is the graphic measurement of the action potential of skeletal muscles. An EMG is done by inserting a sterile needle electrode into the muscle being tested. The resulting electrical activity generated by the muscle during various rates of flexion is amplified and displayed on an oscilloscope.

The EMG can determine the following conditions:

- myopathic muscle wasting versus neuropathic muscle wasting
- muscle denervation
- the level or area of nerve injury
- the occurrence of nerve regeneration

An EMG is useful in planning individualized rehabilitation programs, differentiating myopathies from neuropathies or hysterical reactions, and in the management of peripheral nerve injuries. Serial studies may be done to determine recovery of peripheral nerve function.

Normal Results
Normal nerve conduction status

Nursing Implications
Preprocedure

Explain the procedure to the patient: insertion of needle electrode, muscular aching during needle manipulation, and electrical stimulation of needles causes tingling and possible painful sensation.

During the Procedure

Ask the patient to cooperate and follow commands during exam; the patient will be asked to flex the muscle being tested at varying speeds.

Postprocedure
No specific poststudy care

Signed Consent
Consent form advisable but not required

EPIDURAL LUMBAR VENOGRAM

The epidural lumbar venogram is an invasive radiologic special procedure. A catheter is inserted into the femoral vein, usually the right, and threaded into either one of the sacral veins or an ascending lumbar vein. A contrast media is injected and films are made of the venous plexus in the lumbar region.

The examination is useful in diagnosing herniated or ruptured discs, spinal stenosis, arterio-venous malformations and tumors. Prior lumbar surgery is considered a contraindication for this procedure since the surgery may distort or interrupt the venous structures.

In some institutions lidocaine is mixed with the contrast material to prevent patient discomfort during the procedure. If the patient is allergic to caine products, plain contrast material is used, and the patient may experience a warm feeling in the low back area or mild pain such as cramping, during the contrast injection.

Normal Results

Normal appearance of the venous plexus

Nursing Implications

Preprocedure

1. Check for allergies, especially to caine products. Inform consulting radiologist of caine allergies.
2. Reinforce the explanation of the procedure to the patient as given by the radiologist.
3. Shave and prep the lumbar region as ordered.
4. Keep the patient NPO after midnight the evening before the procedure.

During the Procedure

1. Enforce the activity limitations as ordered following the study: Complete bedrest for 12 hr, then bathroom privileges for 12 hr, then activity as tolerated.
2. Observe the groin puncture site for development of hematoma or hemmorrhage.
3. Check vital signs as follows:
   every 15 min × 2 hr,
   then every 30 min × 2 hr,
   then every hr × 4 hr,
   then QID for 2 dy.
4. Apply pressure and ice to the puncture site if bleeding occurs. Notify physician STAT.
5. Instruct the patient not to cross the legs for at least 48 hr following the study.
6. Serve a diet as tolerated by the patient.
7. Medicate the patient for pain or nausea as ordered.

Signed Consent

Required

MYELOGRAM

During a myelogram, a radiopaque contrast medium is injected into the subarachnoid space of the lumber spine. A myelogram is used to visualize discogenic or neoplastic lesions.

The two most common contrast media used are Pantopaque and Amipaque. Pantopaque is a thick, oily nonabsorbable constrast media. An 18-gauge needle is used to instill the material. Following the procedure, Pantopaque must be removed. Amipaque (Metrizamide) is a water soluble, absorbable contrast material. Instillation can be done with a 22-gauge needle. Because Amipaque is absorbable, it does not require removal after the study. The material slowly mixes with the spinal fluid and rises to the head where it works its way into the cerebral cortex. The material is ultimately absorbed into the blood stream by way of the pacchonian granulations. Peak concentrations in the cerebral cortex occur within 6 to 8 hr and the Amipaque is completely gone from the circulation within 24 hr. Some patients will experience nausea, vomiting. These symptoms are felt to be associated with the cerebral phase of absorption. Allergic reactions to either agent are rare.

Poststudy headaches may be seen with either agent. Headaches occurring after 24 hr are related to the loss of cerebrospinal fluid and are called spinal headaches regardless of the agent used. Poststudy hypotension is a risk for all patients with poorly controlled cardiovascular disease, regardless of the agent used.

Both agents, but especially Amipaque, may have the side effect of convulsions. The high-risk patient for such a complication has a past medical history of seizure activity, alcoholism, dehydration, or phenothiazide or MAO inhibitor drug therapy. Compazine is the most frequently indicated phenothiazide involved.

Normal Results
Normal appearance of the lumbar structures

Nursing Implications
Preprocedure
1. Be sure that the consult to the radiologist includes the reason for the study.
2. Reinforce the explanation of the procedure to the patient as given by the radiologist.
3. Note allergies, especially to iodine or seafoods.
4. Shave and prep the lumbar area as ordered.
5. Cancel any physical therapy the day of the study.
6. Note whether MAO inhibitors have been discontinued for at least 2 wk prior to Amipaque myelogram. Ensure that all other drugs have been stopped 24 hr before the study.

If Pantopaque is to be used
1. Allow the patient to have a liquid breakfast but keep the patient NPO for at least 3 hr prior to the study.
2. Pre-medicate the patient as prescribed, usually Valium and Atropine.
3. Perform and document basic neurologic assessment for baseline information.

If Amipaque is to be used
1. Keep the patient NPO after 4 A.M.
2. Maintain adequate patient hydration. Intravenous fluids are generally given before and after the study. Suggested regime:

Evening before: 1000 cc Ringers Lactate at the rate of 100 cc per hr

Day of test: 1 to 2 hr prior to the study, the radiologist will generally increase the infusion rate to 200 cc per hr.
3. Pre-medicate the patient as ordered.

During the Procedure

1. Patient should know to expect position changes during the study which promote the flow of the contrast media, needle manipulation to inject the dye, removal of the spinal fluid may be painful. Patient must report any unusual sensations that occur during the study to the physician.
2. The spinal fluid is sent to the laboratory from the x-ray department.

Postprocedure

If Pantopaque was used
1. Remember that Pantopaque is removed from the subarachnoid space following the study.
2. Upon return to the room keep the patient on complete bedrest for 12 hr. The first 2 hr of this time period should be in the prone position if possible. The patient should log-roll to change positions. Activity then progresses to bathroom privileges for 12 hr, then activity as tolerated.
3. Unless contraindicated by other disease processes, such as chronic congestive heart failure, push fluids for the first 8 hr following the procedure up to 3000 cc.
4. Perform neurological checks every 2 hr × 24 hr, then daily.

If Amipaque was used
1. Upon return to room, elevate the head of the bed 20 degrees for 8 hr. This will aid in the mixing of Amipaque with the spinal fluid and promote excretion.
2. Keep the patient on bedrest for 12 hr, then bathroom privileges for 12 hr.
3. Force fluids, up to 3000 cc first 8 hr after study.
4. Administer intravenous fluids as prescribed, usually 1000 cc Ringers Lactate at the rate of 100 to 200 cc per hr.
5. Check vital signs
   every 15 min × 2 hr,
   then every 30 min × 2 hr.
   then every hour × 2 hr.
6. Take seizure precautions. High-risk patients may be ordered Valium 10 mg IM every 6 hr × 4 doses.
7. Do not administer phenothiazides, especially Compazine, for 24 hours following the study.
8. Be aware that the patient may have increased low back or leg pain following the study. Paresthesia is generally transient, lasting 2 to 4 hr.
9. Remember that Amipaque is not removed following the study but is absorbed by the body.

Special Consent

Consent form required. The form must indicate which contrast media is to be used.

X-RAYS

X-rays are the most frequently used diagnostic tool. X-rays are made by passing a short wave of radiation through the body tissues. The resulting picture depicts the shadows of structures that block the passage of the x-ray beam. The density of the various structures is reflected by the degree of "whiteness" appearing on the x-ray film.

X-ray films are not three-dimensional pictures and, because of this, different views may be necessary. The most commonly used views are anterior–posterior, posterior–anterior, lateral and oblique.

There is generally a lag between the actual clinical picture and the x-ray film findings. For instance, osteomyelitis may not appear on x-ray for 15 to 20 days after the infection. Findings on chest films are generally 24 hours behind the clinical status of the patient. In addition, initial soft tissue swelling may be severe enough to give false-negative reports. Hairline fractures may not be seen initially on x-ray but will be visible when healing begins.

X-ray films are used to study the following:

- soft tissue for calcification, swelling, unusual shadows
- bone contours
- periosteal reactions
- bone density
- bone destruction

There have been several patterns identified in bone destruction:

- moth-eaten appearance is seen with malignancies and acute infections
- radiolucent areas with smooth borders generally represent cysts
- punched-out areas of bone indicate metastases

Tomograms are special x-rays done at different levels of a structure. They are used when the standard x-ray is inadequate.

Tomograms may be useful in determining more definite locations, questionable cervical or spinal fractures, fracture fragments, bone lesions, and intra-articular loose bodies.

Normal Results

Normal appearance of structures viewed

Nursing Implications

Preprocedure

1. Remove all jewelry and clothing other than patient gown prior to study. Note on the patient's chart where the jewelry and clothing have been stored.
2. Note on the x-ray request pertinent past medical history, that is, pace-

maker insertion, past joint replacement, injury or trauma. A short history of the present health problem is also advisable to aid the radiologist in film interpretation.

3. Notify the physician if the patient expresses undue concern about the amount of radiation during these studies.

4. Permit the parent(s) to accompany the pediatric patient to the radiology department or to assist in holding the child. The parent must wear a protective apron.

During the Procedure

None related to test

Postprocedure

None related to test

Signed Consent

Not required

BIBLIOGRAPHY

Ames Company Division of Miles Lab: Modern Urinalysis, A Guide to Diagnosis of Urinary Tract Disease and Metabolic Disorders, 2nd ed. Chicago, Sterne's Printers, 1974

Armstrong M: McGraw-Hill Handbook of Clinical Nursing. New York, McGraw-Hill, 1979

Chins PL: Child Health Maintenance: Concepts in Family Centered Care. St Louis, CV Mosby, 1979

Donahoo CA, Dimon JH III: Orthopedic Nursing. Boston, Little, Brown & Co., 1977

Donahoo CA, Spichler L: Core Curriculum of Orthopedic Nursing. Orthopedic Nurses Association, Atlanta, Ga.: Dasher & Associates, Inc., 1980

Donahoo KM: Overview of Neuromuscular Disease. Nurs Clin North Am 14, No. 1: 95–106, 1979

Dupont Company: Clinical Significance of Tests Available on Dupont Automatic Clinical Analyzer

Farrell J: Bone structure and function: A self study. ONA J 6, No. 4:141–151, 1979

French RM: The Nurses Guide to Diagnostic Procedures. New York, McGraw–Hill, 1971

Guyton AC: Function of the Human Body, 4th ed. Philadelphia, WB Saunders, 1974

Jones DA, Dunbar CJ, Jirouec MM: Medical Surgical Nursing: A Conceptual Approach. New York, McGraw–Hill, 1978

Marshman GM, Jackson KV: Orthopedic Nursing and Neuromuscular Disease. Nurs Clin North Am 14, No. 1:145–156, 1979

Mook MS: Orthopedics in the emergency room: sprains and strains. ONA J 6, No. 8: 318–319, 1979

Mourod L: Nursing Care of Adults with Orthopedic Conditions. New York, John Wiley & Sons, 1980

Ross AJ, Hurr BE, Norwood ML, Donahoo KM: Neuromuscular Diagnostic Procedures. Nurs Clin North Am 14, No. 1:107–121, 1979

Scipien GM: Comprehensive Pediatric Nursing. New York, McGraw–Hill, 1975

Shafer KN, Sawyer JR, McClusky, Beck E, Phillips, NJ: Medical-Surgical Nursing, 6th ed. St Louis, CV Mosby, 1975

Tilkian SM, Conover MH: Clinical Implications of Laboratory Tests. St Louis, CV Mosby, 1975

Tucker SM, Breeding MA, Canobbio MM, Paquette EV, Wells ME, Williams ME: Patient Care Standards, 2nd ed. St Louis, CV Mosby, 1980

Young DS, Pestaner LC, Gibberman V: Effects of drugs on clinical laboratory tests. Clin Chem 21, No. 5: 1975

Index